CORNEA

COLOR ATLAS

CORNEA
COLOR ATLAS

JAY H. KRACHMER

Professor and Chairman
Department of Ophthalmology
University of Minnesota
Minneapolis, Minnesota

DAVID A. PALAY

Assistant Professor of Ophthalmology
Department of Ophthalmology
Emory University
Atlanta, Georgia

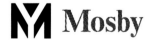 Mosby

St. Louis Baltimore Boston Carlsbad Chicago Naples New York Philadelphia Portland
London Madrid Mexico City Singapore Sydney Tokyo Toronto Wiesbaden

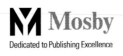

Mosby

Dedicated to Publishing Excellence

A Times Mirror
Company

Publisher: Alison Miller
Acquisition Editor: Laurel Craven
Managing Editor: Kathryn H. Falk
Project Manager: Linda McKinley
Manufacturing Manager: Theresa Fuchs
Book and Cover Designer: Elizabeth Fett

Printed in the United States of America
Composition by: Mosby Electronic Production
Printing/binding by: Buxton & Skinner Printing Co.

Mosby–Year Book, Inc.
11830 Westline Industrial Drive
St. Louis, Missouri 63146

Library of Congress Cataloging in Publication Data

Krachmer, Jay H.
  Cornea color atlas / Jay H. Krachmer, David A. Palay.
    p.   cm.
  Includes index.
  1. Cornea—Diseases—Atlases. I. Palay, David A.   II. Title.
  [DNLM: 1. Corneal Diseases—atlases. 2. Cornea—atlases. 3. Eye Diseases—atlases. WW 17 K885c 1995]
  RE336.K73 1995
  617.7' 19' 00222—dc20
  DNLM/DLC
  for Library of Congress   95-6803
                                                        CIP

95 96 97 98 99 / 9 8 7 6 5 4 3 2 1

With great love and appreciation, I dedicate this book to
My Wife, *Kathryn*, Our Children, *Edward*, *Kara*, and *Jill*
Our Parents, *Paul* and *Rebecca Krachmer*
and *Louis* and *Gertrude Maraist*

Jay H. Krachmer

To my wife *Debra*, my children *Sarah* and *Matthew*,
and my parents *Sandra* and *Bernard*.
Without their love and support this would not have been possible.

David A. Palay

v

Preface

We decided to author this atlas because we felt that using our resources and modern technology, we could produce a book on the cornea with features currently unavailable. We have large slide collections, many generous friends and colleagues (25% of the slides in this book came from others), ample experience in cornea and external eye disease, knowledge in photography and computer imaging, dedicated staffs, generous and cooperative departments of ophthalmology, and most important, loving and supportive families. Finding time was simple—we just slept less.

What does it take to create a good slide depicting its intended features? You must have a patient with those features. The photographer must be either the person requesting the photos or someone carefully informed regarding the location and essential characteristics that should be recorded. In the case of slit lamp photography, the final result is 50% dependent on the photographer's determination, 40% on slit lamp capability, and 10% on photographic knowledge.

Once a slide is obtained, it is no less a first draft than the first draft of a manuscript. In 1995, the first draft of the slide need no more be published than that of the manuscript. A manuscript may undergo many revisions before publication. So too can a slide now be enhanced to better convey its intended meaning.

Slides in this atlas were first carefully selected and then prescanned into a computer by means of a high-quality transparency scanner. They were cropped to maximize final-output resolution. Adjustments were made so that important detail in the dark and light areas of the image would be present in the final scan and the color balance was reasonable. A final scan was then performed, bringing the image into an image-manipulation software program and onto the monitor screen. Changes to the image then included removing artifacts; adjusting brightness, contrast, and color; and increasing saturation, especially for those slides faded with age. The mode had to be changed from the red, green, and blue of the slide to cyan, magenta, yellow, and black for the final printed page, thereby unavoidably losing some of the beautiful blues, especially from slides obtained using the blue light of the slit lamp and those from stained pathologic specimens. Most images were then increased slightly in sharpness.

A high percentage of images then underwent a variety of modifications to augment educational value and emphasize desired features, such as labeling, magnified insets, change to gray-scale mode, and schematic illustrations. All these changes can be accomplished with today's sophisticated but easy-to-use software.

Are we justified in manipulating images? We believe we are as long as the final image either mirrors disease observed by real-life methods of examination or is so stylized as to obviously be recognized as such. An artist's drawing is usually one step removed from reality, yet we easily accept the difference.

In deciding how much detail to include in the accompanying paragraphs and legends, we chose a middle ground, possibly on the short side. The atlas is meant to provide a visual journey through ocular adnexal and anterior segment disease, with brief descriptions of important points along the way. It is not meant to be more. Comprehensive descriptions of disease will be found in the three-volume text, and we encourage the joint use of the text and atlas. By conserving words, we had more space for images. The atlas follows the order of subjects in the second and third volumes of the text. Also, there are pages that draw together findings from various etiologies. An example is the page on iron lines of the cornea.

As we collected slides for the atlas, we continually found better examples and, to a lesser extent, pictorial evidence of entities rarely encountered, even as the deadline for publication approached. If a second edition ensues, we would like for it to be a significant improvement over this one. Therefore we extend an open invitation to all readers who have better slides than those in this atlas or who can fill pictorial gaps to send such slides. Due credit will be given to those contributors whose material is accepted for publication. This invitation goes out everywhere. We would like to include both slides and text relating to those diseases not typically seen in the United States. Wouldn't it be wonderful to include slides from around the world to produce a book depicting conditions that would broaden the experience of all of us?

Throughout this book, reference is made to the value of using various methods of slit lamp examination. We believe that diagnosis begins with observation and the ability to see subtle differences. A differential diagnosis has little benefit if the important signs to be differentiated are not seen. We also believe that many of us were drawn to our field either consciously or subconsciously because we love to observe.

Enjoy our observations. Please let us know what we missed.

JAY H. KRACHMER
DAVID A. PALAY

Acknowledgments

We are extremely grateful to our many colleagues, associates, and friends who helped with the preparation of this book. We would like to credit and thank the following contributors for sending us materials:

W. Lee Alward, M.D., Iowa City, Iowa (9-117)

William Basuk, M.D., Poway, California (6-35)

Allen D. Beck, M.D., Atlanta, Georgia (14-5)

J. Doug Cameron, M.D., Minneapolis, Minnesota (5-6, 9-99, 9-152)

Michael Diesenhouse, M.D., Sun City, Arizona (8-78, 16-8, 16-9)

Claes Dohlman, M.D., Boston, Massachusetts (19-17, 19-18)

Donald Doughman, M.D., Minneapolis, Minnesota (8-77)

Robert S. Feder, M.D., Chicago, Illinois (9-12, 9-13, 9-14, 9-28, 9-29)

Richard K. Forster, M.D., Miami, Florida (6-30, 6-31, 6-34), from the King Khaled Eye Specialist Hospital, Riyadh, Saudi Arabia

W. Richard Green, M.D., Baltimore, Maryland (3-24)

Michael R. Grimmett, M.D., Albuquerque, New Mexico (5-26)

Hans Grossniklaus, M.D., Atlanta, Georgia (2-5, 2-10, 2-12, 2-16, 2-25, 2-28, 2-31, 2-33, 2-35, 5-15, 6-60, 7-6, 7-9, 7-18, 7-21, 7-28, 8-22, 9-3, 9-26, 9-27, 9-38, 9-46, 9-76, 9-79, 9-101, 9-143, 9-155, 10-75)

Edward J. Holland, M.D., Minneapolis, Minnesota (2-34, 2-36, 4-17, 5-5, 5-14, 5-27, 5-36, 6-36, 6-47, 6-48, 6-49, 6-50, 6-61, 6-62, 6-72, 6-79, 6-80, 6-81, 8-10, 8-11, 8-15, 8-26, 8-69, 8-70, 8-71, 8-72, 8-81, 9-39, 9-40, 9-41, 9-49, 9-50, 9-164, 10-6, 10-18, 10-73, 13-21, 13-22, 13-26, 14-77, 14-78, 16-2, 17-3, 17-7, 17-13, 17-14, 17-17, 17-18, 18-16, 18-27, 19-7, 19-8, 19-9, 20-4, 20-5, 20-6, 20-7)

Timothy Johnson, M.D., Ann Arbor, Michigan (17-12)

William H. Knobloch, M.D., Minneapolis, Minnesota (8-8)

Burton J. Kushner, M.D., Madison, Wisconsin (2-8, 2-9)

Peter R. Laibson, M.D., Philadelphia, Pennsylvania (6-12, 6-57, 6-68, 6-69, 6-74, 7-1, 9-2, 9-4, 9-37, 9-131, 10-15, 10-19, 10-22, 10-28, 10-42, 10-50, 10-51, 12-3, 12-4, 12-7, 14-31, 14-75)

Scott Lambert, M.D., Atlanta, Georgia (17-16)

Mary Lynch, M.D., Atlanta, Georgia (7-22, 7-23, 7-24, 7-25)

Marian Macsai, M.D., Morgantown, West Virginia (19-14, 19-15, 19-16)

Mark Mandel, M.D., Hayward, California (14-82)

Mark J. Mannis, M.D., Sacramento, California (3-3, 4-12, 4-14, 6-59, 9-52, 9-53)

Daniel F. Martin, M.D., Atlanta, Georgia (5-2, 13-23)

Jeffrey Nerad, M.D., Iowa City, Iowa (2-15)

John J. Purcell, Jr., M.D., St. Louis, Missouri (9-23, 9-24)

Merlyn Rodrigues, M.D., Ph.D., Baltimore, Maryland (9-68, 9-100, 9-147)

Wendell J. Scott, M.D., Springfield, Missouri (8-14)

Gilbert Smolin, M.D., San Francisco, California (8-9, 8-12, 8-13, 8-60)

Tomy Starck, M.D., San Antonio, Texas (9-119)

Walter Stark, M.D., Baltimore, Maryland (18-46)

Alfred O. Steldt, M.D., Minneapolis, Minnesota (14-56)

Alan Sugar, M.D., Ann Arbor, Michigan (9-77, 9-78)

C. Gail Summers, M.D., Minneapolis, Minnesota (8-7, 8-18)

Keith Thompson, M.D., Atlanta, Georgia (9-35, 20-1, 20-3, 20-10, 20-11)

Gregory L. Thorgaard, M.D., Ottumwa, Iowa (12-20, 12-21)

David Tse, M.D., Miami, Florida (1-15, 1-16)

Arthur W. Walsh, M.D., Minneapolis, Minnesota (8-95, 8-96)

Keith Walter, M.D., Atlanta, Georgia (6-8, 6-9)

George O. Waring III, M.D., Atlanta, Georgia (5-11, 5-16, 7-3, 9-140, 19-19, 20-2)

John Wells III, M.D., Columbia, South Carolina (8-40, 8-41)

Jonathan D. Wirtschafter, M.D., Minneapolis, Minnesota (8-51, 8-52)

Ted H. Wojno, M.D., Atlanta, Georgia (1-1, 1-2, 1-3, 1-5, 1-6, 1-7, 1-8, 1-11, 1-12, 1-14, 2-4, 2-11, 2-13, 2-17, 2-18, 2-19, 2-21, 2-22, 2-23, 2-26, 2-27, 2-29, 2-30, 2-32, 5-29, 5-39, 5-40, 6-3, 14-22)

Martha M. Wright, M.D., Minneapolis, Minnesota (9-118, 9-138, 9-139)

Drs. Doug Cameron, Hans Grossniklaus, Ed Holland, Peter Laibson, and Ted Wojno made large contributions of photographs and provided editorial assistance. Dr. Jules Baum helped with the writing of the preface.

Many of the photographs were taken by the photography departments at Emory University and the University of Minnesota and the cornea fellows at the University of Iowa. We would like to thank Jim Gilman and Ray Swords of Emory University and Bill McMichael of the University of Minnesota for their photographic expertise.

We are indebted to Jill Fishbaugh and Deb Strike, who helped with the gathering of patient histories for many of the legends.

We would especially like to express our gratitude to Janet Kenney (Atlanta) and Kari Graham (Minneapolis). Janet expeditiously typed and retyped the text in her off hours and coordinated many of the day-to-day activities related to this project. Kari catalogued the slides, organized the book, and facilitated proofing of the illustrations.

Finally, we wish to thank our patients, who gave their time to be photographed so that others could learn from their pathology.

Contents

CORNEA

COLOR ATLAS

CHAPTER 1

Diseases of the Lid
ANATOMIC ABNORMALITIES

The eyelids protect the eyes and redistribute the tear film over the ocular surface. Anatomic abnormalities of the eyelids are often associated with corneal exposure and, in severe cases, corneal ulceration.

Ectropion

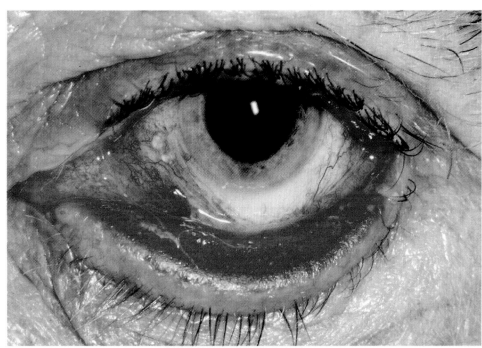

FIGURE 1-1 ***Involutional ectropion.*** This disorder is caused by laxity of the lid tissue associated with aging. It is almost always seen in the lower lids. The laxity specifically affects the lower lid retractors and/or canthal tendons.

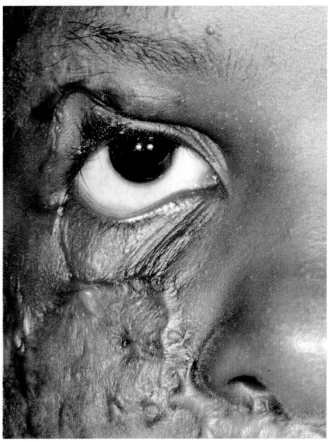

FIGURE 1-2 ***Cicatricial ectropion.*** This disorder is caused by scarring of the lid tissue or periocular skin. Eversion of the lid results from traction caused by the scar. In this case a burn injury to the skin resulted in lower lid ectropion.

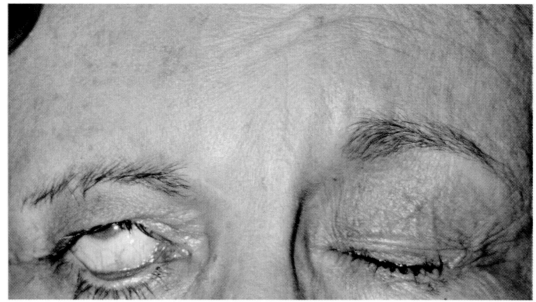

FIGURE 1-3 **Paralytic ectropion.** This disorder is caused by damage to the seventh cranial nerve. Weakness of the orbicularis muscle leads to an out-turning of the lower eyelid. This patient exhibits a paralytic ectropion and a poor Bell's phenomenon caused by a seventh nerve palsy. Normal furrowing of the brow is absent. Exposure keratitis may occur, and these patients require aggressive topical lubrication and, occasionally, a tarsorrhaphy.

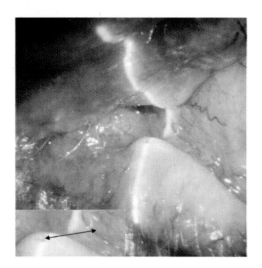

FIGURE 1-4 **Punctal ectropion.** This disorder may occur in an otherwise normally positioned lid. The arrow indicates an abnormal space between the lid and the eye *(inset)*. Repair may be needed in patients with epiphora.

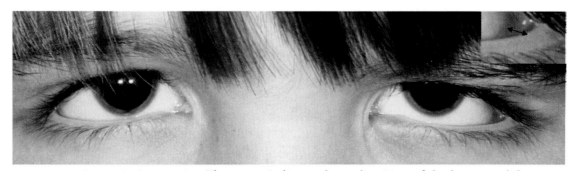

FIGURE 1-5 **Congenital ectropion.** The arrow indicates the malposition of the lower eyelid *(inset)*. This patient also has features of blepharophimosis syndrome, including telecanthus, epicanthus, ptosis, and a poorly developed nasal bridge.

Entropion

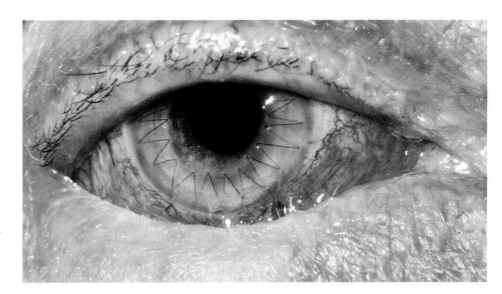

FIGURE 1-6 *Involutional entropion.* This occurred after penetrating keratoplasty. The lower eyelid is turned in and the eyelashes rub on the conjunctiva and cornea.

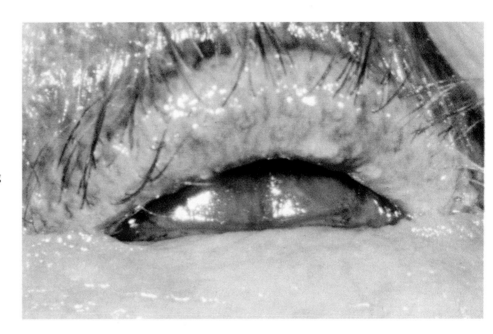

FIGURE 1-7 *Cicatricial entropion.* This disorder is caused by scarring of the palpebral conjunctiva, with resultant in-turning of the lid margins. In this case the conjunctival scarring results from Stevens-Johnson syndrome. Cicatricial entropion is also seen in ocular cicatricial pemphigoid, trachoma, herpes zoster ophthalmicus, and severe burns.

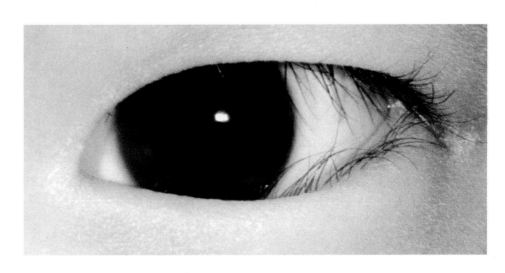

FIGURE 1-8 *Epiblepharon.* This is caused by an overriding of the skin and pretarsal muscle above the lid margin, which causes an in-turning of the lid margin and lashes. Epiblepharon usually resolves with aging and rarely requires treatment.

Trichiasis

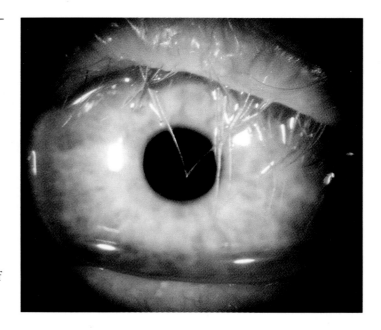

FIGURE 1-9 *Trichiasis.* This is an acquired malposition of the eyelashes. In this patient the eyelashes rub on the superior cornea.

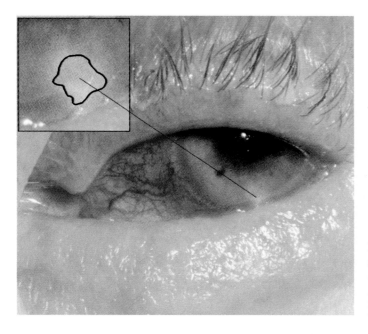

FIGURE 1-10 *Spastic entropion.* This can be caused by acute ocular inflammation or irritation in a patient with a previously unrecognized involutional entropion. Here the lashes rub on the lower cornea and have caused a corneal erosion *(inset).*

Distichiasis

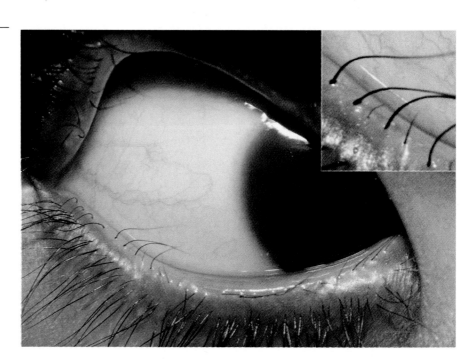

FIGURE 1-11 *Distichiasis.* In this rare condition an extra row of eyelashes exits from the meibomian orifices *(inset).* The eyelashes may rub on the conjunctiva or cornea.

Lagophthalmos

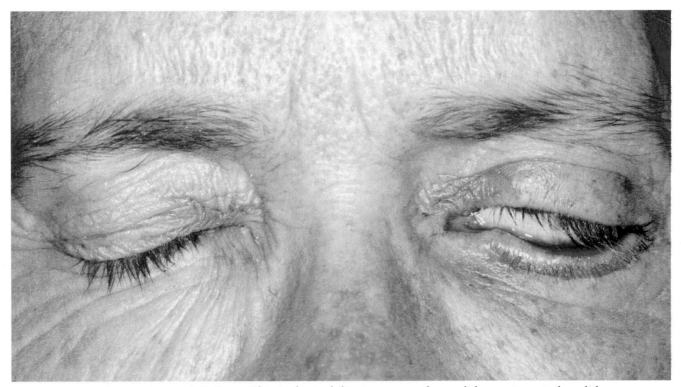

FIGURE 1-12 *Lagophthalmos.* This is the inability to appose the eyelids on attempted eyelid closure. In this case a left seventh nerve palsy has caused a lower lid paralytic ectropion and lagophthalmos.

Ptosis

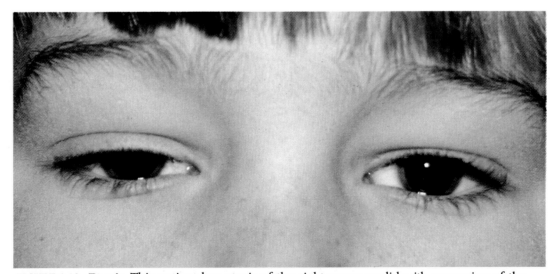

FIGURE 1-13 *Ptosis.* This patient has ptosis of the right upper eyelid with narrowing of the palpebral fissure. The right brow is elevated in an attempt to raise the abnormally low right upper eyelid. The abnormal lid position has induced astigmatism in the right eye. Results of keratometry in the right eye are 47.00 × 87/42.25 × 174; in the left eye, results are nearly spherical.

Floppy Eyelid

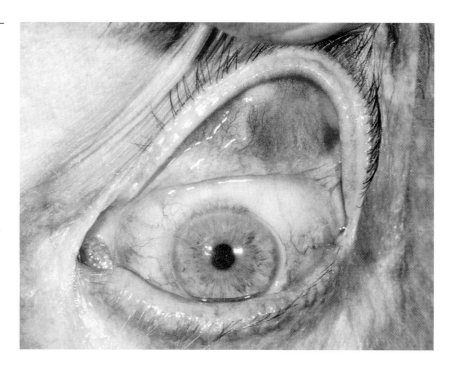

FIGURE 1-14 *Floppy eyelid syndrome.* This syndrome is associated with excessive laxity of the upper eyelid. The eyelid is easily everted with superior traction. Patients often complain of redness, irritation, and mucoid discharge. The symptoms are worse in the morning and may be related to nocturnal eversion of the eyelids leading to corneal exposure.

Lower Lid Imbrication

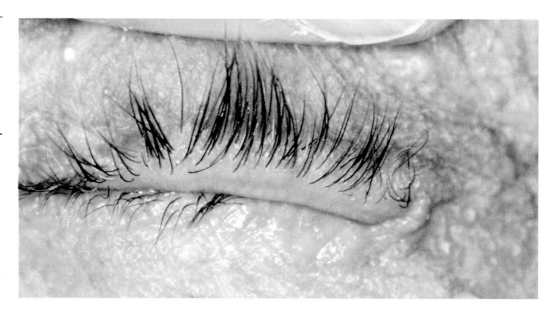

FIGURE 1-15 *Eyelid imbrication syndrome.* The upper eyelid rides over the lower eyelid. This syndrome shares many features with floppy eyelid syndrome, including redness, irritation, and a mucoid discharge. Nocturnal eversion of the eyelids may also occur.

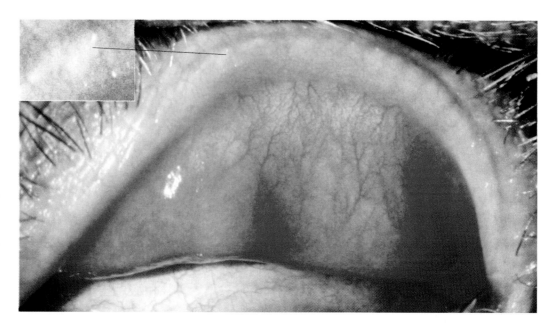

FIGURE 1-16 *Eyelid imbrication syndrome.* Keratinization of the upper palpebral conjunctiva *(inset)* and papillary conjunctivitis with lower lid imbrication. The keratinization is caused by chronic rubbing of the upper lid over the lower lid.

CHAPTER 2

Diseases of the Lid
TUMORS

Patients with abnormal growths on their eyelids are often initially seen by the general practitioner. It is important to differentiate benign lid tumors from malignant lid tumors. Occasionally, a biopsy is needed to establish the diagnosis.

Benign Lid Tumors

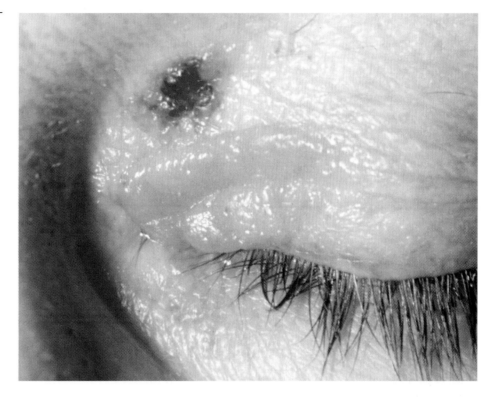

FIGURE 2-1 *Amyloid deposits.* These appear as elevated, waxy-yellow deposits in the skin. The deposits are usually bilateral and symmetric. They are occasionally associated with a superficial hemorrhage, as seen in this case.

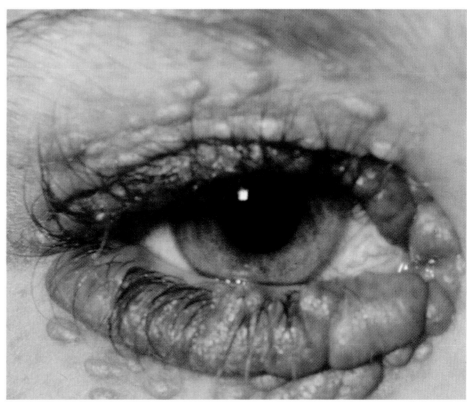

FIGURE 2-2 *Xanthogranuloma deposits in the eyelid of an 8-year-old boy.* Xanthogranulomas can also occur on the cornea (see Figure 5-37) and iris. Children with iris xanthogranulomas may initially come to the ophthalmologist with spontaneous hyphemas.

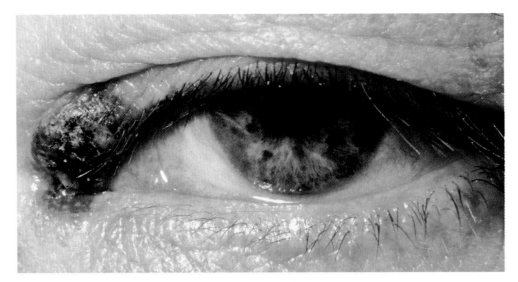

FIGURE 2-3 **Nevus of the lids.** Nevi may be congenital or acquired and pigmented or nonpigmented. This split nevus or "kissing nevus" occurs when the tumor involves both upper and lower eyelids.

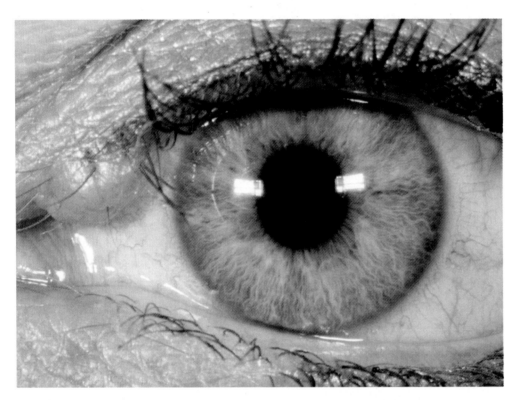

FIGURE 2-4 **Intradermal nevus.** The nevus cells are located exclusively within the dermis, as seen on the upper eyelid in this patient. These nevi are often nonpigmented and elevated.

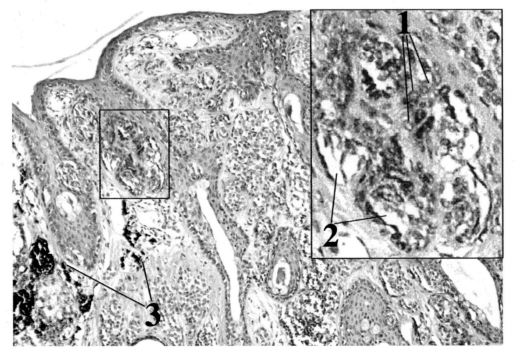

FIGURE 2-5 **Histopathology of a compound nevus.** Nests of nevus cells (1) are lined by clear melanocytes (2). Melanophages (3) are at the junction of the epidermis and dermis and in the dermis.

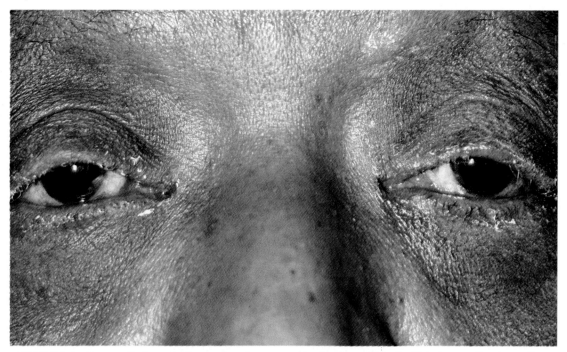

FIGURE 2-6 *Congenital oculodermal melanocytosis (nevus of Ota).* This is a collection of melanocytes in the periocular skin associated with melanosis oculi (see Figure 2-7). It most commonly occurs in Asian and African-American patients.

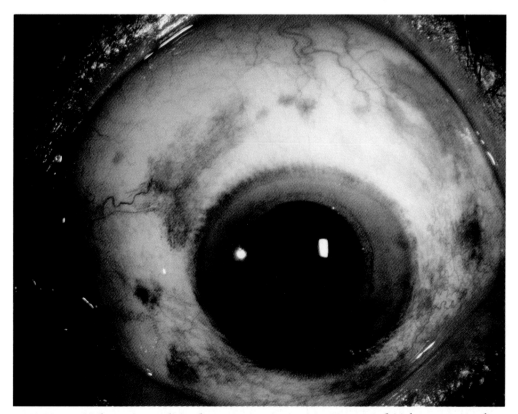

FIGURE 2-7 *Melanosis oculi in the same patient as in Figure 2-6.* Melanocytes in the episclera and sclera are responsible for the slate-blue discoloration. The conjunctiva over these lesions is mobile. The risk of uveal malignant melanomas is increased in Caucasian patients with this lesion.

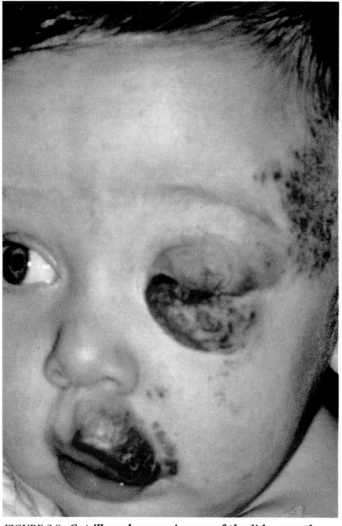

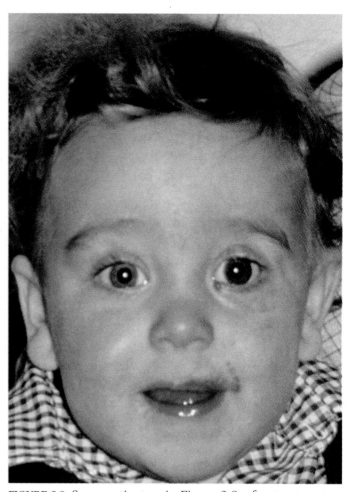

FIGURE 2-8 *Capillary hemangiomas of the lids, mouth, and temporal skin.* These tumors are first seen several weeks after birth and grow rapidly during the first year of life. They often resolve spontaneously, but treatment is needed when severe disfigurement, anisometropia, strabismus, or amblyopia occurs.

FIGURE 2-9 Same patient as in Figure 2-8, after treatment with intralesional corticosteroids.

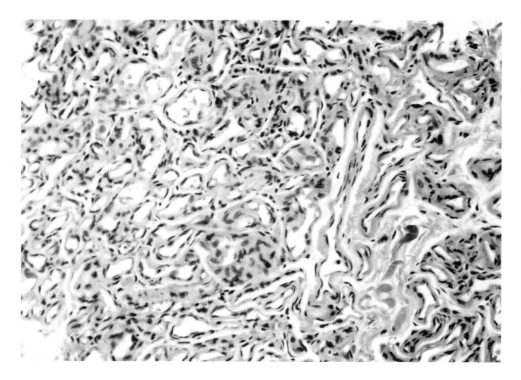

FIGURE 2-10 *Histopathology of a capillary hemangioma.* Multiple small capillary channels lined with endothelial cells are seen.

FIGURE 2-11 *A seborrheic keratosis.* This elevated, oily, crusted lesion appears to be stuck onto the surrounding skin. The lesion is common in older persons and is not premalignant.

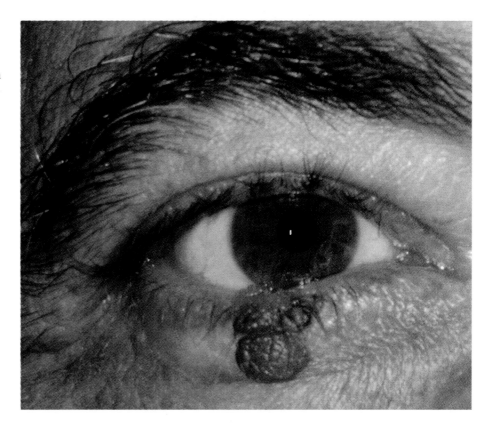

FIGURE 2-12 *Histopathology of a seborrheic keratosis.* A nodule of elevated epithelium is seen. Pseudocysts with keratin *(1)* are found within the lesion.

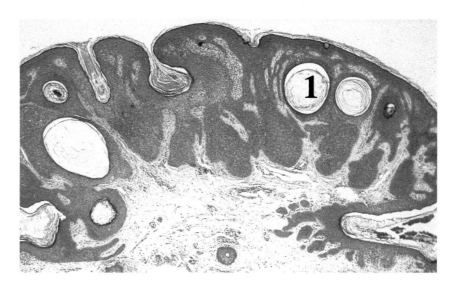

FIGURE 2-13 *Actinic keratoses.* These flat, scaly lesions arise in sun-exposed areas. They are premalignant and may develop into basal or squamous cell carcinoma.

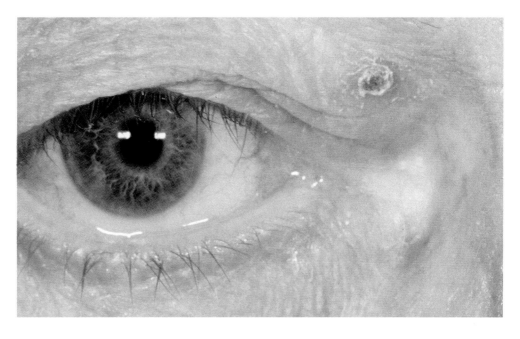

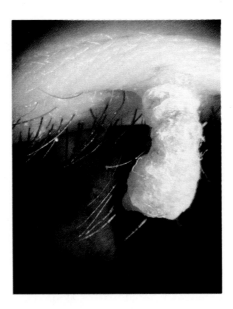

FIGURE 2-14 *An actinic keratosis.* This may enlarge and form a cutaneous horn, as seen on the upper eyelid of this patient.

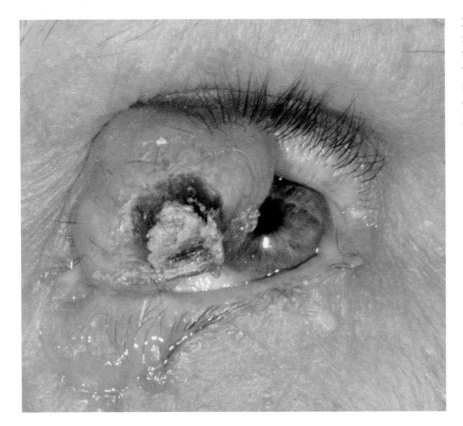

FIGURE 2-15 *A keratoacanthoma.* This rapidly enlarging growth may be seen on the eyelids. There is a central crater filled with keratin. These lesions may spontaneously involute but are often excised for cosmetic concerns and to exclude the possibility of a malignant lesion.

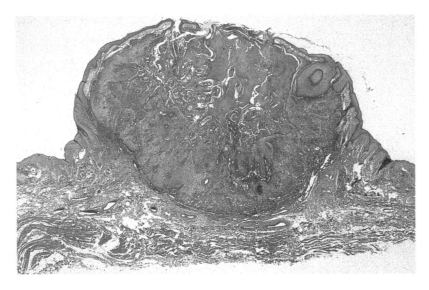

FIGURE 2-16 *Histopathology of a keratoacanthoma.* The central crater of keratin is buttressed by normal epithelium on both sides.

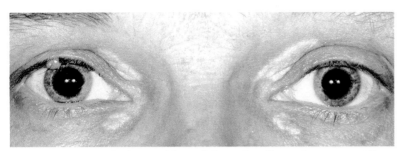

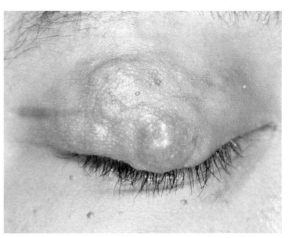

FIGURE 2-17 *Xanthelasma.* These bilateral yellow plaques usually occur in the medial canthal regions. These lesions may be associated with hypercholesterolemia, particularly if they occur in a young patient. In addition, this patient has a probable intradermal nevus on the right upper eyelid margin.

FIGURE 2-18 *Varices.* Varices composed of dilated venous channels are seen in the upper eyelid. It gives a blue discoloration to the overlying skin.

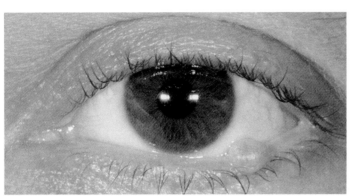

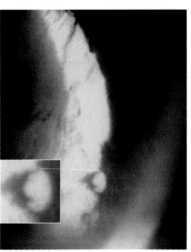

FIGURE 2-19 *Neurofibromas.* Composed of proliferating Schwann cells, they may be seen as elevated nodules and found on the skin anywhere in the body. Here the neurofibroma is on the lower lid margin.

FIGURE 2-20 *A Lisch nodule.* This elevated iris lesion is often seen in neurofibromatosis. They are multiple and tan and composed of nevus cells (*inset*).

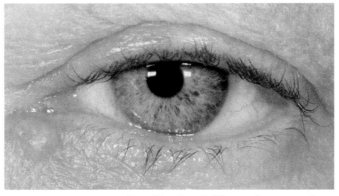

FIGURE 2-21 *Cysts of Moll's gland.* These slow-growing tumors are usually found on the lower lid near the puncta.

Malignant Lid Tumors

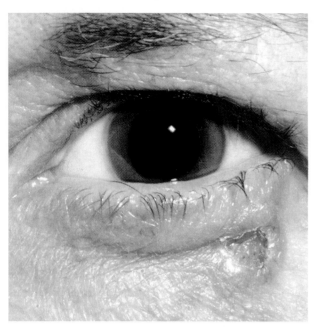

FIGURE 2-22 *Basal cell carcinomas.* These slow-growing tumors are found in sun-exposed areas. They are the most common eyelid malignancy and are usually located on the lower eyelid.

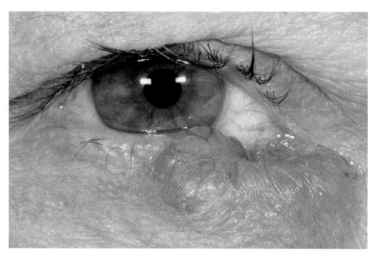

FIGURE 2-23 *A large, nodular, basal cell carcinoma.* The edges are raised and pearly, with a central ulceration.

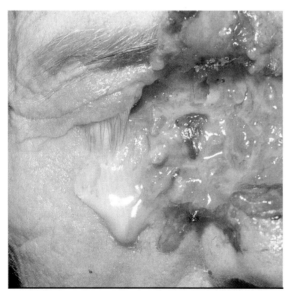

FIGURE 2-24 *A large basal cell carcinoma.* This lesion has invaded deep into the periorbital tissue. Basal cell carcinomas rarely metastasize but may exhibit extensive local invasion if neglected.

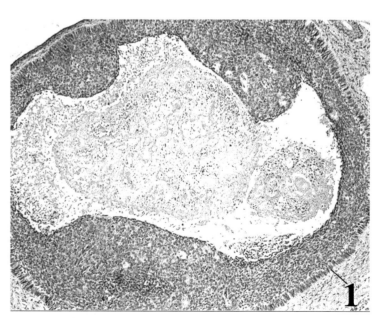

FIGURE 2-25 *Histopathology of a basal cell carcinoma.* Basophilic nests of cells with peripheral palisading *(1)* are seen.

FIGURE 2-26 *A squamous cell carcinoma.* This is a rare malignancy of the eyelids. It commonly arises in sun-exposed areas and may resemble other lesions of the eyelid, such as keratoacanthoma, basal cell carcinoma, and seborrheic keratosis. The inset shows pearly raised margins of a small squamous cell carcinoma.

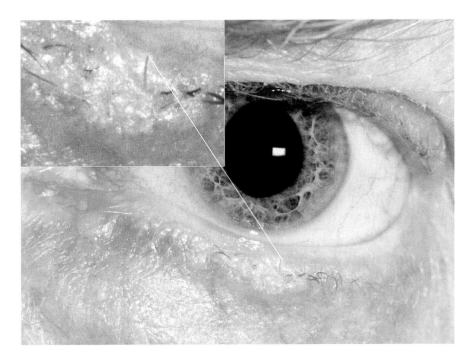

FIGURE 2-27 An extensive squamous cell carcinoma of the upper eyelid.

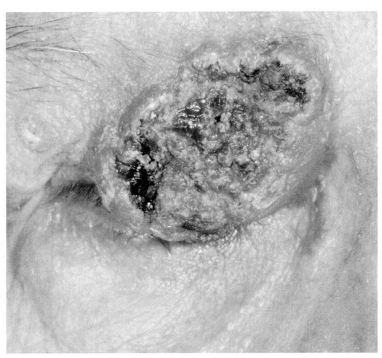

FIGURE 2-28 *Histopathology of squamous cell carcinoma.* Eosinophilic cells with large cytoplasms are shown. Keratin pearls *(1)* and dyskeratotic cells *(2)* are seen within the lesion. Dyskeratotic cells have small, dark nuclei and produce keratin.

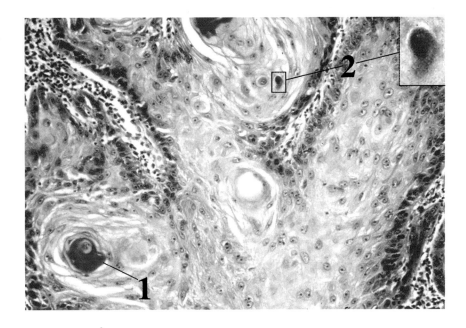

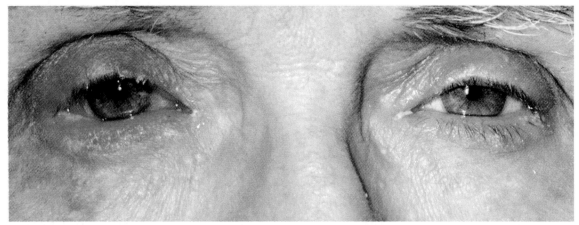

FIGURE 2-29 *A sebaceous cell carcinoma of the right eyelids.* A unilateral or asymmetric chronic blepharitis in an older patient should always raise the suspicion of sebaceous cell carcinoma.

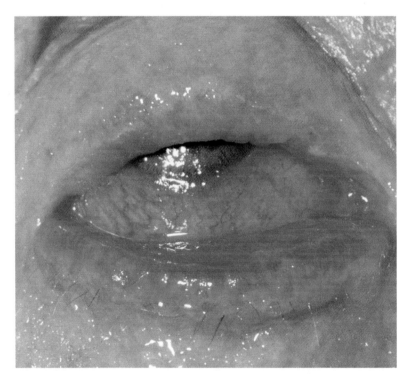

FIGURE 2-30 *Lid margin in sebaceous cell carcinoma.* It is thickened and erythematous and has extensive lash loss. This tumor is highly malignant and may spread by direct extension, lymphatics, or blood vessels.

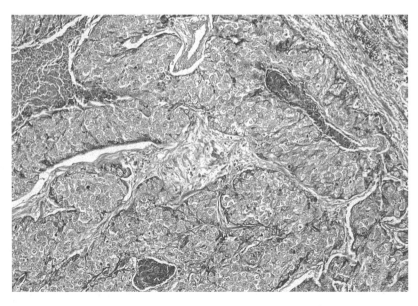

FIGURE 2-31 *Histopathology of sebaceous cell carcinoma.* Cells in nests and cords with vacuolated, foamy cytoplasms are shown. When the diagnosis is suspected, a full-thickness lid biopsy should be performed.

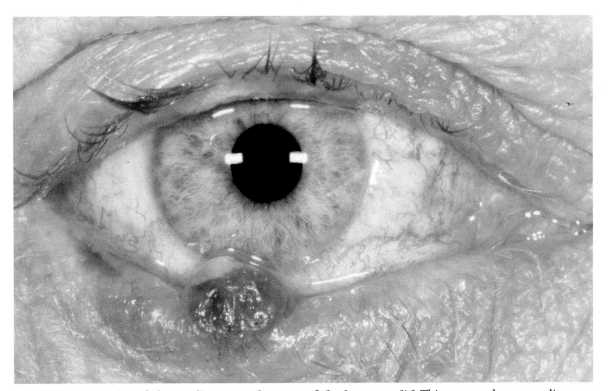

FIGURE 2-32 *A nodular malignant melanoma of the lower eyelid.* This extremely rare malignancy of the eyelid may arise de novo or from preexisting nevi. The prognosis depends on the depth of tumor invasion. This tumor can spread hematogenously and through lymphatic channels.

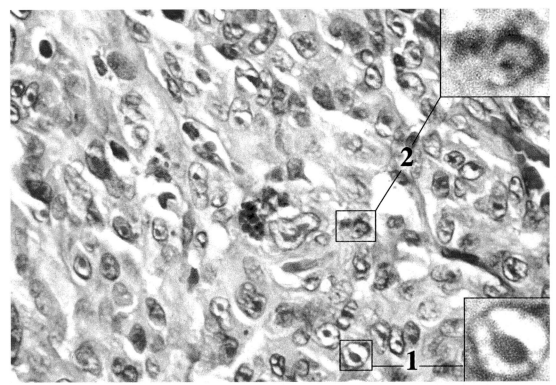

FIGURE 2-33 *Histopathology of a malignant melanoma of the eyelid.* Epithelioid cells with pleomorphic nuclei and eosinophilic nucleoli *(1)* are shown. Clumps of melanin are seen within the cytoplasm *(2)*.

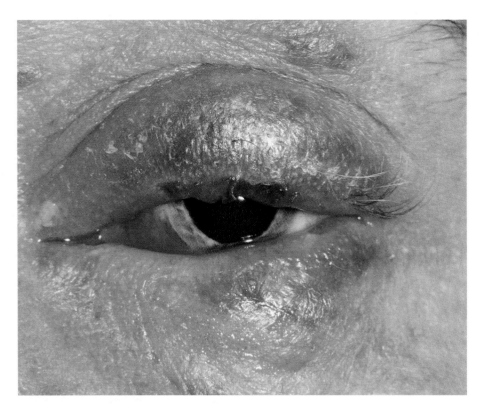

FIGURE 2-34 **Kaposi's sarcoma of the eyelids.** This lesion diffusely infiltrates the lid and has a reddish or purple discoloration. This tumor is found almost exclusively in immunocompromised patients.

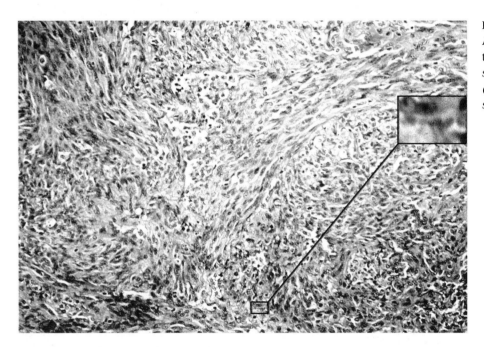

FIGURE 2-35 **Histopathology of Kaposi's sarcoma.** There is proliferation of spindle cells with slit-like spaces between the cells. Erythrocytes *(inset)* can be seen within the slit-like spaces.

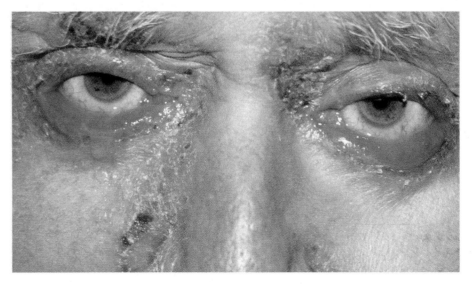

FIGURE 2-36 **Mycosis fungoides.** This is a cutaneous T-cell lymphoma that occasionally involves the periocular skin. Early in the disease process the lesions are eczematoid; they later progress to indurated plaques.

CHAPTER 3

Diseases of the Lid
INFLAMMATION AND INFECTION

Infectious and inflammatory diseases of the eyelids are often associated with conjunctivitis and symptoms of ocular discomfort. These patients are commonly seen in clinical practice.

Blepharitis

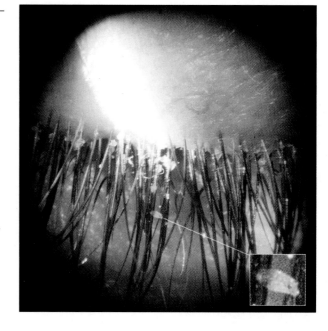

FIGURE 3-1 *Seborrheic blepharitis.* This disorder is often associated with seborrheic dermatitis. Patients complain of redness, burning, and mattering of the eyelids. It is usually bilateral and often associated with meibomian gland dysfunction. The lashes are covered with yellow, greasy scales. The scales are translucent and easily removed *(inset)*.

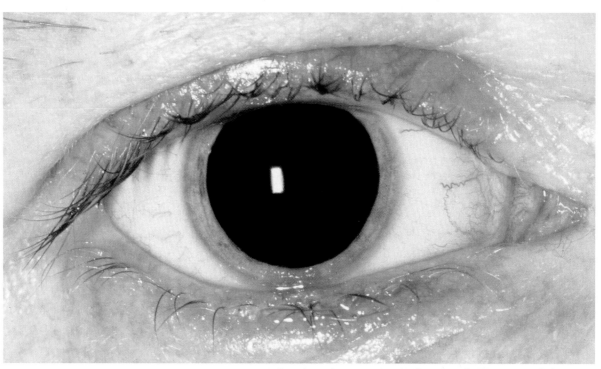

FIGURE 3-2 *Staphylococcal blepharitis.* This disorder is associated with inflammation of the anterior lid lamella and is usually not seen with meibomian gland dysfunction. Erythema of the anterior lid margin, lash loss, misdirected lashes, and ocular discharge are common findings.

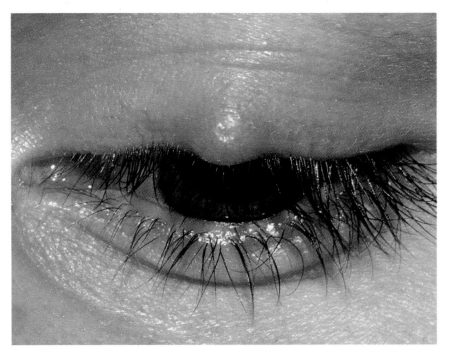

FIGURE 3-3 *A hordeolum (stye).* This is an acute inflammation of the lid margin. An internal hordeolum originates in the meibomian glands, and an external hordeolum originates in Moll's glands, Zeis' glands, or lash follicles. This external hordeolum is on the upper eyelid.

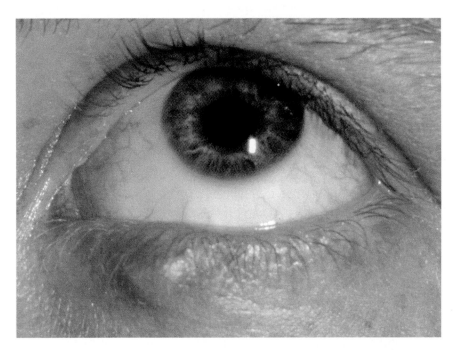

FIGURE 3-4 *A chalazion.* This is an acute inflammation of the eyelid caused by a localized obstruction of meibomian glands. The histopathology shows sebaceous secretions surrounded by a granulomatous reaction.

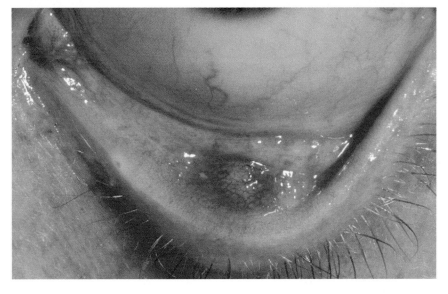

FIGURE 3-5 *Same patient as in Figure 3-4.* The lower lid is everted, and a focal nodular conjunctivitis is seen overlying the chalazion.

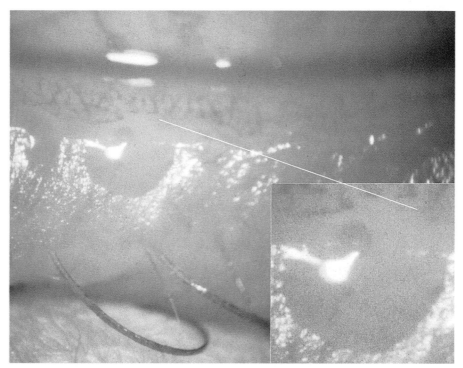

FIGURE 3-6 *Meibomitis.* The lid margin is erythematous, and a loose, oily discharge is easily expressed from the meibomian orifices *(inset).* This condition is often associated with seborrheic blepharitis.

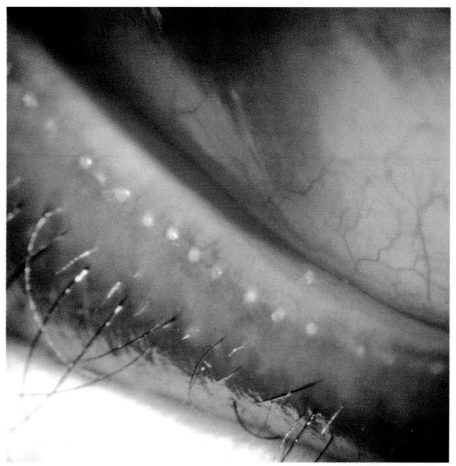

FIGURE 3-7 *Meibomitis.* In contrast to Figure 3-6, here the disorder is associated with a thick, toothpastelike secretion. The glands are plugged, and the secretions can be expressed with moderate pressure on the lid margin.

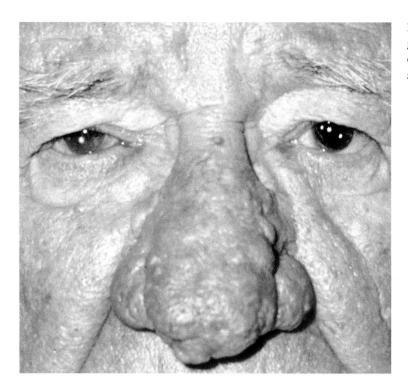

FIGURE 3-8 ***Rosacea.*** This is a chronic sebaceous gland dysfunction of the skin. This male patient exhibits rhinophyma, an enlargement of the nose secondary to sebaceous gland hypertrophy.

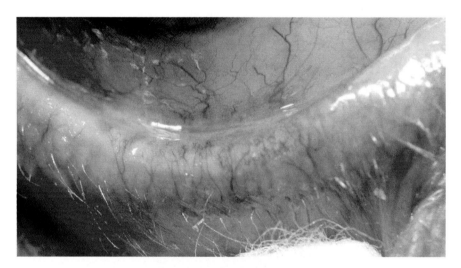

FIGURE 3-9 ***Rosacea.*** It is often associated with blepharitis and meibomian gland dysfunction.

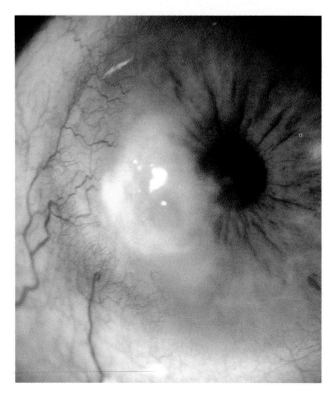

FIGURE 3-10 ***Chronic rosacea.*** Corneal vascularization and scarring can result.

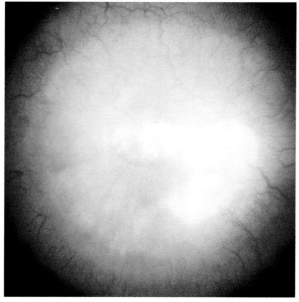

FIGURE 3-11 **Chronic rosacea keratitis.** This patient has severe corneal scarring, vascularization, and lipid degeneration.

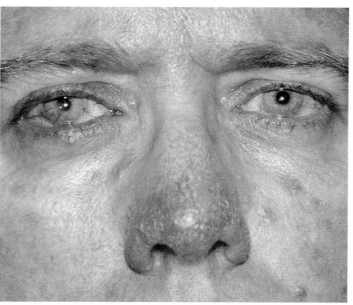

FIGURE 3-12 **Rosacea.** Occurring with greater frequency in females, as in this patient, rosacea often involves erythema, telangiectasia, and acne as common skin findings.

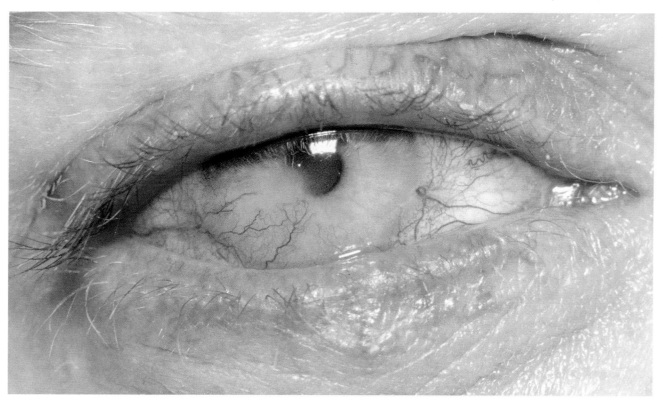

FIGURE 3-13 **Same patient as in Figure 3-12.** The lid margins and conjunctiva are inflamed, and there is corneal pannus and scarring.

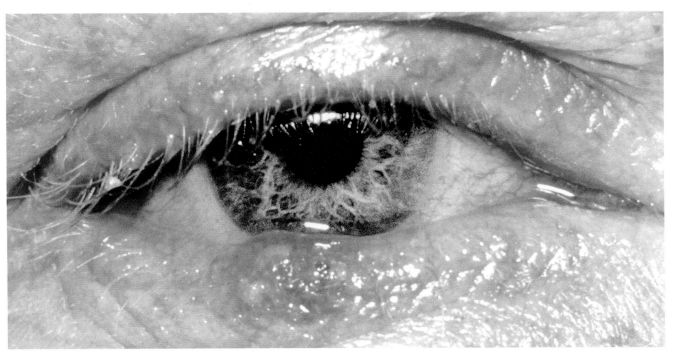

FIGURE 3-14 Mixed anterior and posterior lid margin disease.

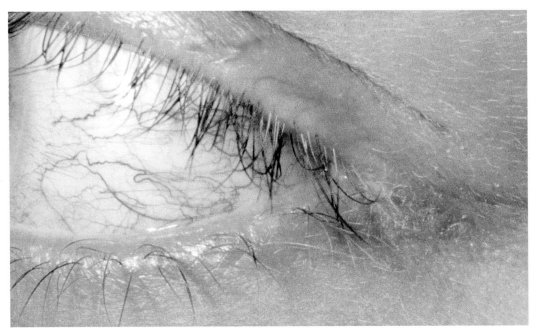

FIGURE 3-15 *Angular blepharitis.* This is an inflammation of the lateral lid margins and canthal region. If it is infectious, it is often associated with bacterial infection from *Moraxella* or *Staphylococcus* species.

Bacterial Infections

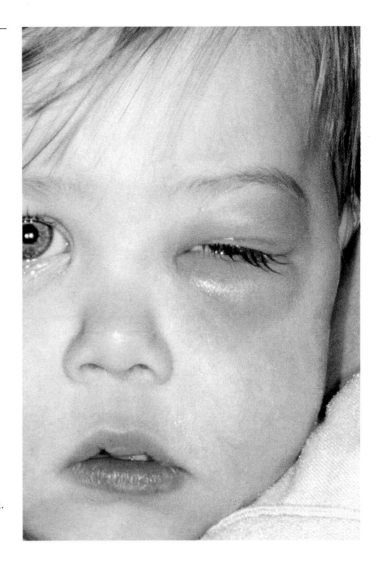

FIGURE 3-16 *Preseptal cellulitis.* This is an infection of the periorbital tissue anterior to the orbital septum. Visual acuity, pupil reactivity, and ocular motility are normal.

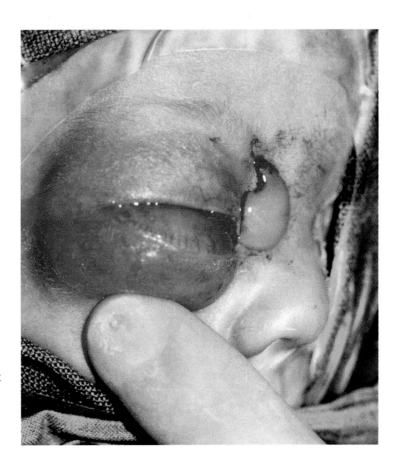

FIGURE 3-17 *Orbital cellulitis.* This infection of the orbital tissues usually extends from an infection in the paranasal sinuses. Here an ethmoid sinusitis has extended into the orbital tissues. Clinical features that distinguish an orbital cellulitis from a preseptal cellulitis include fever, proptosis, severe chemosis, ocular motility disturbances, pupillary abnormalities, and decreased vision.

Viral Infections

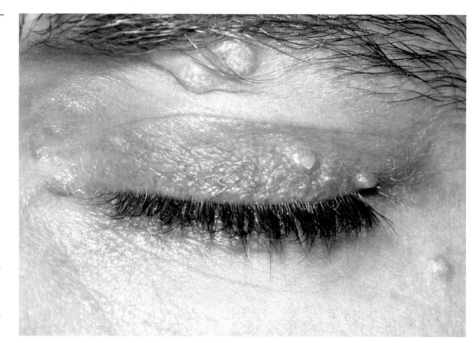

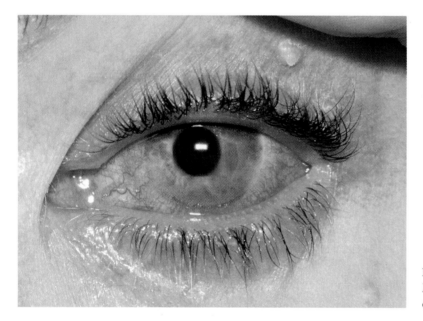

FIGURE 3-18 *Multiple molluscum contagiosum lesions on the periocular lid in a patient with AIDS.* The small elevated lesions with a central umbilicated core are caused by a pox virus.

FIGURE 3-19 *Same patient as in Figure 3-18.* Molluscum lesions near the lid margin can produce a toxic follicular conjunctivitis.

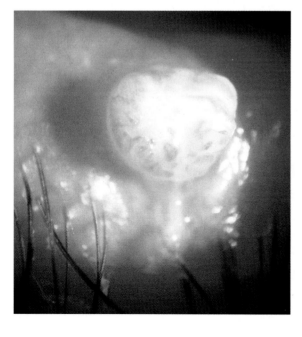

FIGURE 3-20 *A papilloma.* This is a hyperkeratotic lesion with multiple small vascular loops. It is a benign lesion caused by the papilloma virus.

Parasitic Infections

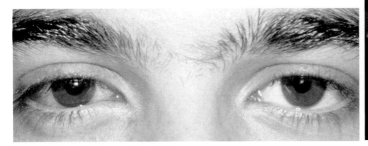

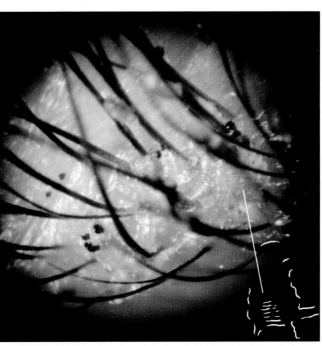

FIGURE 3-21 *Lid infestation with the crab louse (Phthirus pubis).* Chronic conjunctivitis is seen in this patient's right eye. Symptoms include itching, redness, and irritation.

FIGURE 3-22 *Phthirus pubis infestation of the eyelashes.* The adult louse has six legs and appears transparent with direct illumination. The schematic *(lower right)* shows the outline of a louse.

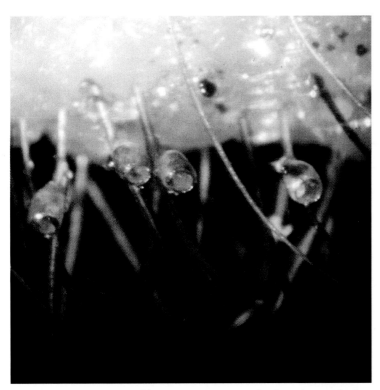

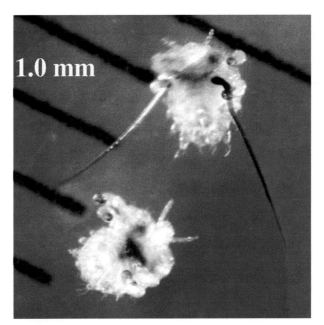

FIGURE 3-23 *Nits.* Ovoid eggs are seen attached to the eyelashes. They hatch 1 to 2 weeks after they are laid. The reddish-brown granular material on the lid seen here and in Figure 3-22 is feces from the lice.

FIGURE 3-24 *Lice.* Two lice are seen after removal from the eyelid. The upper louse is clinging to cilia. Crab lice usually measure 2 mm or less, whereas head and body lice are usually 2 to 4 mm long.

Allergic Inflammations

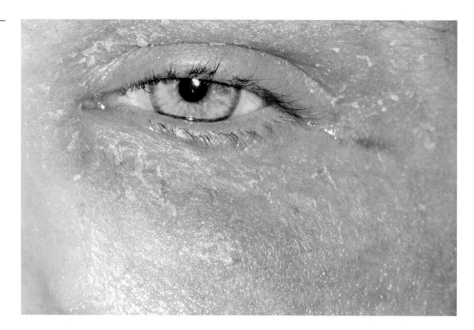

FIGURE 3-25 *Contact dermatitis.* This may develop after prolonged use of a topical medication. Clinically, an eczematous reaction of the lid margin and redness of the periocular skin occur. Symptoms include itching and irritation. This patient developed a reaction to tape after several days of pressure patching a corneal abrasion.

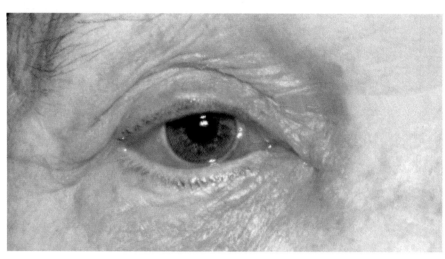

FIGURE 3-26 *Hypersensitivity reaction.* Thimerosal is believed to cause a type-IV hypersensitivity reaction of the conjunctiva. Here the thimerosal was a preservative in a contact lens solution. It is now used less frequently in a contact lens solution because of this type of reaction.

Foreign Body Abscess

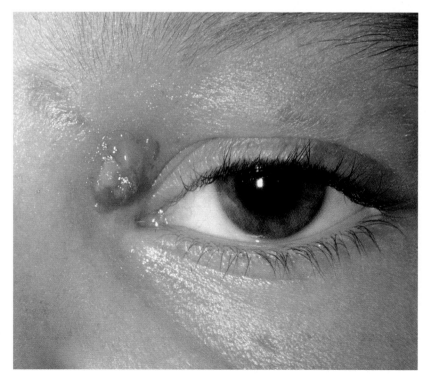

FIGURE 3-27 *Foreign body reaction.* A retained foreign body may present as a localized area of eyelid inflammation. Here an occult wood foreign body was surgically removed.

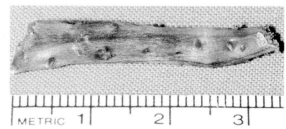

FIGURE 3-28 *Foreign body.* The wood foreign body was approximately 3.5 cm long.

CHAPTER 4

Disorders of Tear Production and the Lacrimal System

The tear film is composed of three layers: the mucous layer, the aqueous layer, and the lipid layer. The mucous layer is produced by conjunctival goblet cells and is in direct contact with the corneal epithelium. The aqueous layer is produced by the main lacrimal gland and the accessory lacrimal glands. The most anterior layer is the lipid layer, which is produced by the meibomian glands.

Dry Eye

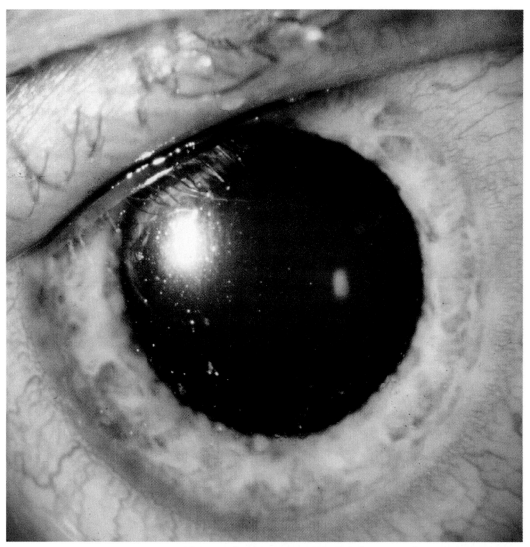

FIGURE 4-1 *Dry eye syndrome.* This is often associated with lid margin disease. Dry eyes can occur as both quantitative and qualitative disorder of tear production. In this example, the upper lid margin is inflamed and shows lash loss. The corneal surface is dry, and there is an irregular light reflex. Mucus is evident on the corneal surface.

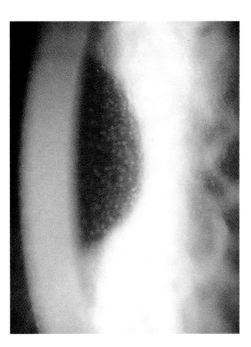

FIGURE 4-2 *Superficial punctate keratopathy.* This is a common finding in patients with dry eye syndrome. The irregular epithelial surface can be appreciated without special stains.

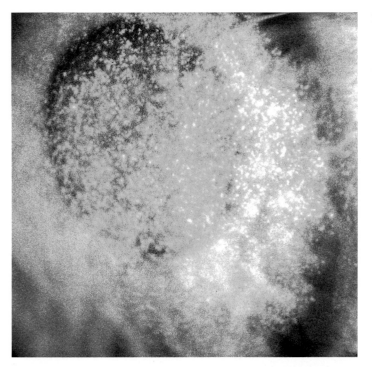

FIGURE 4-3 *Fluorescein staining in the same patient as in Figure 4-2.* Fluorescein is a water-soluble dye that stains in areas of missing epithelium.

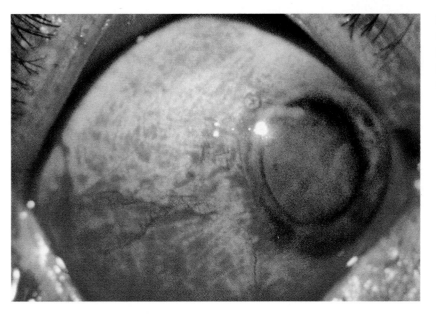

FIGURE 4-4 *Rose bengal stain of conjunctival epithelial cells in dry eyes.* Recent evidence suggests that rose bengal stains cells devoid of an overlying mucin layer as opposed to degenerated or dead cells.

FIGURE 4-5 *Dry eye syndrome.* Rose bengal may also stain corneal epithelial cells. In addition, rose bengal stains a mucous filament inferiorly (*inset*). Mucus does not stain well with fluorescein.

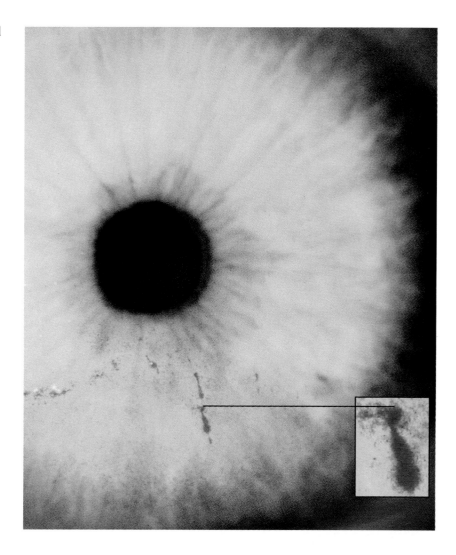

FIGURE 4-6 *Lacrimal gland tumor resulting in a dry eye.* In this patient with pseudotumor of the lacrimal gland, the corneal surface is irregular and there are mucous filaments.

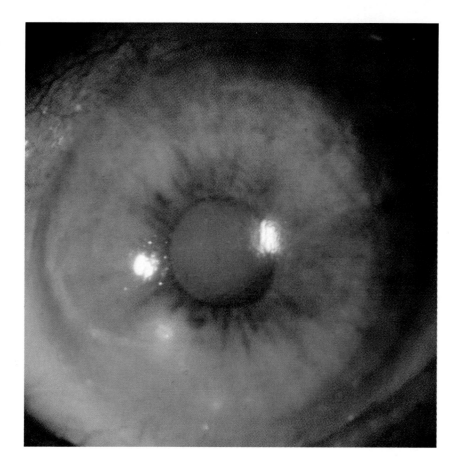

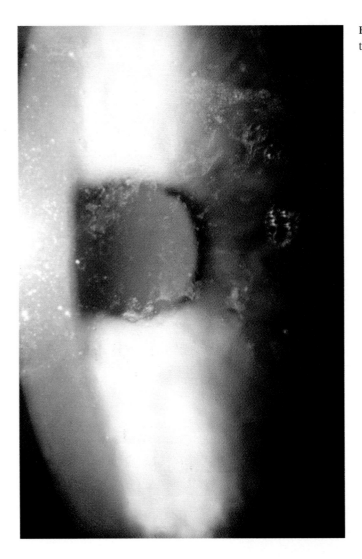

FIGURE 4-7 *Dry eye syndrome.* Mucous debris is stuck on the epithelium.

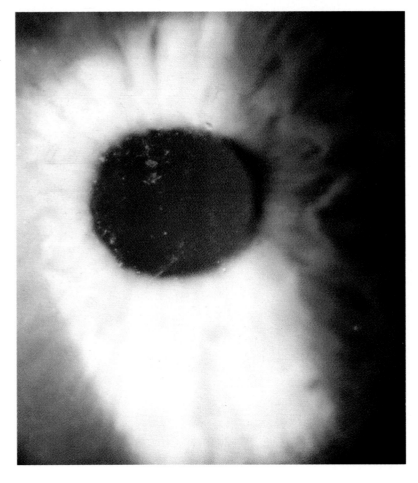

FIGURE 4-8 *Same patient as in Figure 4-7.* Several minutes after administration of 10% acetylcysteine (Mucomyst), this was the appearance of the eye. Acetylcysteine is a mucolytic agent that is effective in the treatment of excessive mucus.

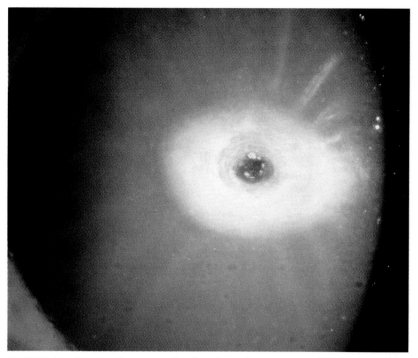

FIGURE 4-9 **Severe dry eyes.** Sterile ulceration can result.

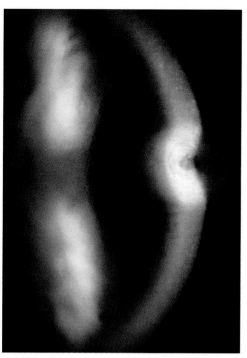

FIGURE 4-10 **Dry eye syndrome.** Slit beam examination of this patient's cornea shows extensive tissue loss with a descemetocele.

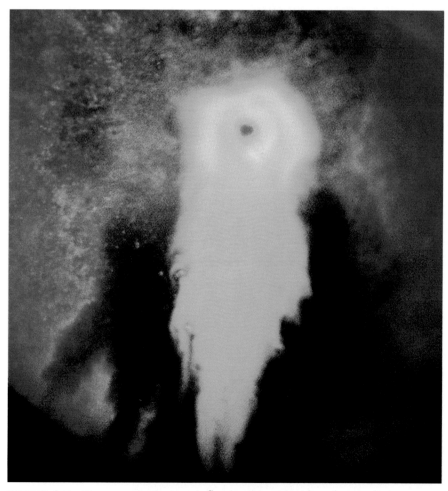

FIGURE 4-11 **Dry eye syndrome.** A fluorescein strip placed over the descemetocele indicates an active leak (positive Seidel's test).

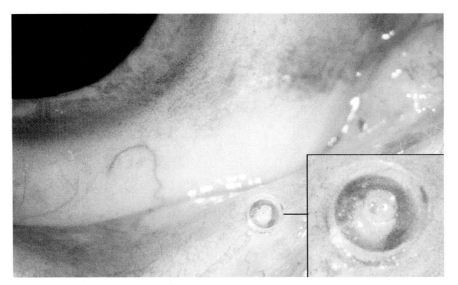

FIGURE 4-12 *Dry eye syndrome.* A silicone punctal plug *(inset)* has been placed in the right inferior punctum. The plug increases the volume of the tear film by decreasing tear outflow.

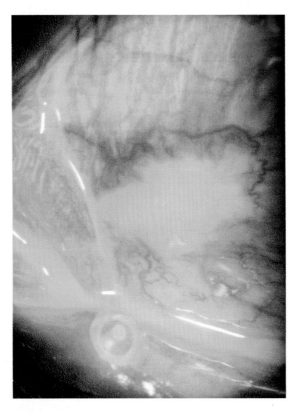

FIGURE 4-13 *Dry eye syndrome.* Silicone plugs can rub on the conjunctiva. Fluorescein stains an area of conjunctival erosion.

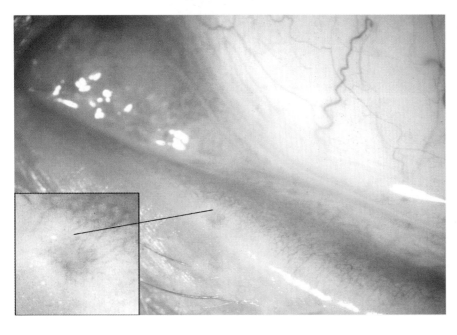

FIGURE 4-14 *Dry eye syndrome.* Permanent punctal occlusion can be performed with cautery. The left lower punctum has been occluded, and fluorescein pools in the occluded area *(inset).*

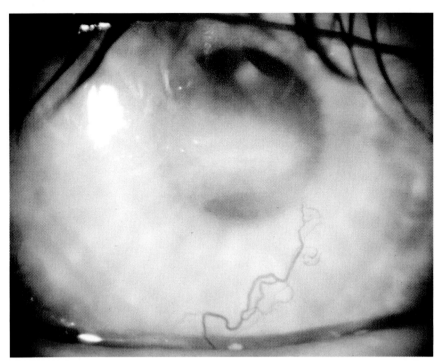

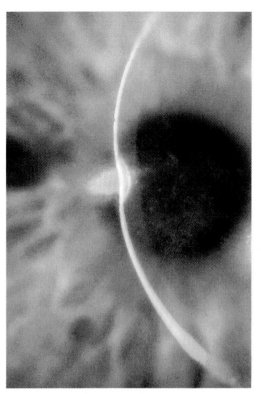

FIGURE 4-15 *Dry eye syndrome.* Familial dysautonomia (Riley-Day syndrome) causes systemic autonomic instability. Here the cornea is scarred from a previous corneal ulcer. These patients have corneal hypesthesia and dry eyes.

FIGURE 4-16 *Severe dry eye syndrome with graft-versus-host disease.* Here a sterile corneal ulceration is seen.

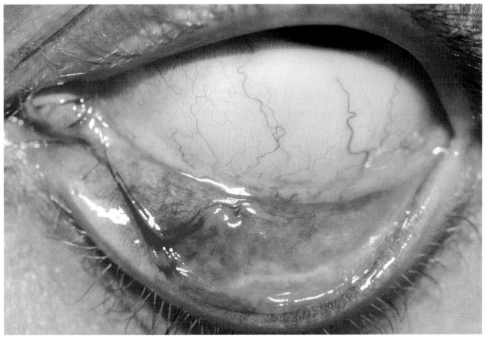

FIGURE 4-17 *Dry eye syndrome with graft-versus-host disease.* This patient has a severe dry eye and membranous conjunctivitis.

Dacryoadenitis, Dacryocystitis, and Canaliculitis

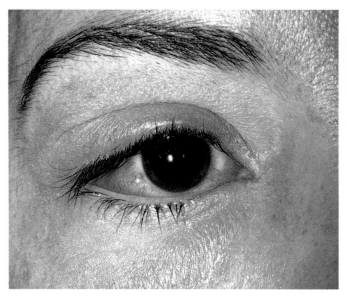

FIGURE 4-18 *Dacryoadenitis.* This is an inflammation of the lacrimal gland. The superior temporal lid is erythematous, and the lid margin is S-shaped as a result of the underlying enlargement of the lacrimal gland.

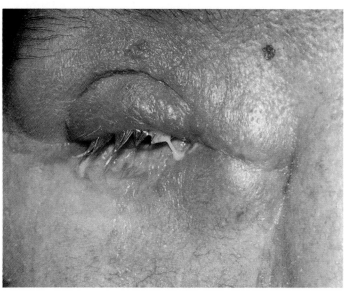

FIGURE 4-19 *Dacryocystitis.* This is an inflammation of the lacrimal sac. Here an acute infection is seen, with erythema and enlargement lateral to the nasal bridge. Mucopurulent conjunctivitis is also present.

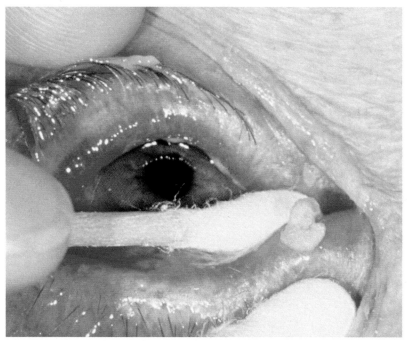

FIGURE 4-20 *Acute canaliculitis.* This includes conjunctivitis, inflamed and pouting punctum, and expressible discharge from the canaliculus. This case of canaliculitis was caused by *Actinomyces israelii.*

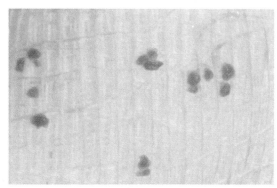

FIGURE 4-21 *Canaliculitis.* Sulfur granules composed of mycelial filaments are found within the discharge.

CHAPTER 5

Conjunctival Disease
TUMORS

Conjunctival tumors can be divided into squamous neoplasms, melanocytic neoplasms, and subepithelial neoplasms. It is often possible to differentiate benign lesions from malignant lesions based on the appearance of the lesion; however, in some cases a biopsy is necessary.

Squamous Neoplasms of the Conjunctiva

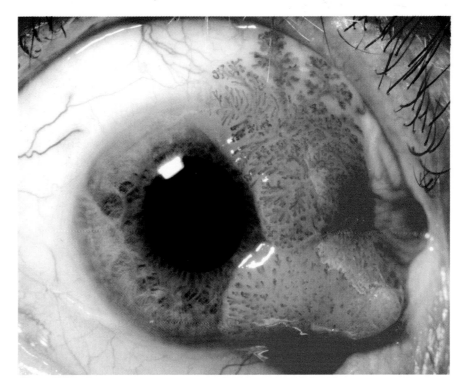

FIGURE 5-1 *A papilloma.* This benign lesion of the conjunctiva consists of multiple fibrovascular connective tissue cores with an overlying epithelium. Lesions may be sessile or pedunculated. They are caused by a papilloma virus, and in older adults, these lesions can be premalignant.

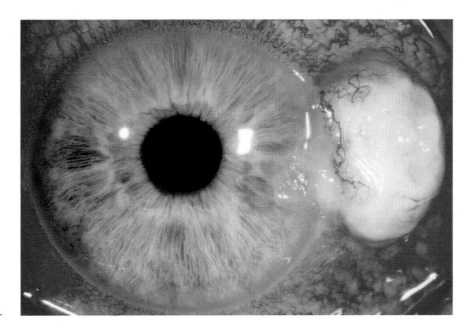

FIGURE 5-2 *A conjunctival keratoacanthoma.* This exceedingly rare lesion is similar to the keratoacanthoma on the skin. The lesions arise rapidly, are elevated, and contain a central keratin core.

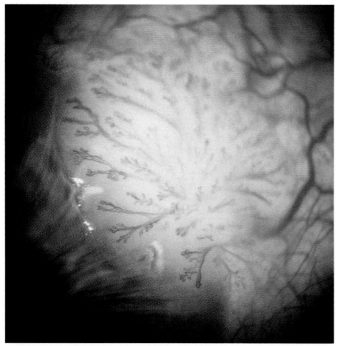

FIGURE 5-3 *Conjunctival intraepithelial neoplasia.* This occurs predominantly in older Caucasians. It usually begins at the limbus in the interpalpebral region and is associated with chronic sun exposure. The lesions are characteristically elevated and have a gelatinous appearance. The conjunctiva is diffusely injected around the lesion, and within the lesion, there are loops of vessels that often point anteriorly. The lesion may resemble a papilloma.

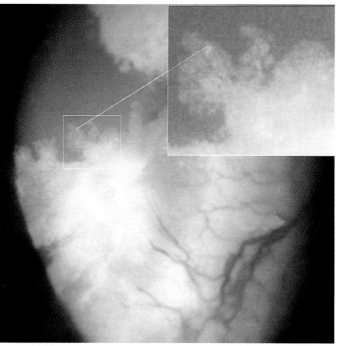

FIGURE 5-4 *Conjunctival intraepithelial neoplasia.* In many cases, the lesion extends onto the cornea and has waxy, scalloped extensions *(inset)*.

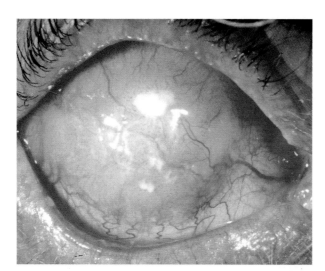

FIGURE 5-5 *Extensive conjunctival intraepithelial neoplasia with severe corneal vascularization and scarring.* The neoplasia in this case was confined to the epithelium.

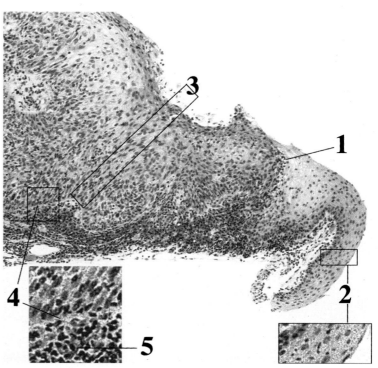

FIGURE 5-6 *Conjunctival intraepithelial neoplasia.* There is a junction between normal epithelium on the right and neoplastic epithelium on the left *(1)*. Normal cells show a maturation continuum from immature cells in the basal layer to mature anterior cells *(2)*. In contrast, on the neoplastic side, immature cells extend through the full thickness of the epithelial layers *(3)*. The basement membrane underlying the neoplastic cells is intact *(4)*. Beneath it are chronic inflammatory cells *(5)*.

FIGURE 5-7 *Extensive squamous cell carcinoma of the conjunctiva.* Initially the patient refused resection and then returned with this advanced lesion.

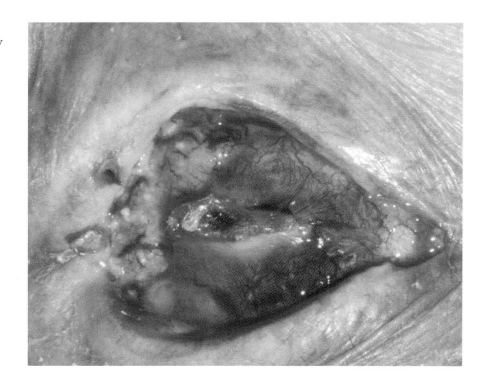

FIGURE 5-8 *Same patient as in Figure 5-7.* The lesion has metastasized to the preauricular nodes circled. The nodes are firm, raised, and immobile.

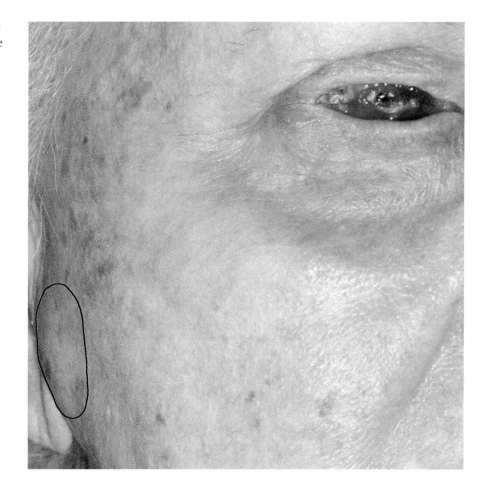

Melanocytic Neoplasms and Other Pigmented Lesions of the Conjunctiva

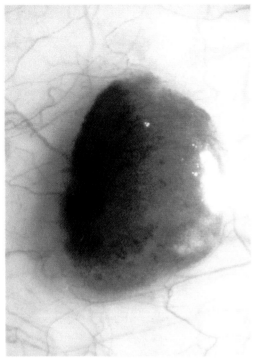

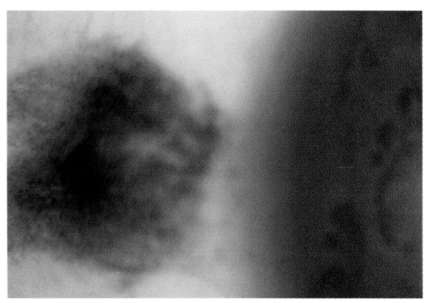

FIGURE 5-9 **Nevi.** These are benign pigmented lesions of the conjunctiva. They usually occur on the bulbar conjunctiva and are freely mobile over the sclera. This is an elevated conjunctival nevus.

FIGURE 5-10 A flat conjunctival nevus.

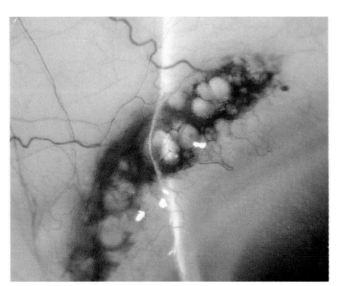

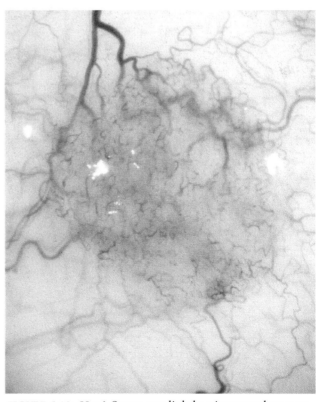

FIGURE 5-11 **Nevi.** Occasionally, they develop clear cystic spaces.

FIGURE 5-12 **Nevi.** Some are lightly pigmented or nonpigmented.

FIGURE 5-13 *Primary acquired melanosis (PAM).* This is a flat, golden-brown or tan pigmentation of the conjunctiva; its appearance may change with time. This acquired lesion usually occurs in the fourth decade of life or later, primarily in Caucasians. PAM with atypia may progress to malignant melanoma.

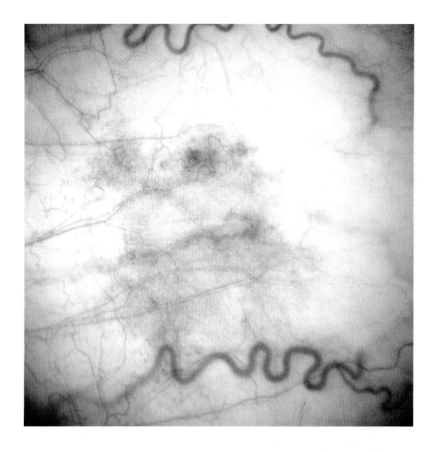

FIGURE 5-14 *Malignant melanoma of the conjunctiva.* This lesion can arise de novo, from a preexisting nevus, or from preexisting PAM with atypia. This tumor may appear on the palpebral conjunctiva or the bulbar conjunctiva and commonly occurs at the limbus. It is elevated and highly vascular and is occasionally accompanied by a hemorrhagic component, as in this case.

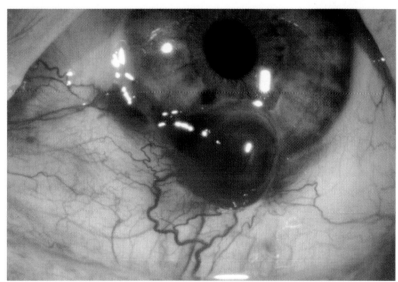

FIGURE 5-15 *Histopathology of a conjunctival malignant melanoma.* There is invasion of the substantia propria with pleomorphic melanocytes *(1)* and melanophages *(2)* with pigment.

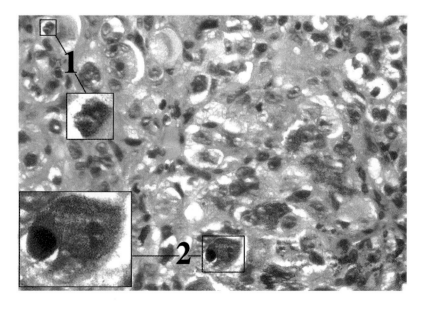

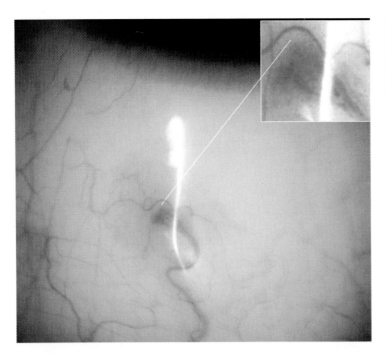

FIGURE 5-16 *Melanosis.* Pigmentation can occur around an Axenfeld's intrascleral nerve loop. The pigmentation is found near the limbus and is benign and nonmobile, since it is located within the sclera. These areas of pigmentation are more common in African-American patients.

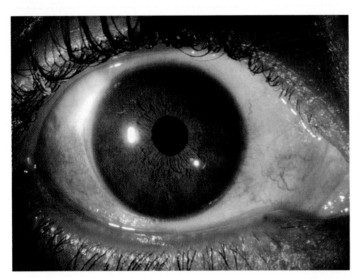

FIGURE 5-17 *Racial melanosis.* This flat, deeply pigmented lesion of the conjunctiva is commonly found near the limbus and in the interpalpebral area. It develops early in life, is uninflamed, and rarely changes in appearance. It occurs primarily in darkly pigmented patients and has no malignant potential.

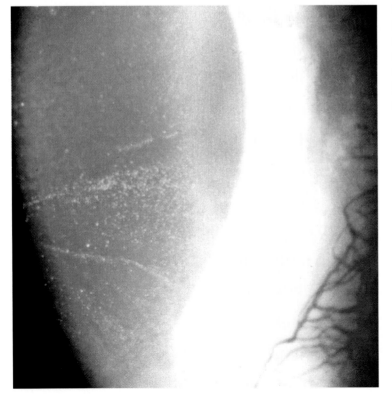

FIGURE 5-18 *Striate melanokeratosis.* This can be associated with pigmented limbal lesions, such as racial melanosis. Chronic irritation of the corneal epithelium results in migration of pigmented stem cells from the limbus onto the cornea. The corneal lesion appears whorl-like, which represents the path of epithelial cell migration.

Subepithelial Neoplasms and Other Lesions

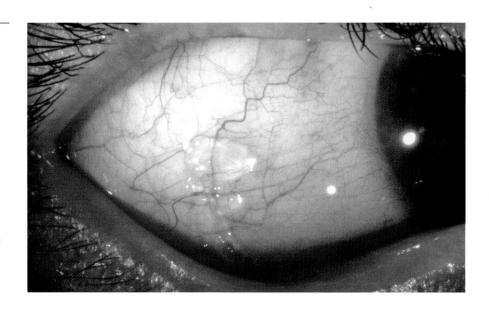

FIGURE 5-19 *Lymphangiectasis.* There is a collection of dilated lymphatic channels within the conjunctiva. They are clear, elevated, and cystic.

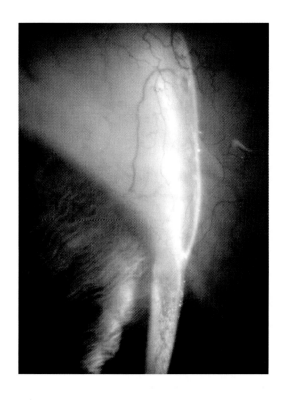

FIGURE 5-20 *Lymphangiectasis.* A thin slit view shows the lymphatic channels to be cystic and elevated.

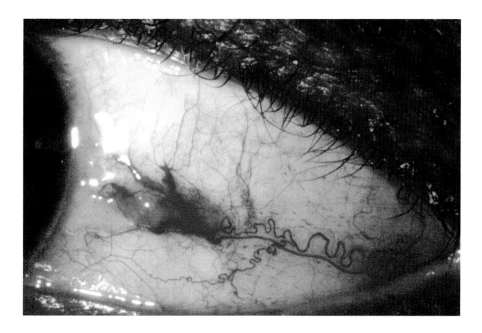

FIGURE 5-21 *Lymphangiectasis.* Occasionally, this disorder has a hemorrhagic component.

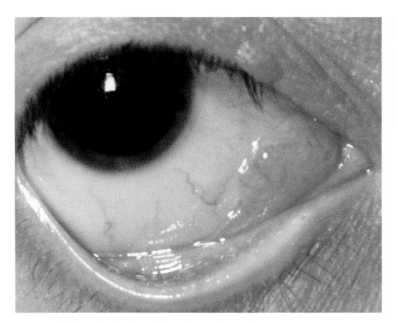

FIGURE 5-22 *Lymphangioma within the conjunctiva.* These rare tumors usually occur during the first decade of life and often enlarge with upper respiratory tract infections. In contrast to lymphangiectasis, these lesions are composed of a proliferation of lymphatic channels and lymphoid tissue. They are solid, pinkish tumors.

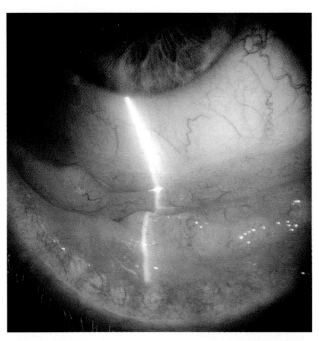

FIGURE 5-23 *Benign lymphoid hyperplasia.* Lymphoid lesions of the conjunctiva are typically elevated and salmon colored. The surrounding tissue is uninflamed. A local biopsy is necessary to establish the diagnosis.

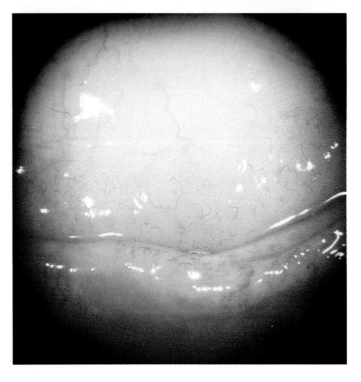

FIGURE 5-24 *Localized lymphoma on the bulbar conjunctiva.* A biopsy was consistent with B-cell lymphoma, and there was no evidence of systemic lymphoma.

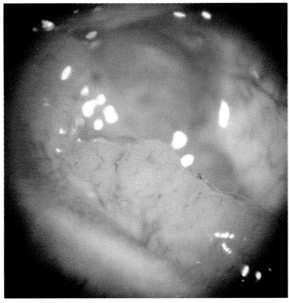

FIGURE 5-25 Localized lymphoma involving both the bulbar and palpebral conjunctivae.

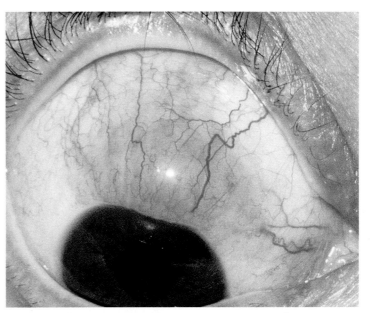

FIGURE 5-26 *Conjunctival lesion in a patient with systemic lymphoma.* Similar to the lesions already noted, this is elevated and salmon colored; the surrounding tissue is uninflamed.

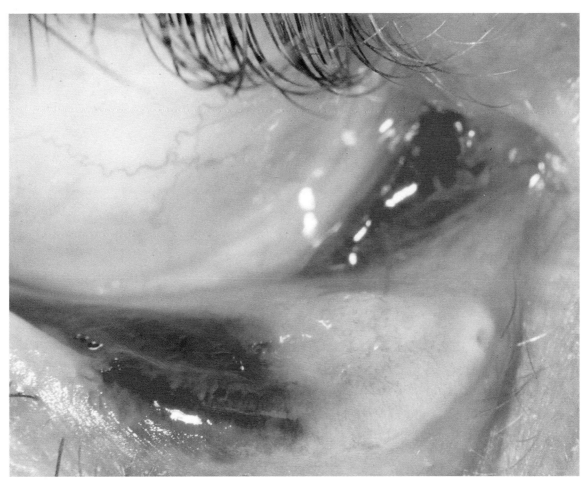

FIGURE 5-27 *Kaposi's sarcoma of the conjunctiva and lower lid in a patient with AIDS.* The lesion is elevated and highly vascular.

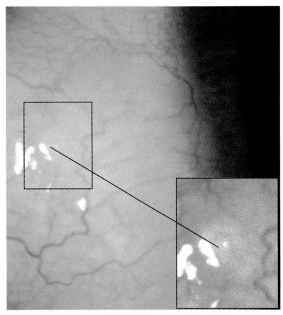

FIGURE 5-28 A limbal sarcoid nodule (*inset*).

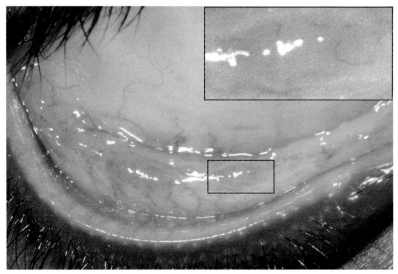

FIGURE 5-29 *Multiple sarcoid nodules in the inferior fornix.* These solid, raised lesions (*inset*) may resemble follicles.

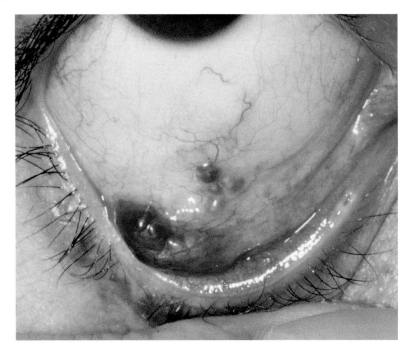

FIGURE 5-30 *Hemangiomas.* These lesions rarely occur in the conjunctiva.

FIGURE 5-31 A conjunctival hemangioma in a patient with Osler-Weber-Rendu disease.

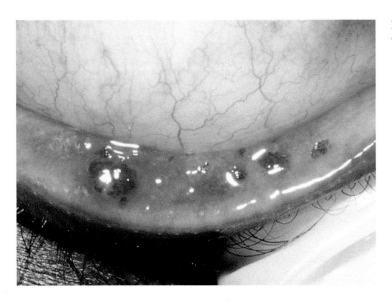

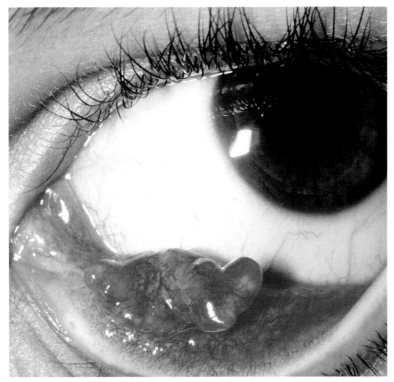

FIGURE 5-32 *A pyogenic granuloma.* This lesion arises after inflammation of the conjunctiva and is often seen after a surgical procedure. It is composed of granulation tissue (fibroblasts, capillaries, and inflammatory cells) and does not contain granulomas.

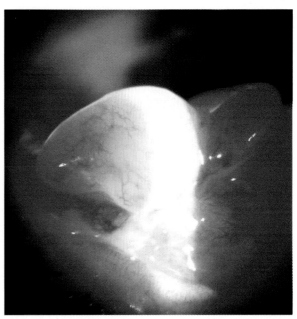

FIGURE 5-33 *Pyogenic granulomas.* These lesions grow rapidly, are pedunculated, and have a beefy red or fleshy appearance. They can resolve with topical corticosteroid treatment; however, excision may be necessary.

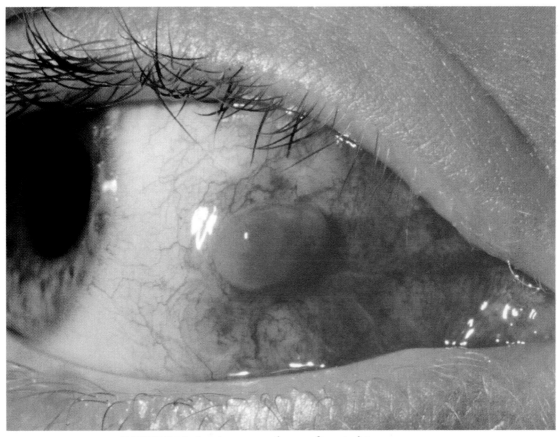

FIGURE 5-34 A suture granuloma after strabismus surgery.

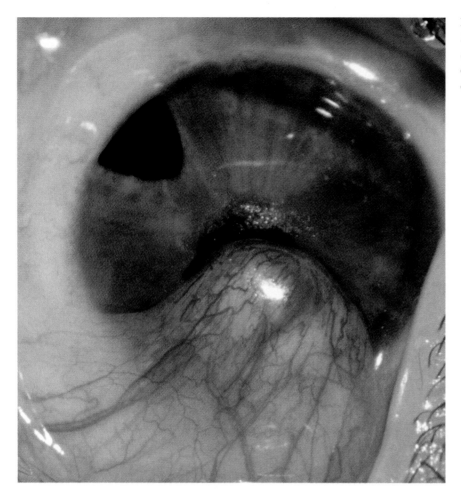

FIGURE 5-35 *A recurrent keloid on the left cornea in a patient with Lowe syndrome.* Unlike a pterygium, this lesion extends from the inferior limbus onto the cornea and deep into the corneal stroma.

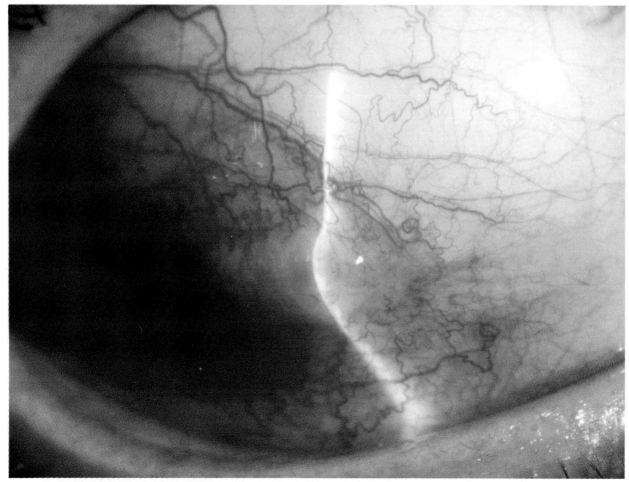

FIGURE 5-36 *Nodular fasciitis.* This lesion is an acute proliferation of sheets of immature fibroblasts. It occurred in response to multiple self-inflicted needle punctures to the conjunctiva.

FIGURE 5-37 *A xanthogranuloma on the cornea of an 8-year-old boy.* Xanthogranulomas can also occur on the skin (see Figure 2-2) and the iris. Children with iris xanthogranulomas may come to the ophthalmologist with spontaneous hyphemas.

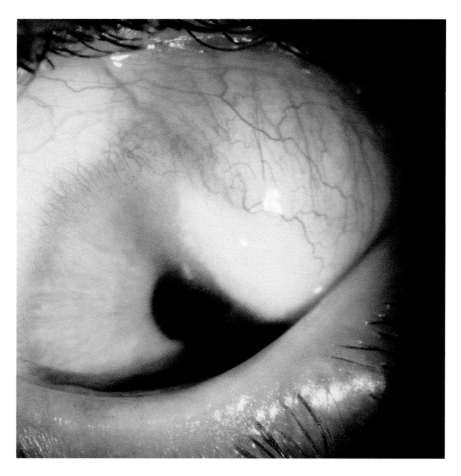

FIGURE 5-38 A presumed xanthogranuloma in a 9-year-old boy.

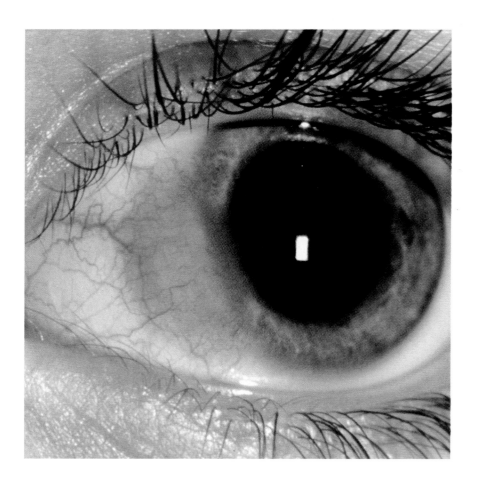

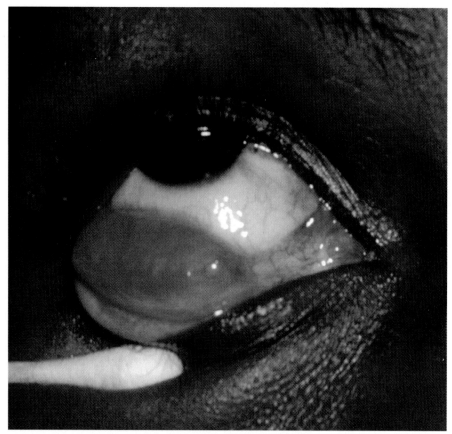

FIGURE 5-39 *A large conjunctival cyst arising from the palpebral conjunctiva.* The central cyst is clear, and the margins of the cyst are easily seen.

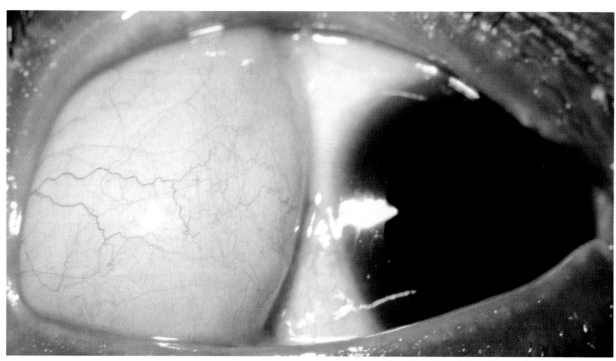

FIGURE 5-40 *Prolapsed orbital fat mistaken for a conjunctival cyst.* In contrast to the conjunctival cyst in Figure 5-39, this lesion is not clear and the margins cannot be easily seen. With digital pressure, the prolapsed fat can be pushed back into the orbit, but it returns when the pressure is removed.

CHAPTER 6

Conjunctivitis

Conjunctivitis is one of the more common conditions seen in general practice. Certain signs of conjunctival inflammation, such as follicles, giant papillae, membranes, and symblepharon, may be helpful in establishing a definitive diagnosis.

Clinical Features

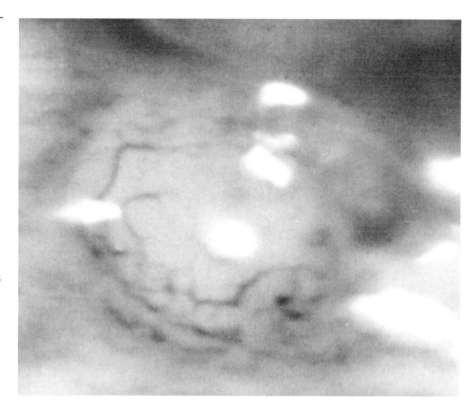

FIGURE 6-1 *A conjunctival follicle.* This is a lymphocytic response in the conjunctiva. Vessels are on the surface and especially around the base of the follicle, but they lack the central vascular core seen in a papilla. Follicles are more rounded and deeper than papillae.

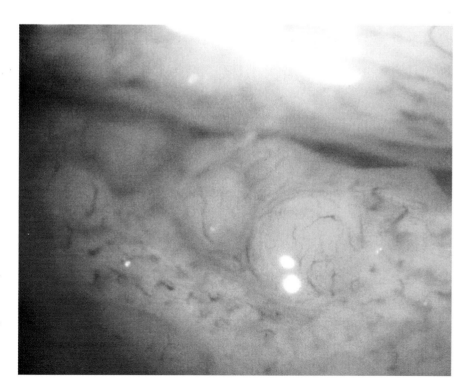

FIGURE 6-2 *Conjunctival follicles in the inferior palpebral conjunctiva.* Causes of acute follicular conjunctivitis include adenoviral keratoconjunctivitis, adult inclusion conjunctivitis, and primary herpes simplex keratoconjunctivitis. Causes of chronic follicular conjunctivitis include adult inclusion conjunctivitis, trachoma, toxic response to medications or molluscum contagiosum lesions, and Parinaud's oculoglandular syndrome.

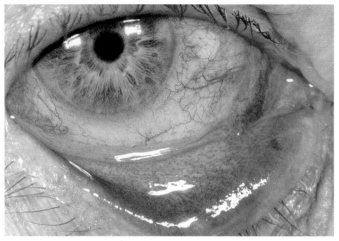

FIGURE 6-3 *Chronic conjunctival inflammation.* A papillary response is a nonspecific response to chronic conjunctival inflammation and can occur along with a follicular response. In contrast to follicles, papillae are smaller and contain a central fibrovascular core.

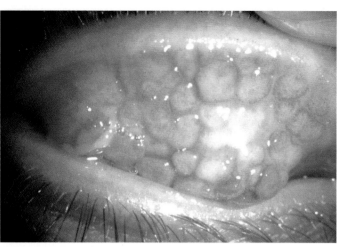

FIGURE 6-4 *Giant papillary conjunctivitis.* This is seen in vernal keratoconjunctivitis or as a response to chronic irritation from a contact lens, an ocular prosthesis, or an exposed suture.

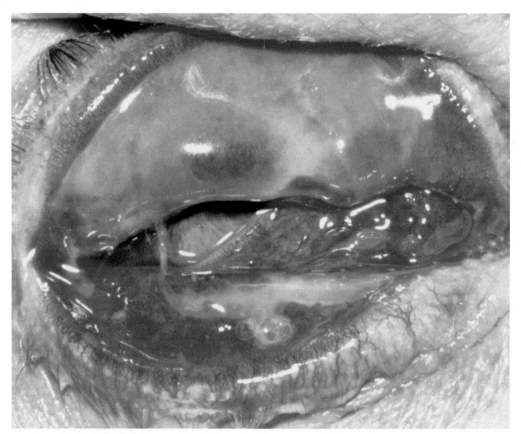

FIGURE 6-5 *Membranous conjunctivitis.* A transudation of protein and fibrin from the conjunctiva can cause a membranous or pseudomembranous conjunctivitis. Pseudomembranes can be easily stripped from the conjunctiva, whereas membranes are more adherent to the underlying conjunctiva.

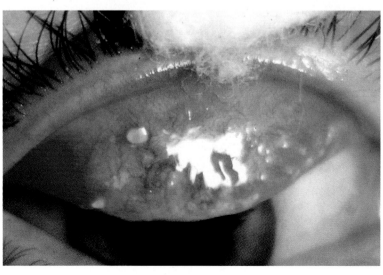

FIGURE 6-6 *Conjunctival concretions.* These are benign lesions of the palpebral conjunctiva. Occasionally, they are extensive and can cause ocular irritation. Surgical excision is usually curative.

Bacterial Conjunctivitis

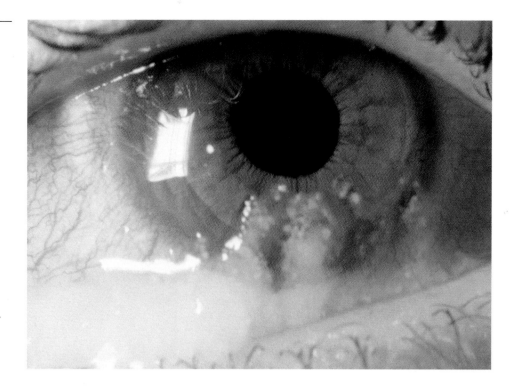

FIGURE 6-7 **Bacterial conjunctivitis.** There may be a prominent purulent or mucopurulent discharge.

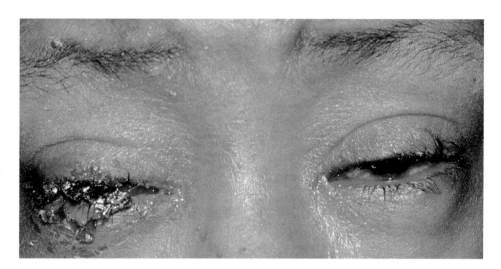

FIGURE 6-8 **Hyperacute conjunctivitis.** This disorder is characterized by a rapidly progressing conjunctivitis. Chemosis and conjunctival membranes are often present. This type of conjunctivitis can be unilateral or bilateral and is often associated with a prominent preauricular node. Here the right eye is infected by *Neisseria gonorrhoeae. N. meningitidis* may produce a similar clinical picture.

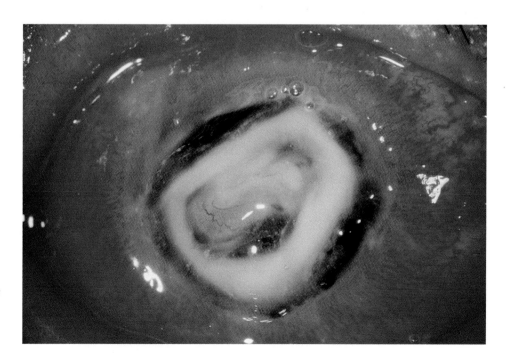

FIGURE 6-9 **Extensive corneal ulcer with a perforation of the right eye of the patient in Figure 6-8.** The patient experienced an expulsive hemorrhage, and retina plugs the perforation site.

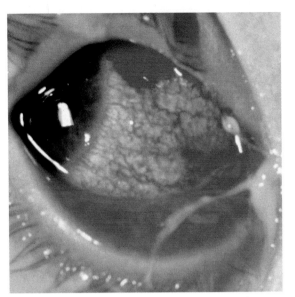

FIGURE 6-10 *Gonococcal conjunctivitis.* There is a prominent mucopurulent discharge.

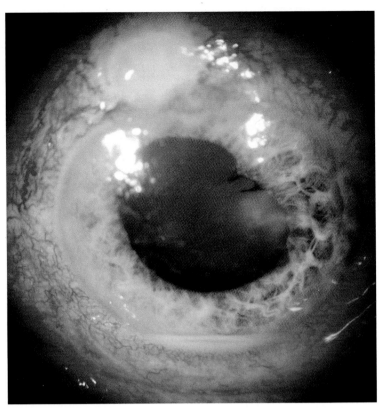

FIGURE 6-11 *Infection in a filtering bleb leading to endophthalmitis.* The bleb is white as compared with the surrounding conjunctiva. A hypopyon is present.

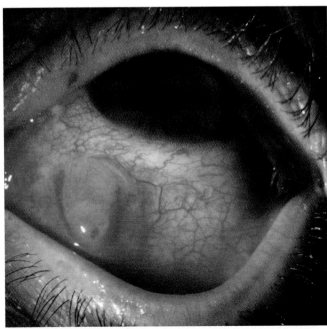

FIGURE 6-12 Chronic conjunctivitis caused by an extruding scleral buckle.

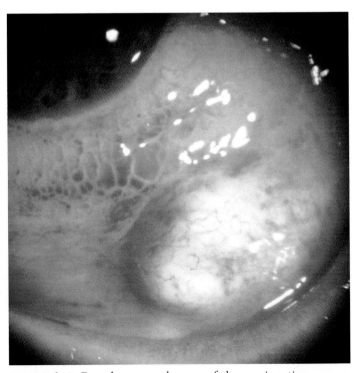

FIGURE 6-13 *Pseudomonas* abscess of the conjunctiva.

Viral Conjunctivitis

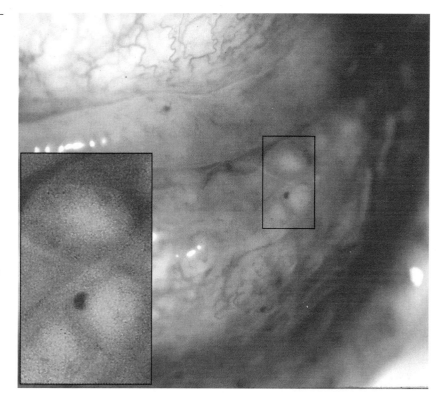

FIGURE 6-14 *Epidemic keratoconjunctivitis (EKC).* Extremely contagious, EKC is usually associated with adenoviral serotypes 8 and 19, although many other serotypes can cause conjunctivitis. EKC is usually bilateral, with the second eye infected 3 to 7 days after the first. It causes a follicular conjunctivitis, as seen here. Often there are small petechial hemorrhages present *(inset).*

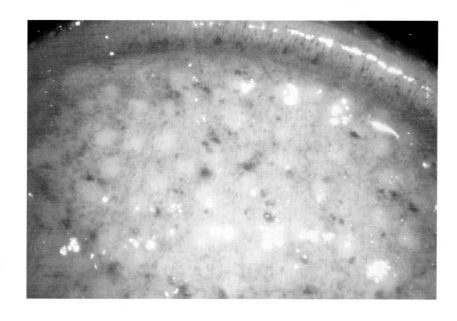

FIGURE 6-15 *EKC.* Follicles are typically found on the palpebral conjunctiva of both the upper and lower lids. Small petechial hemorrhages are often present.

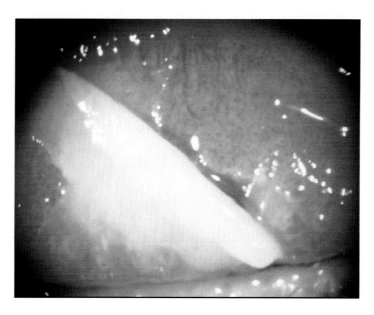

FIGURE 6-16 *EKC.* In severe cases, transudation of protein and fibrin can result in a pseudomembrane. As noted in Figure 6-5, a pseudomembrane, as opposed to a membrane, can be easily stripped from the underlying conjunctiva.

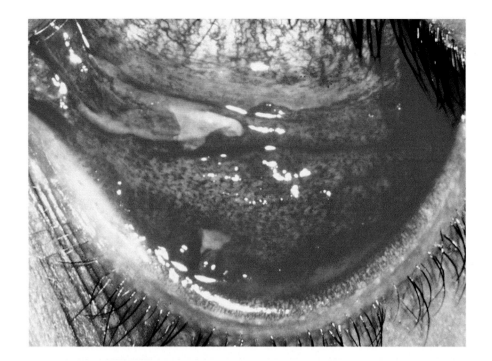

FIGURE 6-17 *Same patient as in Figure 6-16, after removal of the pseudomembrane.* There is a diffuse papillary response in the conjunctiva and a small residual piece of the pseudomembrane in the inferior fornix.

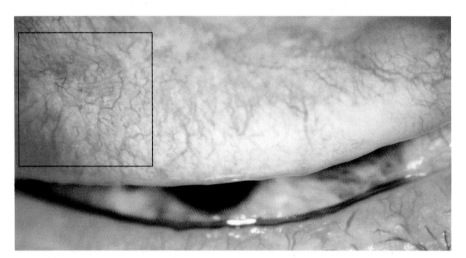

FIGURE 6-18 *EKC.* After the lesion has resolved, an unusual complication can be scarring of the conjunctiva *(box).*

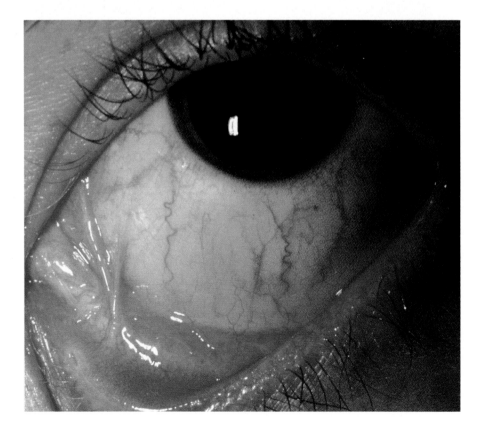

FIGURE 6-19 *EKC.* Rarely, symblepharon develop after a severe case of EKC.

FIGURE 6-20 **EKC.** Subepithelial infiltrates may develop 10 to 14 days after the acute infection. Histologically, they are composed of lymphocytes and may be an immunologic reaction to viral proteins in the cornea.

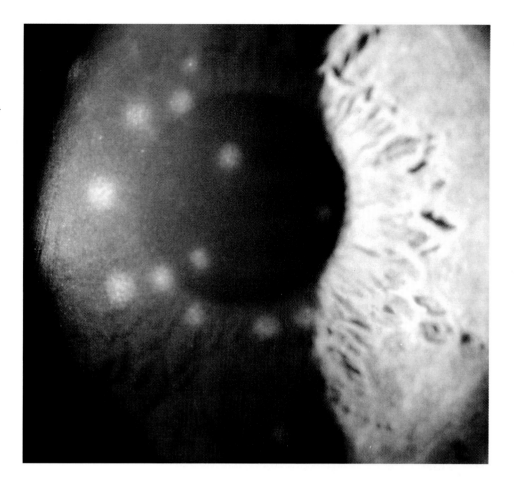

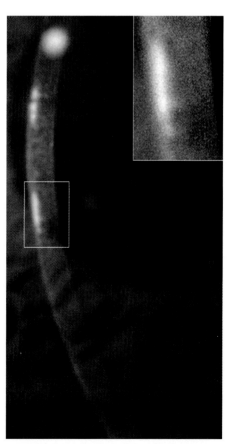

FIGURE 6-21 **EKC.** A thin slit beam view demonstrates that subepithelial infiltrates are located in the anterior stroma (*inset*).

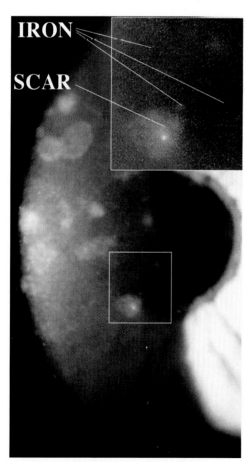

FIGURE 6-22 **EKC.** Rarely, severe cases cause corneal scarring. A change in the tear distribution over the corneal surface has resulted in iron deposition in the corneal epithelium (*box*).

Chlamydial Infections—Adult Inclusion Conjunctivitis

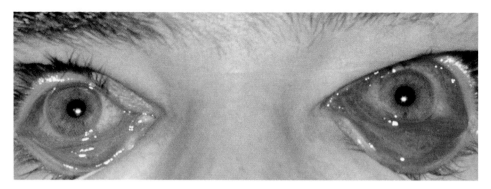

FIGURE 6-23 **Adult inclusion conjunctivitis.** This chlamydial infection is associated with serotypes D through K. The source of infection is usually the genitalia. This is a bilateral case, but unilateral cases are more prevalent. Enlarged preauricular nodes are often present in acute cases.

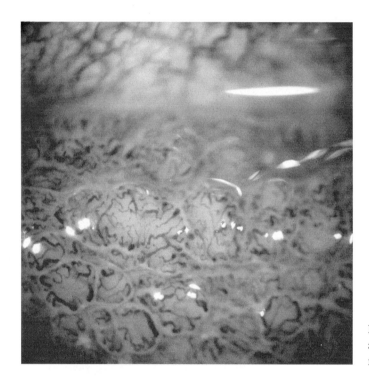

FIGURE 6-24 **Adult inclusion conjunctivitis.** During an acute infection, prominent follicular conjunctivitis and moderate injection of the conjunctiva occur.

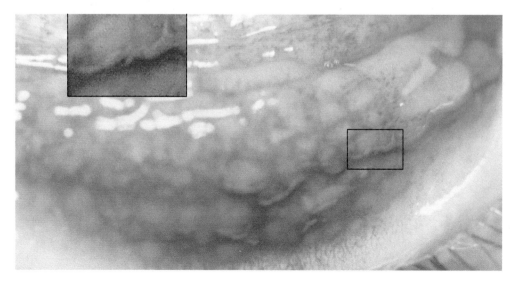

FIGURE 6-25 **Chronic adult inclusion conjunctivitis.** The follicles remain but are associated with less injection of the conjunctiva. Scant mucopurulent discharge is present **(inset).**

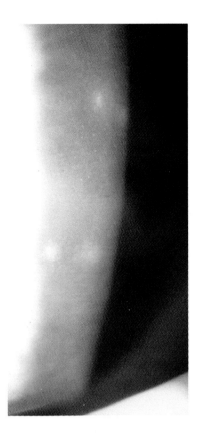

FIGURE 6-26 *Adult inclusion conjunctivitis.* Peripheral subepithelial infiltrates can occur 2 to 3 weeks after the initial infection. These are believed to be an immunologic response to chlamydial antigens.

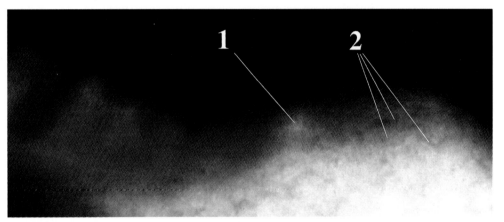

FIGURE 6-27 *Adult inclusion conjunctivitis.* Subepithelial infiltrate *(1)* and superficial vascularization *(2)* in the peripheral cornea.

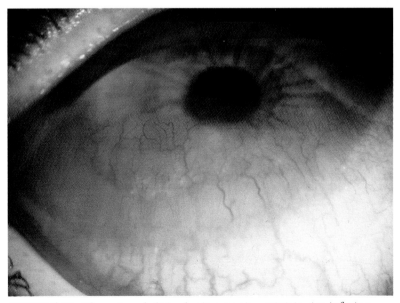

FIGURE 6-28 *Chronic adult inclusion conjunctivitis.* An inferior vascular pannus may develop.

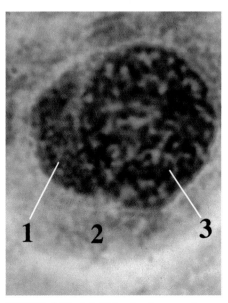

FIGURE 6-29 *Adult inclusion conjunctivitis.* An epithelial cell from a conjunctival scraping shows basophilic inclusion bodies *(1)*, the cell cytoplasm *(2)*, and the cell nucleus *(3)*.

Chlamydial Infections—Trachoma

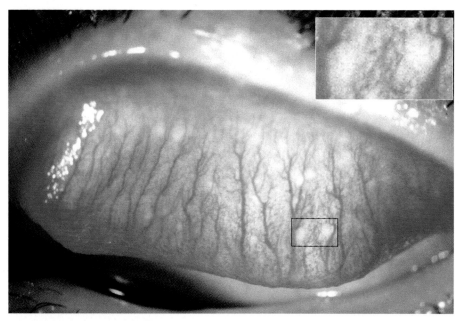

FIGURE 6-30 *Trachoma.* This chlamydial infection is caused by serotypes A through C. The disease is extremely rare in the United States, although it is epidemic in some Native American tribes. In acute trachoma, there is a follicular response of the conjunctiva, which is more prominent on the superior tarsal conjunctiva *(inset).* World Health Organization classification is as follows: trachomatous inflammation—follicular (TF).

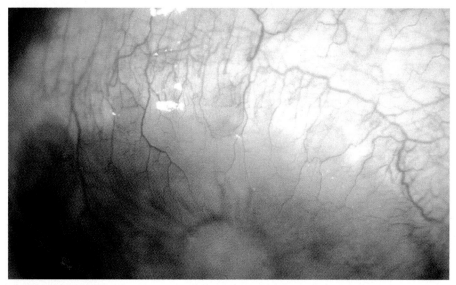

FIGURE 6-31 *Trachoma.* A corneal pannus may be seen in advanced disease. In addition, Herbert's pits are seen at the superior limbus.

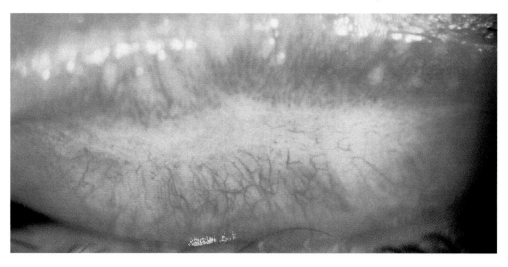

FIGURE 6-32 *Trachoma.* Arlt's lines are horizontal bands of conjunctival scarring on the upper tarsal conjunctiva and are associated with advanced trachoma. World Health Organization classification is as follows: trachomatous scarring (TS).

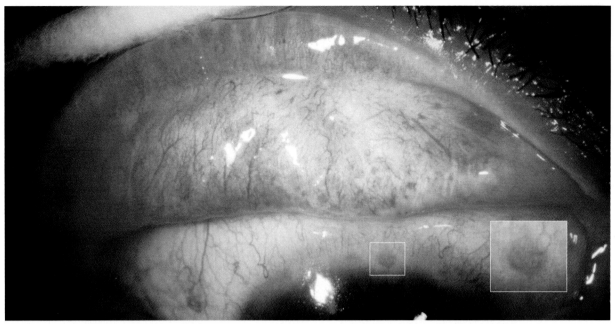

FIGURE 6-33 *Trachoma.* Herbert's pits are round, depressed, limbal scars with an overlying thickened epithelium *(inset).* These pits are formed from limbal follicles that leave a scar when they resolve. This patient also has significant scarring on the upper tarsal conjunctiva.

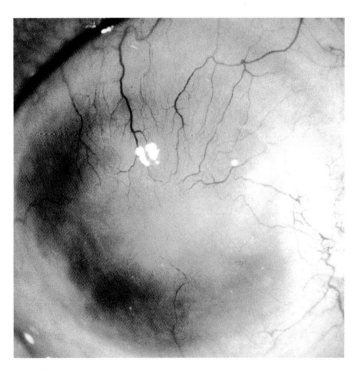

FIGURE 6-34 *Trachoma.* This patient with inactive trachoma has extensive corneal vascularization and scarring. World Health Organization classification is as follows: corneal opacity (CO).

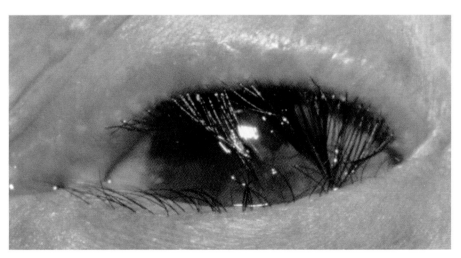

FIGURE 6-35 *Trachoma.* Cicatricial entropion and trichiasis have developed. World Health Organization classification is as follows: trachomatous trichiasis (TT).

Ophthalmia Neonatorum

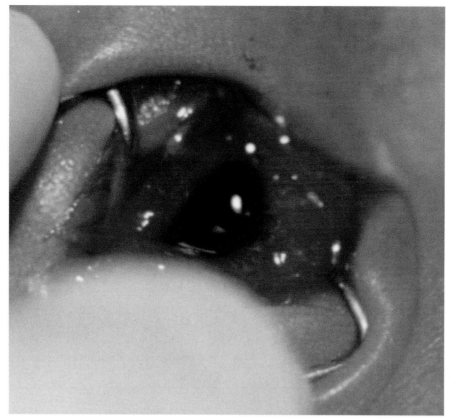

FIGURE 6-36 *Neonatal inclusion conjunctivitis (inclusion blennorrhea).* This is acquired during passage through the birth canal and occurs several days after birth. In contrast to adult inclusion conjunctivitis, the response is papillary rather than follicular. The conjunctivitis is more intense, it may be associated with chemosis or pseudomembranes, and a mucopurulent discharge may be present.

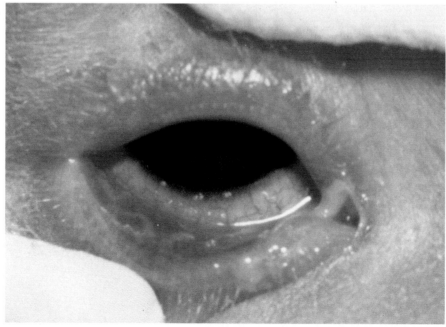

FIGURE 6-37 *Gonococcal conjunctivitis of the newborn.* This is acquired during passage through the birth canal and occurs a few days after birth. A mucopurulent discharge is usually present. Gram stain reveals intraepithelial gram-negative diplococci. Aggressive treatment with systemic and topical antibiotics is indicated, since severe corneal ulceration can occur.

Parinaud's Syndrome

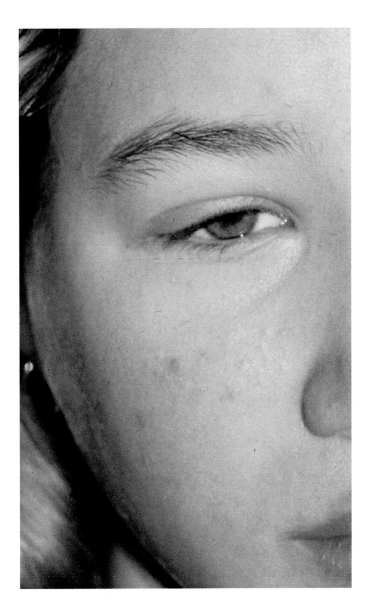

FIGURE 6-38 *Parinaud's oculoglandular syndrome.* This group of diseases is characterized by localized conjunctival granulomas and regional lymphadenopathy. The most common etiology is cat scratch disease, which has recently been attributed to the bacterium ***Bartonella henselae.*** This patient had a conjunctival granuloma on the palpebral conjunctiva of the upper lid with resultant ptosis. Prominent preauricular adenopathy is present.

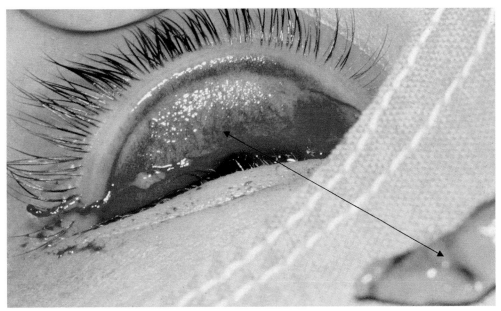

FIGURE 6-39 *Parinaud's oculoglandular syndrome.* The granuloma was excised. The arrow points to the site of the excision.

Parasitic Conjunctivitis

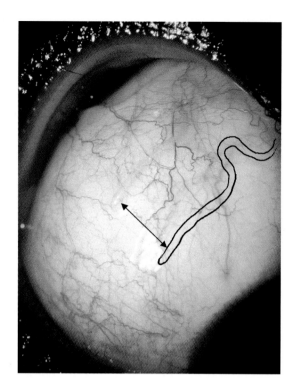

FIGURE 6-40 *Loiasis.* This parasitic infection is primarily confined to Africa. The microfilariae are inoculated into the subcutaneous tissue by the bite of the mango fly. In this patient, the *Loa loa* worm is located beneath the conjunctiva *(above and left of the drawn outline).*

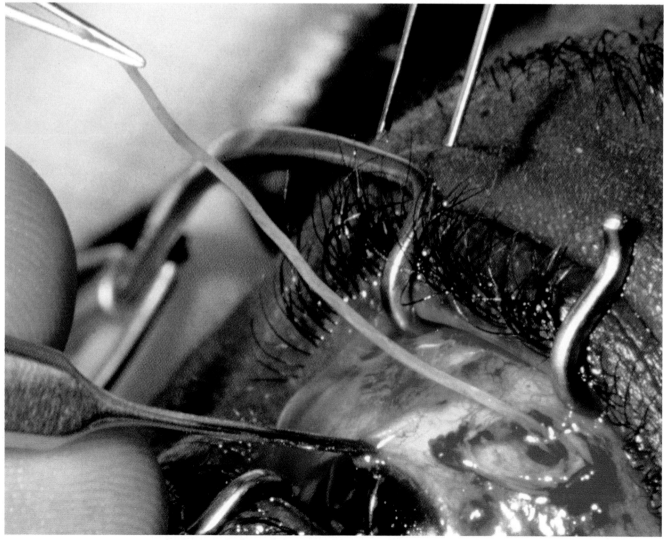

FIGURE 6-41 *Loiasis.* Surgical removal of the worm from the patient in Figure 6-40.

Allergic Conjunctivitis

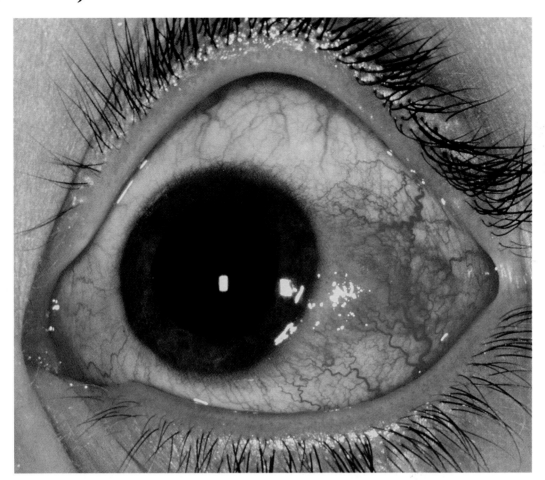

FIGURE 6-42 Localized allergic conjunctivitis resulting from poison ivy.

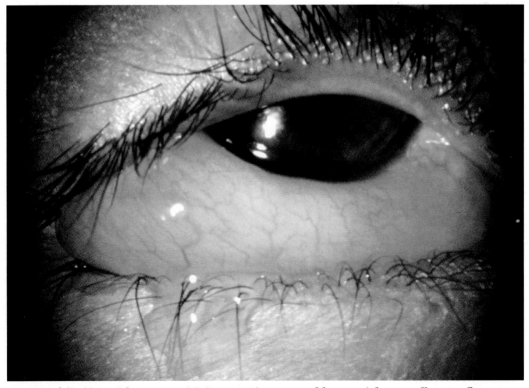

FIGURE 6-43 *Type-I hypersensitivity reaction caused by an airborne allergen.* Common inciting agents include animal dander, dust, plant pollens, ragweed, and mold spores. Symptoms of itching and irritation occur shortly after exposure. Ocular signs include a diffuse conjunctivitis accompanied (in this case) by severe chemosis.

Vernal and Atopic Keratoconjunctivitis

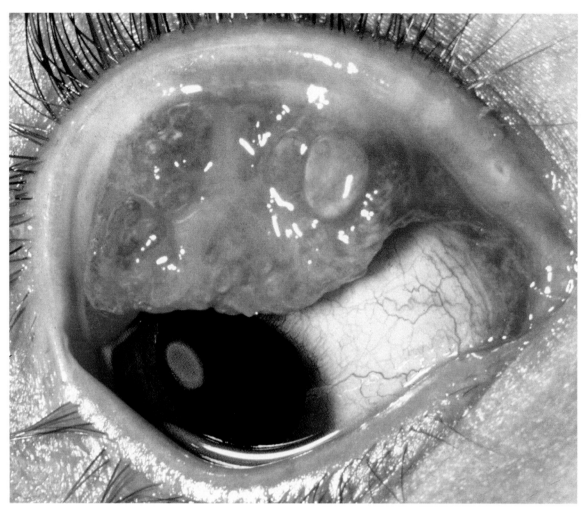

FIGURE 6-44 *Vernal keratoconjunctivitis.* This seasonal conjunctivitis is usually seen in children and adolescents. Symptoms include itching, irritation, and mucoid discharge. Prominent giant papillae with a mucoid discharge are present on the upper palpebral conjunctiva. A shield ulcer is seen on the superior cornea. Mechanical irritation from the giant papillae and eye rubbing may predispose to shield ulcers.

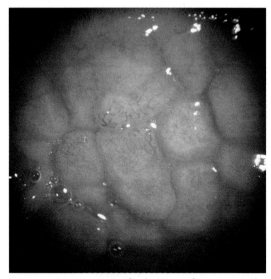

FIGURE 6-45 A magnified view of giant papillae in a patient with vernal keratoconjunctivitis.

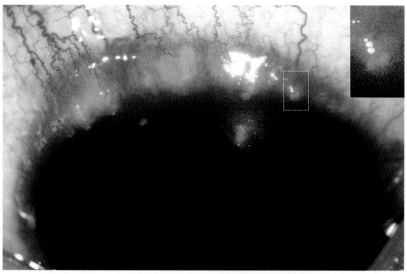

FIGURE 6-46 *Limbal vernal keratoconjunctivitis.* This type is more common in African-Americans and Native Americans and is characterized by large gelatinous elevations at the corneal limbus. It is often associated with Horner-Trantas' dots *(inset)*. Horner-Trantas' dots are collections of eosinophils usually present for less than 1 week.

FIGURE 6-47 *Atopic keratoconjunctivitis.*
In contrast to vernal keratoconjunctivitis, atopic keratoconjunctivitis occurs in young adults, has no seasonal preference, and is characterized by small-to medium-sized papillae, usually more prominent in the lower fornix. In its severe form, it is associated with more advanced conjunctival and corneal scarring. This patient has a chronic atopic blepharokeratoconjunctivitis with thickened lid margins.

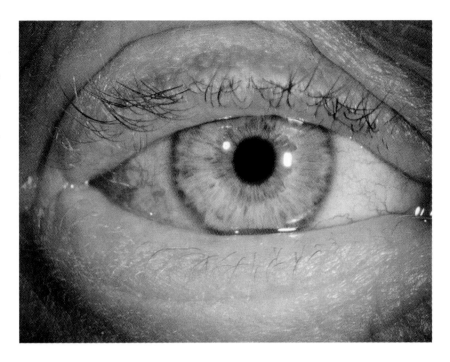

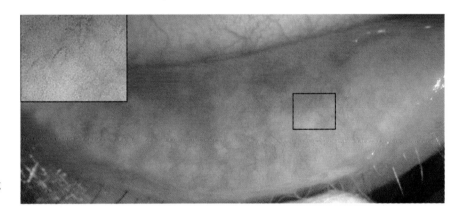

FIGURE 6-48 *Same patient as in Figure 6-47.* There is vascularization and scarring of the conjunctiva *(inset).*

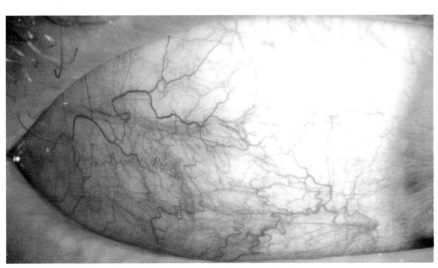

FIGURE 6-49 Chronic conjunctival inflammation in the same patient as in Figures 6-47 and 6-48.

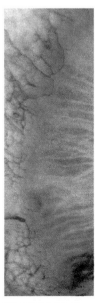

FIGURE 6-50 *Same patient as in Figures 6-47 to 6-49.* A magnified section of cornea reveals a peripheral corneal pannus.

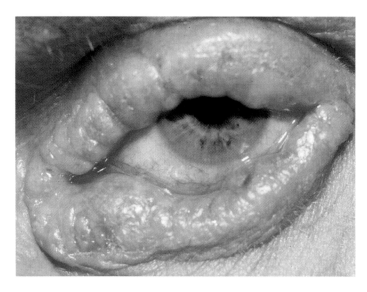

FIGURE 6-51 *Severe atopic eye disease.* Markedly thickened lid margins, chronic conjunctival inflammation, and peripheral corneal scarring are seen.

Giant Papillary Conjunctivitis

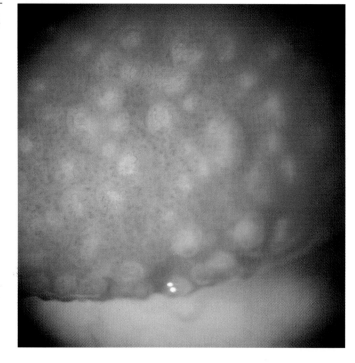

FIGURE 6-52 *Giant papillary conjunctivitis.* This is thought to be a type-IV hypersensitivity reaction that is exacerbated by chronic conjunctival irritation. It is most commonly seen in contact lens wearers (see Figure 15-1). Patients complain of itching, irritation, and a slight mucoid discharge. Giant papillae are seen on the upper palpebral conjunctiva. In this case the conjunctivitis was associated with an ocular prosthesis.

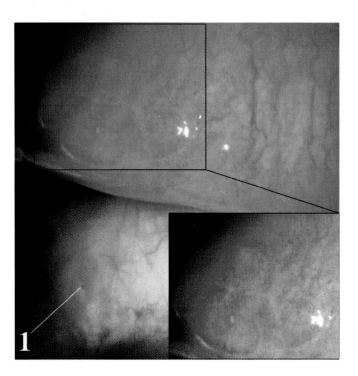

FIGURE 6-53 Giant papillary conjunctivitis *(inset)* induced by a nylon suture *(1)*.

Ocular Cicatricial Pemphigoid

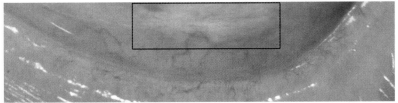

FIGURE 6-54 *Ocular cicatricial pemphigoid (OCP).* This bilateral progressive scarring disease of the conjunctiva is rarely seen before age 50. It is more common in females. Subepithelial fibrosis is the earliest stage of this disease. Subtle subepithelial fibrotic bands are seen in the inferior fornix (*box*). This patient had a chronic relapsing blepharoconjunctivitis previously attributed to meibomian gland dysfunction.

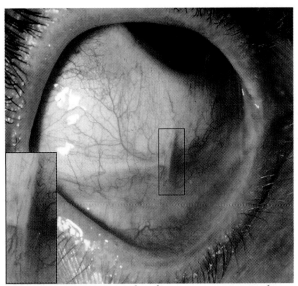

FIGURE 6-55 *OCP.* As the disease progresses, the fornices shorten and symblepharon form *(inset).*

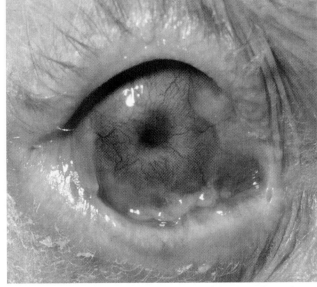

FIGURE 6-56 *OCP.* The fornices are obliterated, and severe vascularization and scarring of the cornea occurs.

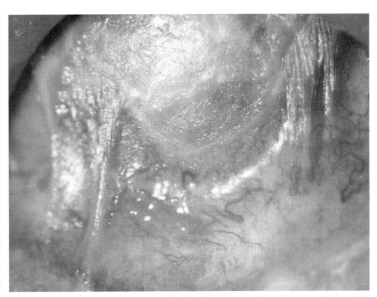

FIGURE 6-57 *OCP.* In the final stages, the conjunctiva and cornea become keratinized.

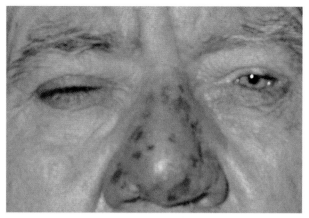

FIGURE 6-58 **OCP.** Approximately 25% of patients have bullous lesions of the skin.

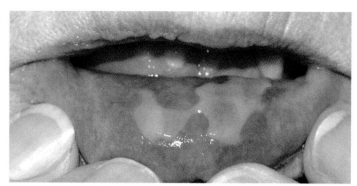

FIGURE 6-59 **OCP.** Approximately 90% of patients have mucosal lesions in the oropharynx.

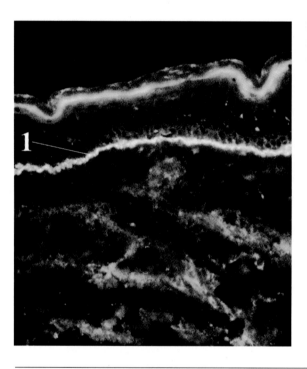

FIGURE 6-60 **OCP.** Immunoglobulin is deposited in the basement membrane tissue *(1)*, as demonstrated by this immunofluorescent stain.

Linear IgA Disease

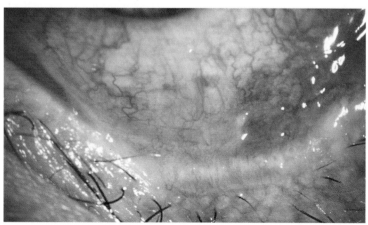

FIGURE 6-61 **Linear IgA disease.** This disorder results in conjunctival scarring and symblepharon formation. The predominant immunoglobulin deposited is IgA, and the prognosis is better than with ocular cicatricial pemphigoid.

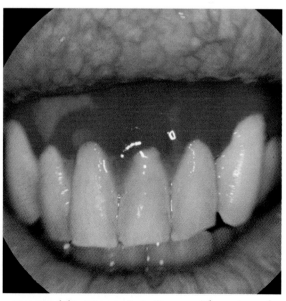

FIGURE 6-62 **Linear IgA disease.** There is oral mucosal involvement.

Stevens-Johnson Syndrome

Stevens-Johnson syndrome is a severe inflammatory disease of the skin and mucous membranes. It can be associated with medications or infectious agents and is believed to be an autoimmune disorder.

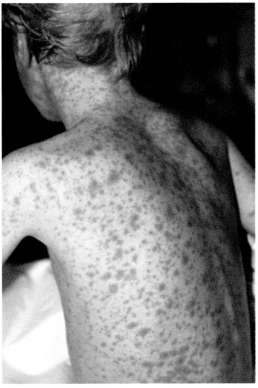

FIGURE 6-63 **Stevens-Johnson syndrome.** This patient has bullous skin lesions on the skin of the back.

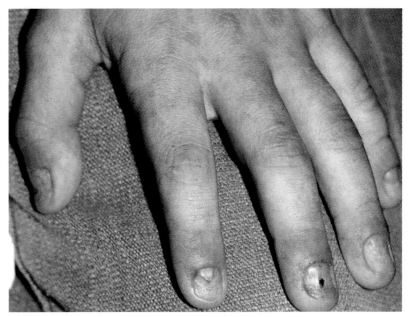

FIGURE 6-64 **Stevens-Johnson syndrome.** Scarring of the hands and fingernails can occur.

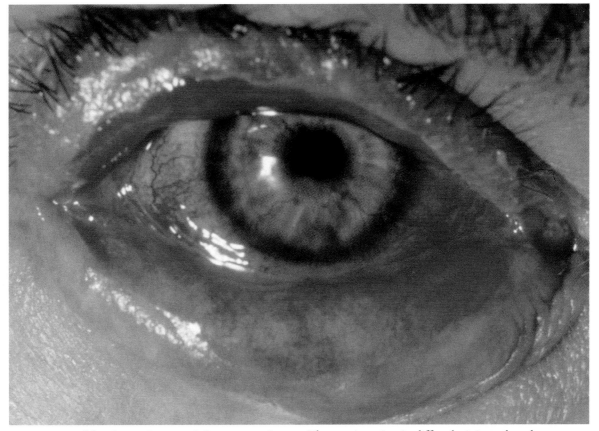

FIGURE 6-65 **Acute Stevens-Johnson syndrome.** The conjunctiva is diffusely injected and thickened. Corneal vascularization occurs in severe cases.

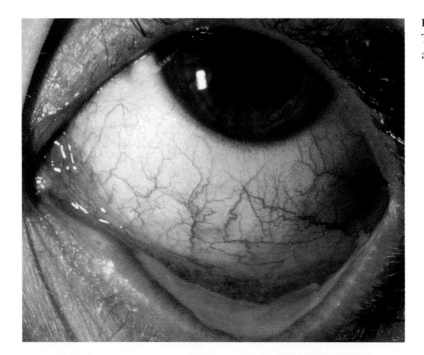

FIGURE 6-66 *Stevens-Johnson syndrome.*
Transudation of proteins and fibrin can result in a membranous conjunctivitis.

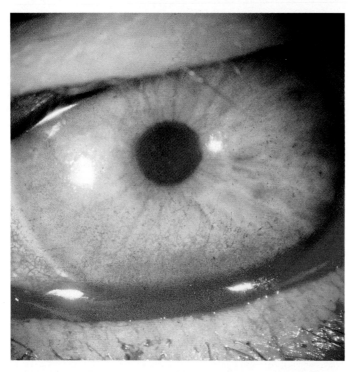

FIGURE 6-67 *Stevens-Johnson syndrome.* Mucin production is altered. This patient has an adequate tear meniscus but demonstrates rose bengal staining of epithelial cells devoid of an overlying mucin layer.

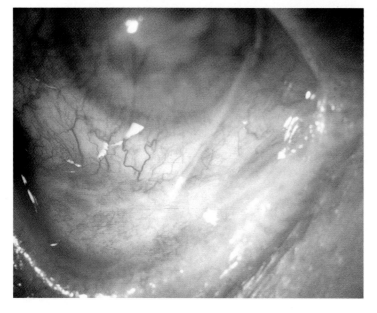

FIGURE 6-68 *Stevens-Johnson syndrome.* Corneal scarring, conjunctival scarring, and symblepharon formation may occur after the acute stage.

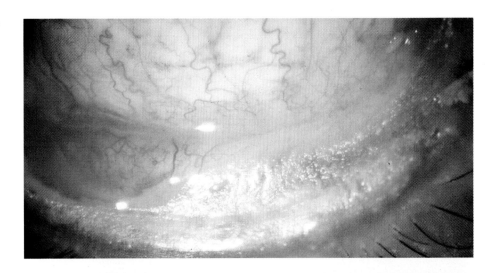

FIGURE 6-69 *Severe Stevens-Johnson syndrome.* There is keratinization of the conjunctiva.

FIGURE 6-70 *Stevens-Johnson syndrome.* There is moderate corneal vascularization and scarring.

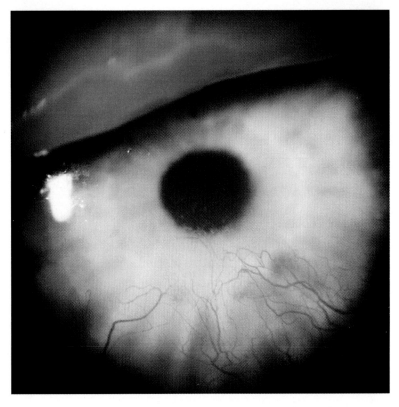

FIGURE 6-71 *Advanced Stevens-Johnson syndrome.* The cornea can become totally vascularized and opaque.

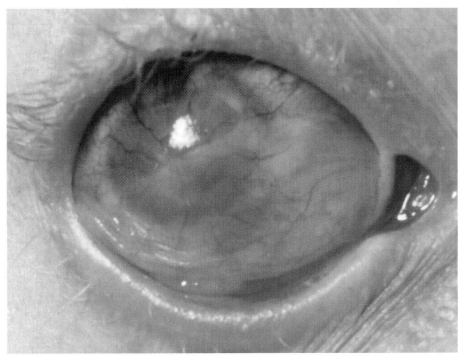

Reiter's Syndrome

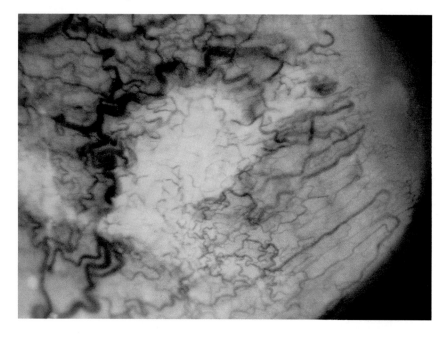

FIGURE 6-72 ***Reiter's syndrome.*** This syndrome consists of arthritis, urethritis, and conjunctivitis and primarily occurs in young males. Nonspecific papillary conjunctivitis with a mucopurulent discharge is common. Occasionally, these patients have ulcerations of the conjunctiva (as seen here) or buccal mucosa.

Toxic Conjunctivitis

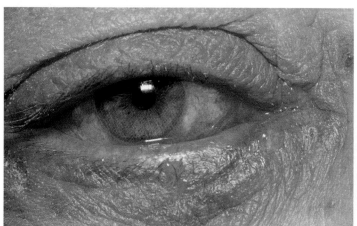

FIGURE 6-73 ***Toxic follicular conjunctivitis.*** This case occurred after several weeks of Viroptic therapy. Other agents causing a toxic follicular conjunctivitis include miotics, Propine, and atropine.

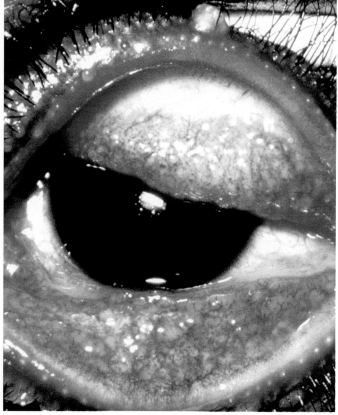

FIGURE 6-74 ***Toxic follicular conjunctivitis.*** This was caused by products from a molluscum lesion on the upper eyelid margin.

Theodore's Superior Limbic Keratoconjunctivitis

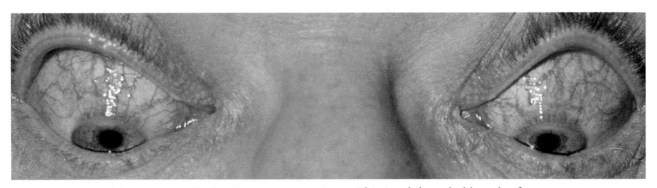

FIGURE 6-75 *Superior limbic keratoconjunctivitis.* This is a bilateral although often asymmetric inflammation of the superior bulbar conjunctiva. There is focal injection of the superior conjunctiva, and rose bengal staining is often positive in this region. The superior conjunctiva is redundant, and the inflammation may result from chronic rubbing of the superior tarsal conjunctiva with the superior bulbar conjunctiva. Many of these patients have systemic thyroid abnormalities.

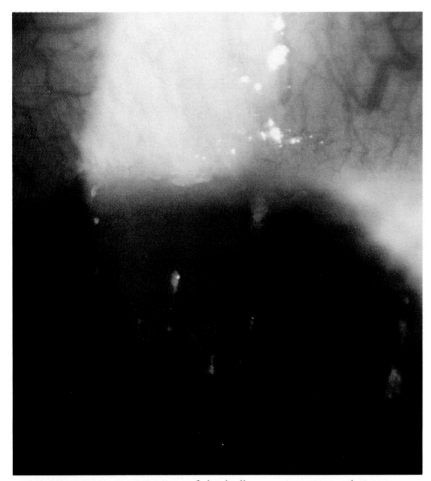

FIGURE 6-76 Superior injection of the bulbar conjunctiva, gelatinous hypertrophy of the limbal tissue, and superior filaments on the cornea.

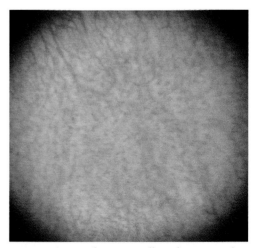

FIGURE 6-77 Velvety papillary hypertrophy on the upper tarsal conjunctiva.

Ligneous Conjunctivitis

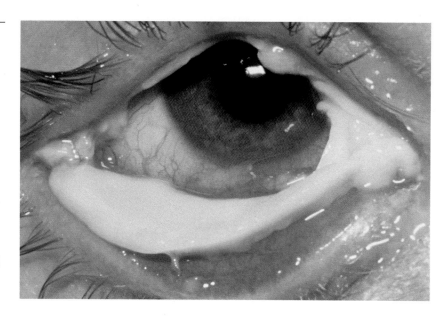

FIGURE 6-78 *Ligneous conjunctivitis.* This is a bilateral chronic conjunctivitis of unknown etiology. The condition usually begins in early childhood and may be precipitated by local injury or a systemic process. It is characterized by exuberant fibrinous conjunctival membranes, which recur despite mechanical removal.

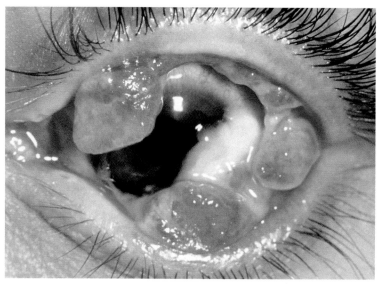

FIGURE 6-79 *Ligneous conjunctivitis.* Appearance of the eye before treatment with topical cyclosporin A.

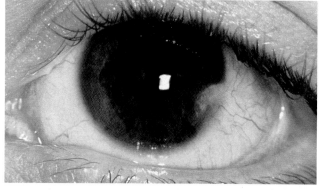

FIGURE 6-80 *Ligneous conjunctivitis.* Same patient as in Figure 6-79, after treatment with topical cyclosporin A. The conjunctivitis has resolved, and there is slight corneal scarring temporally.

Factitious Conjunctivitis

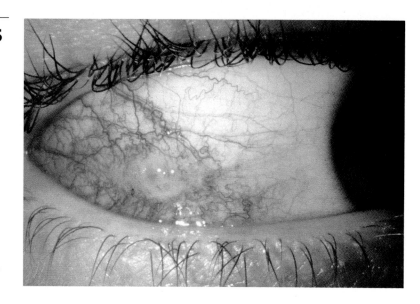

FIGURE 6-81 *Factitious conjunctivitis.* Rarely, conjunctivitis is due to factitious causes. This patient repeatedly stabbed the conjunctiva with a straight pin.

CHAPTER 7

Developmental Abnormalities Of The Cornea

Developmental abnormalities of the cornea result from a complex interaction of genetic and environmental influences. These abnormalities are present at birth, in contrast to other genetic disorders, which develop later in life. Many of these disorders develop during the sixth to eighteenth week of gestation, when differentiation of the anterior segment occurs.

Developmental Corneal Opacities and Abnormalities of Size and Shape

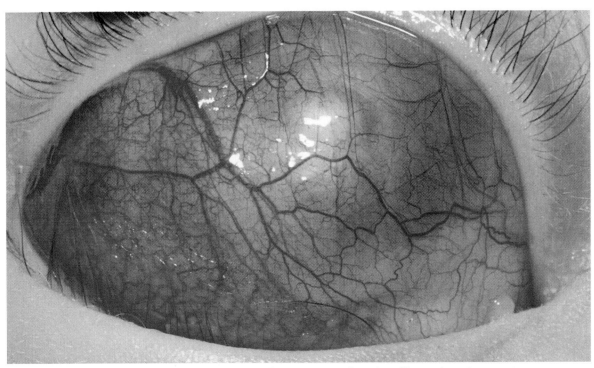

FIGURE 7-1 *Microphthalmos with cyst.* The eye is small and malformed, and a cyst is contiguous with the globe. The cyst is formed from proliferating retina. This abnormality occurs when the embryonic (choroidal) fissure fails to close.

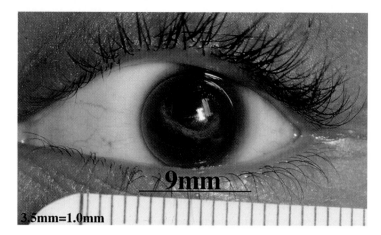

FIGURE 7-2 **Microcornea.** This is defined as a corneal diameter less than 10 mm in an eye of normal size. If the entire eye is small, the condition is termed ***nanophthalmos.*** This patient with microcornea had congenital cataracts removed and is wearing an aphakic contact lens.

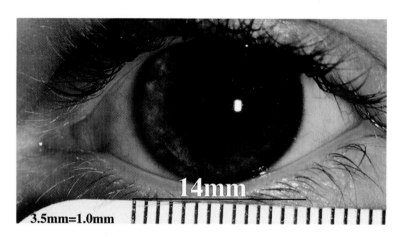

FIGURE 7-3 **Megalocornea.** The corneal diameter is greater than or equal to 13 mm. It is most commonly transmitted as an X-linked recessive disorder, and for that reason, 90% of affected patients are males. It is associated with numerous ocular and systemic disorders. The relative corneal diameter difference between Figures 7-2 and 7-3 is the actual difference; the same scale is used for both figures.

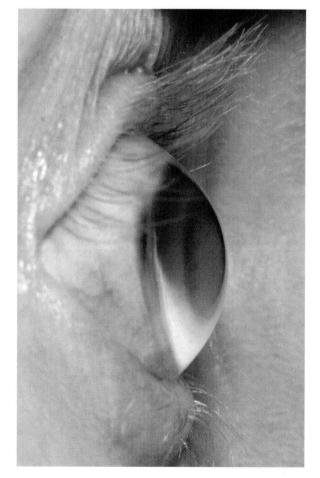

FIGURE 7-4 **Megalocornea.** The corneas in this disorder are often steep, and the patients are usually myopic.

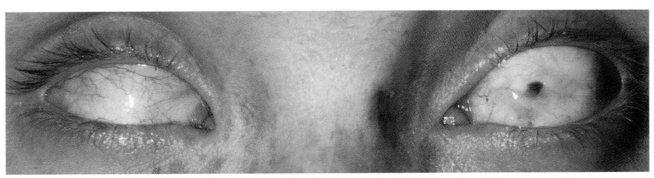

FIGURE 7-5 *Sclerocornea.* There is peripheral whitening or scleralization of the cornea. The cornea may be totally opaque, as in the right eye of this patient, or there may be a central relatively clearer area, as seen in the left eye. The central cornea is flat because it reflects the curvature of the sclera. There are usually associated ocular abnormalities, and the prognosis for vision with keratoplasty is poor.

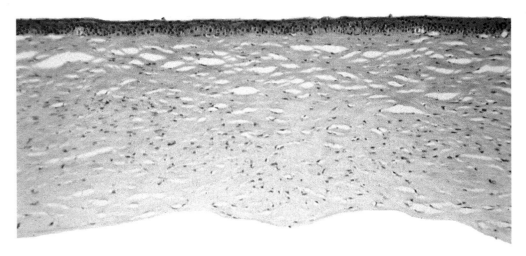

FIGURE 7-6 *Histopathology of sclerocornea.* The absence of Bowman's layer, increased cellularity of the corneal stroma, and loss of the normal collagen lamellar architecture can be seen.

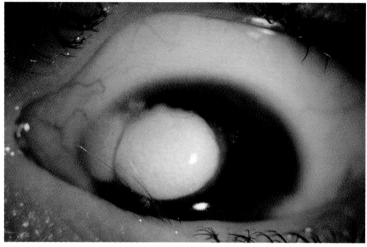

FIGURE 7-7 **Corneal dermoid.** A corneal dermoid is a collection of ectodermal elements such as sweat glands, hair follicles, and sebaceous glands on the corneal surface. These lesions are well circumscribed and elevated. In this case, abnormal lashes from the lower lid are rubbing on the cornea; however, in some cases, lashes are found exiting from the substance of the dermoid.

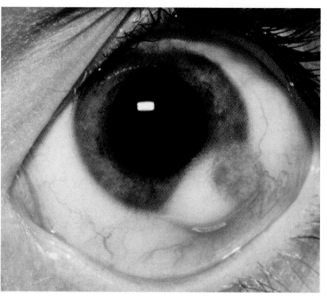

FIGURE 7-8 **Limbal dermoid.** Although this tumor does not extend into the visual axis, it can induce astigmatism and resultant amblyopia.

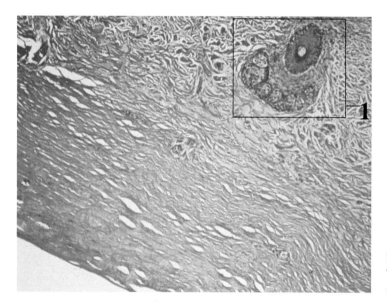

FIGURE 7-9 **Histopathology of a corneal dermoid.** The dermis and dermal-like appendages in the corneal stroma are shown. Pilosebaceous unit (1).

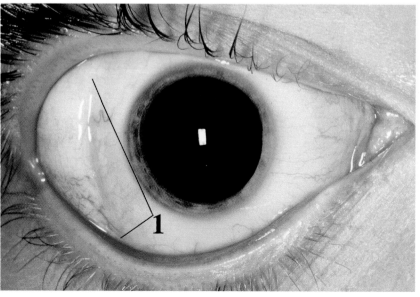

FIGURE 7-10 **Lipodermoid.** These tumors are composed primarily of fatty tissue and are usually located beneath the conjunctiva on the lateral aspect of the globe (1). The posterior aspect of the lesion often extends far posteriorly and cannot be identified in this patient. These tumors can be removed for cosmetic reasons, but it is important to excise only the anterior aspect of the tumor and not to attempt excision of the entire lesion.

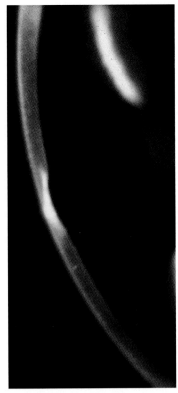

FIGURE 7-11 *Circumscribed posterior keratoconus.* This developmental defect is usually unilateral. There is a focal indentation of the posterior cornea with overlying stromal scarring. The vision is usually not greatly affected.

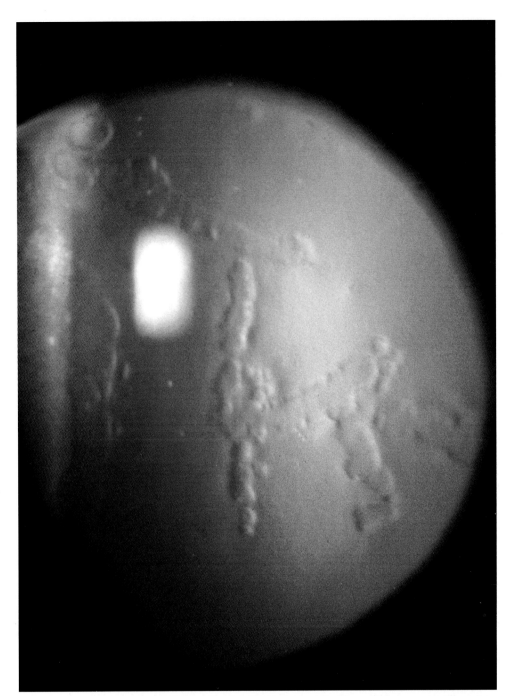

FIGURE 7-12 *Posterior corneal vesicles.* These are typically noted as an incidental finding. They are unilateral, and vision is not affected. They appear as singular or grouped vesicular lesions at the level of Descemet's membrane and endothelium. They should be distinguished from vesicular lesions in posterior polymorphous dystrophy, which are bilateral, and associated with ocular abnormalities in other family members (see Figures 9-59 through 9-68).

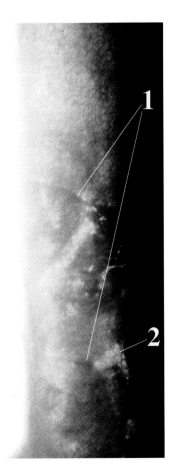

FIGURE 7-13 *Specular photomicrograph of posterior corneal vesicles.* The vesicles *(1)* are surrounded by normal endothelial cells *(2).*

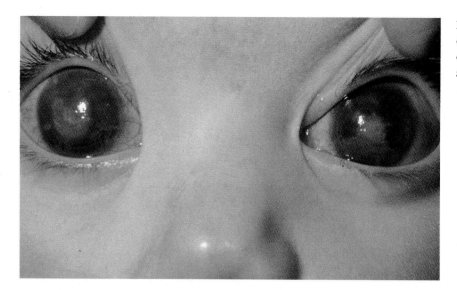

FIGURE 7-14 *Congenital glaucoma.* This child was initially misdiagnosed and developed severe buphthalmos. Central corneal scarring is present.

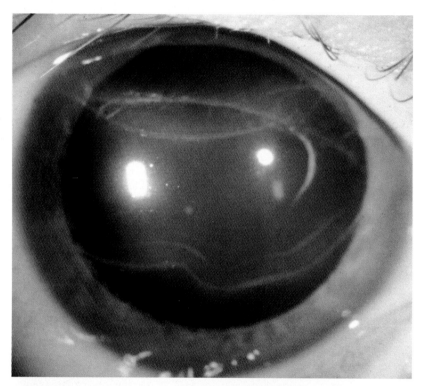

FIGURE 7-15 *Congenital glaucoma.* Breaks in Descemet's membrane (Haab's striae) may occur. The breaks are usually horizontal in the central cornea and become concentric near the limbus. These should be contrasted with breaks in Descemet's membrane occurring from birth trauma, which are usually more vertical (see Figures 14-27 through 14-34).

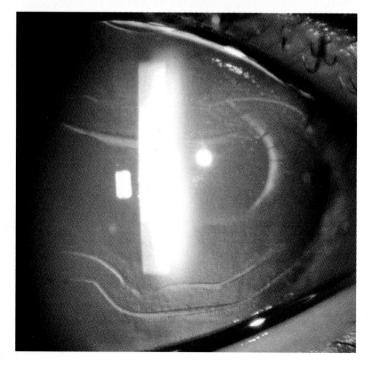

FIGURE 7-16 *Red reflex view of Haab's striae.* The breaks in Descemet's membrane have a railroad track appearance, which is the result of scrolling of Descemet's membrane on both sides of the break.

Anterior Chamber Cleavage Syndromes

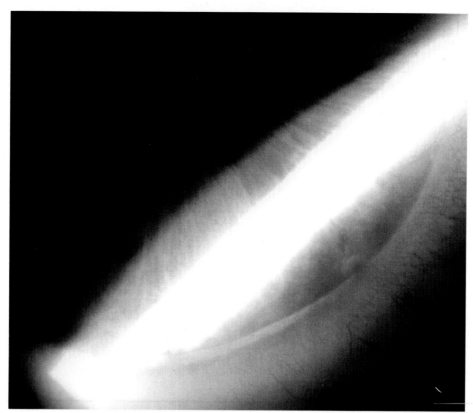

FIGURE 7-17 **Posterior embryotoxon.** This is an enlargement and anterior displacement of Schwalbe's line. It is a common finding, present in as many as 30% of normal eyes.

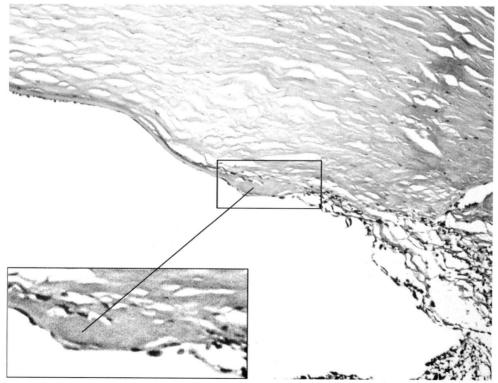

FIGURE 7-18 **Histopathology of posterior embryotoxon.** Schwalbe's line is enlarged at the junction of Descemet's membrane and the nonpigmented trabecular meshwork.

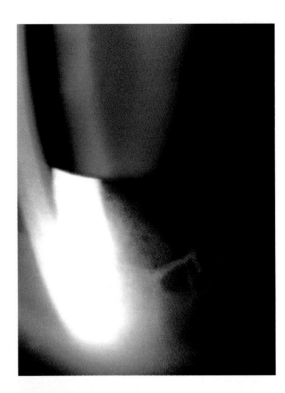

FIGURE 7-19 *Axenfeld's anomaly.* Fine iris strands adhere to an enlarged Schwalbe's line. If the disorder is associated with glaucoma, it is termed *Axenfeld's syndrome.*

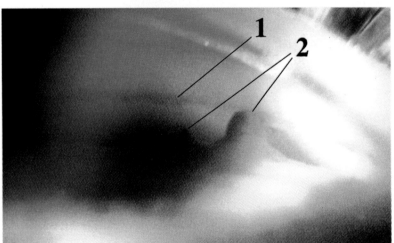

FIGURE 7-20 *Axenfeld's anomaly.* Gonioscopy reveals an enlarged Schwalbe's line *(1)* with adherent iris strands *(2).*

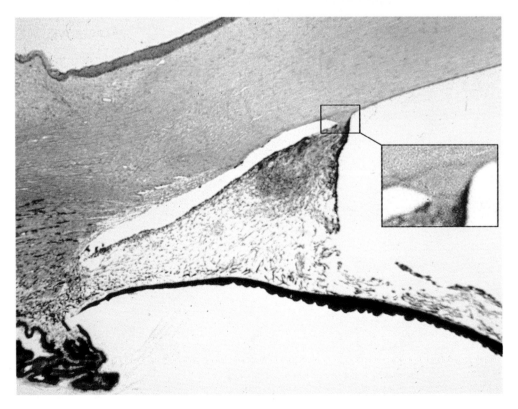

FIGURE 7-21 *Histopathology of Axenfeld's anomaly.* There is an area of adherence between the iris and Schwalbe's line *(inset).*

FIGURE 7-22 **Rieger's anomaly.** There is hypoplasia of the iris stroma and mild corectopia. Iris abnormalities are more extensive in Rieger's anomaly as compared with Axenfeld's anomaly, although both anomalies probably represent a spectrum of disease.

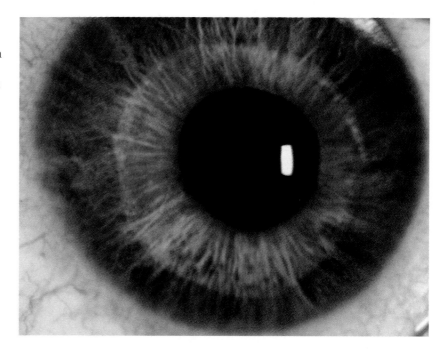

FIGURE 7-23 **Rieger's anomaly.** Similar to Axenfeld's anomaly, there is a prominent Schwalbe's line *(1)* with adherent iris strands *(2)*.

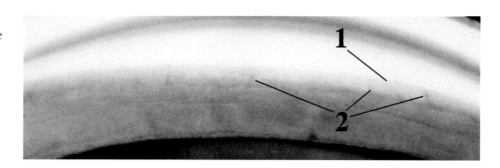

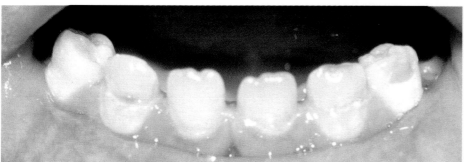

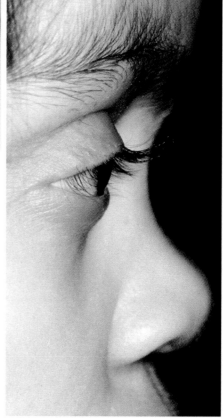

FIGURES 7-24 AND 7-25 **Rieger's syndrome.** This is a combination of Rieger's anomaly and systemic abnormalities, which include microdontia (Figure 7-24, *above*) and a flat nasal bridge with maxillary hypoplasia (Figure 7-25, *right*). Inheritance is usually autosomal dominant.

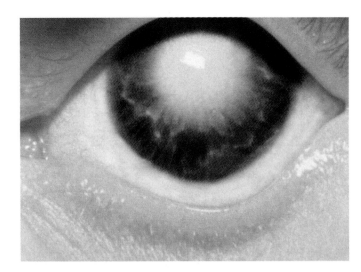

FIGURE 7-26 *Peter's anomaly.* There is central opacification of the corneal stroma with relative clearing in the corneal periphery. In mild cases, adherent strands of iris tissue extend from the pupillary margin to the posterior cornea. In severe cases the iris is markedly abnormal and the lens may adhere to the posterior cornea. Glaucoma is often present.

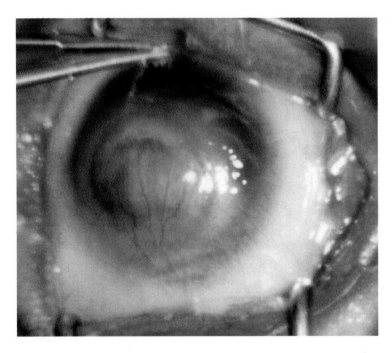

FIGURE 7-27 *Severe Peter's anomaly.* There is marked opacification of the cornea and a superficial vascular pannus.

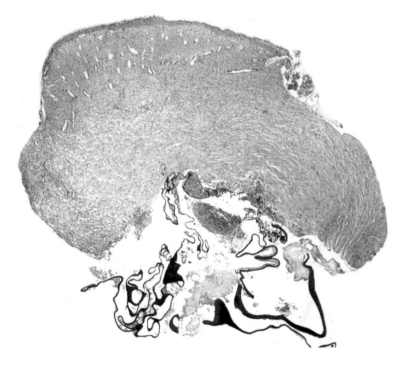

FIGURE 7-28 *Histopathology of Peter's anomaly.* Shown are the increased cellularity and abnormal collagen in the corneal stroma, a loss of normal endothelium and Descemet's membrane, and the adherence of the lens capsule to the posterior cornea.

CHAPTER 8

Corneal Manifestations Of Systemic Disease And Therapies

The corneal manifestations of systemic disease are usually noted in patients with an established systemic diagnosis. Occasionally, however, the clinician has a unique opportunity to diagnose a systemic condition based on the results of the ocular examination. Many of these conditions result in abnormal deposition of material in the cornea. These can easily be discerned because the cornea is normally clear and deposits of any type produce clouding.

Metabolic Disorders

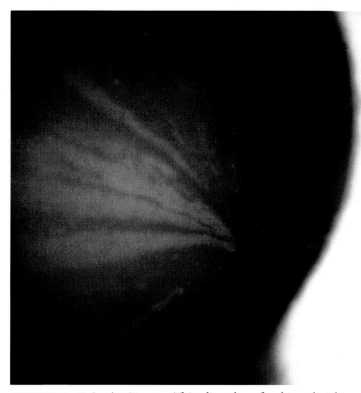

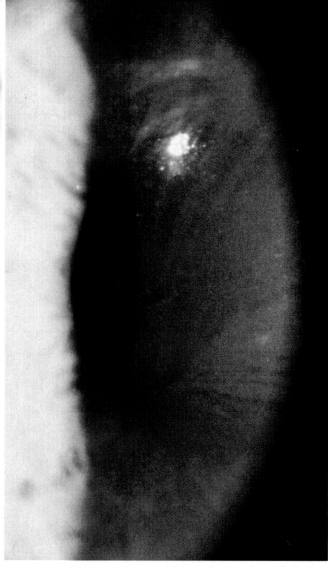

FIGURE 8-1 **Fabry's disease.** This disorder of sphingolipid metabolism results in the deposition of trihexosylceramide in tissues throughout the body. It is transmitted as an X-linked recessive disorder. This male patient has the characteristic deposits in a whorl distribution in the corneal epithelium (cornea verticillata). Nearly all patients with Fabry's disease have this finding.

FIGURE 8-2 **Fabry's disease.** This is the mother of the patient in Figure 8-1. Approximately 90% of female carriers have cornea verticillata.

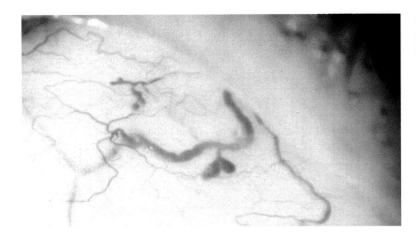

FIGURE 8-3 *Fabry's disease.* Deposits of sphingolipid in the vascular endothelium produce dilated conjunctival vessels with small aneurysms.

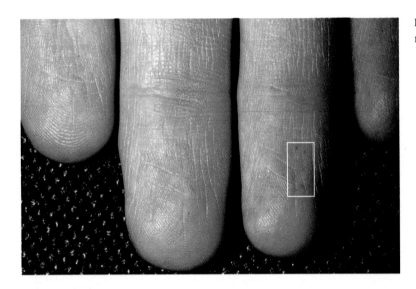

FIGURE 8-4 *Fabry's disease.* Small, punctate, dark-red, vascular lesions appear in the skin *(box).*

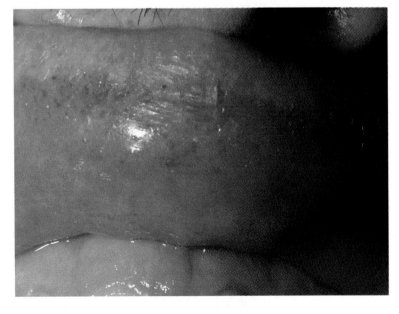

FIGURE 8-5 *Fabry's disease.* There are small telangiectatic vascular abnormalities in the buccal mucosa.

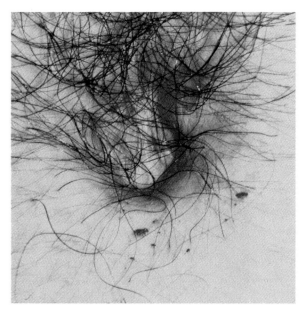

FIGURE 8-6 *Fabry's disease.* Dark red vascular lesions are seen in the periumbilical skin in this patient.

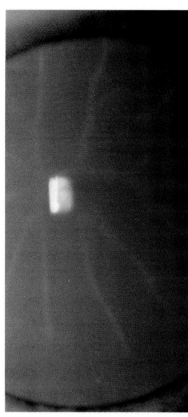

FIGURE 8-7 *Fabry's disease.* Approximately 50% of patients with this disorder have posterior spokelike cataracts, possibly representing deposits of sphingolipid along the lens suture lines.

FIGURE 8-8 *Fabry's disease.* The retinal vessels may be dilated and torturous.

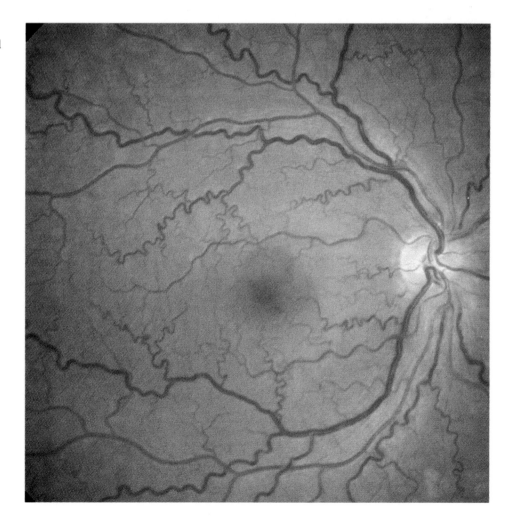

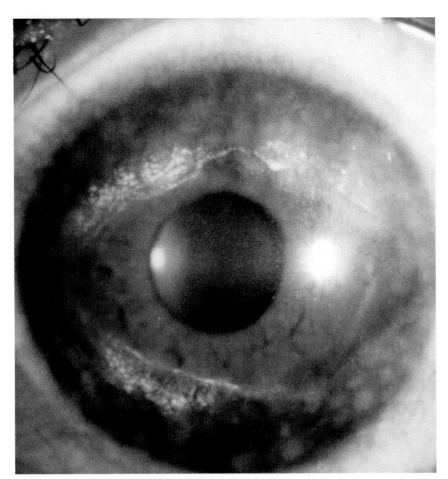

FIGURE 8-9 *Fish eye disease.* This familial condition results in lipid deposition in the cornea. The lipid deposition tends to be denser in the periphery; in advanced forms, diffuse corneal clouding resembling the eyes of boiled fish occurs. Systemically, there is a deficiency in esterification of free cholesterol in high-density α-lipoprotein (HDL). HDL levels are markedly reduced, and triglyceride levels are elevated.

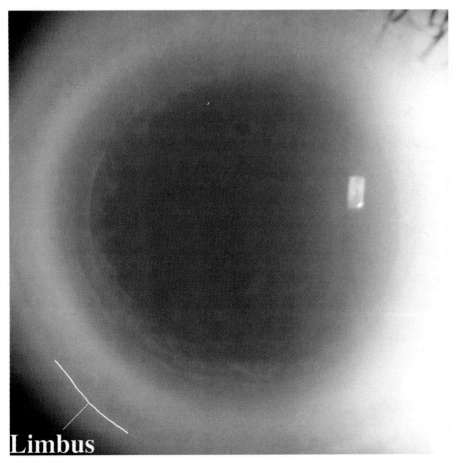

Limbus

FIGURE 8-10 *Lecithin-cholesterol acyltransferase (LCAT) deficiency.* This autosomal recessive disorder results in lipid deposition in the cornea. The plasma demonstrates elevated unesterified cholesterol and lecithin. Systemically, these patients may have renal failure and anemia; however, the corneal findings may precede these manifestations.

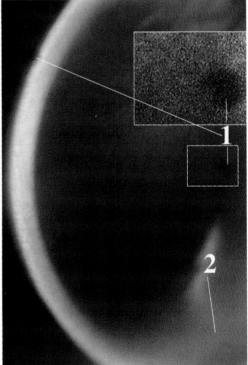

FIGURE 8-11 *LCAT deficiency.* Centrally, the deposits are small white dots, which may surround clear lacunae *(1).* In the peripheral cornea the deposits are denser *(2)* and resemble arcus senilis.

FIGURE 8-12 *Alkaptonuria.* This is an autosomal recessive disorder of phenylalanine and tyrosine metabolism. A metabolic intermediate, homogentisic acid, accumulates throughout the body, causing pigmentary changes. Pigment may accumulate in the eye near the insertion of the recti muscles, particularly the lateral rectus.

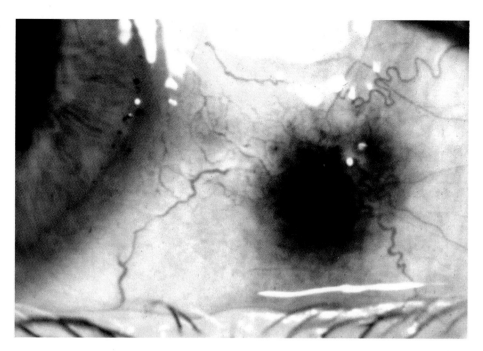

FIGURE 8-13 *Congenital porphyria.* In this disorder of heme biosynthesis, vesicular and ulcerative lesions occur on sun-exposed portions of the skin and eye. In this example the inferior cornea is scarred and vascularized from chronic ulcerations. Other forms of porphyria result in similar blistering and scarring on the conjunctiva and cornea.

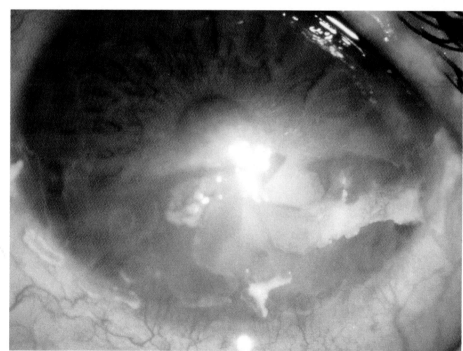

FIGURE 8-14 *Tangier disease.* This systemic abnormality of lipid metabolism is inherited as an autosomal recessive disorder. Systemic abnormalities include an absence of normal HDL in plasma, yellow-orange tonsillar hyperplasia, hepatosplenomegaly, and lymphadenopathy. In this patient, localized lipid deposition in the cornea is associated with vascularization. A white dotlike haze, similar to LCAT deficiency (see Figures 8-10 and 8-11), has also been described. This patient also had multiple lid abnormalities and corrective surgical procedures due to lipid infiltration of the lids. The first patients described with this disorder were from Tangier Island, Virginia.

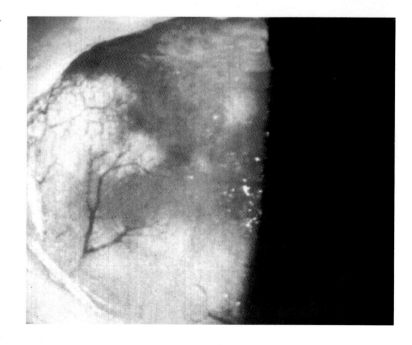

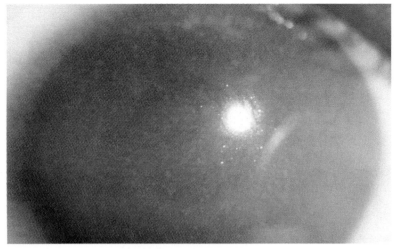

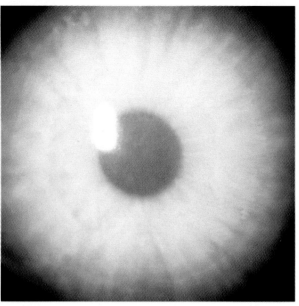

FIGURE 8-15 *Hurler's syndrome.* An autosomal recessive disorder of mucopolysaccharide metabolism, Hurler's syndrome results in the accumulation of dermatan sulfate and heparan sulfate in tissues throughout the body. Corneal clouding begins early in life and is diffuse. The clouding is composed of fine, gray punctate opacities.

FIGURE 8-16 *Scheie's syndrome.* Similar to Hurler's syndrome, this autosomal recessive disorder of mucopolysaccharide metabolism results in the accumulation of dermatan sulfate and heparan sulfate throughout the body. This patient has diffuse corneal clouding.

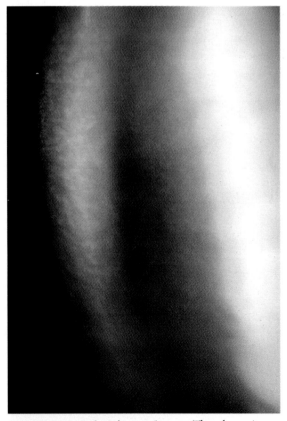

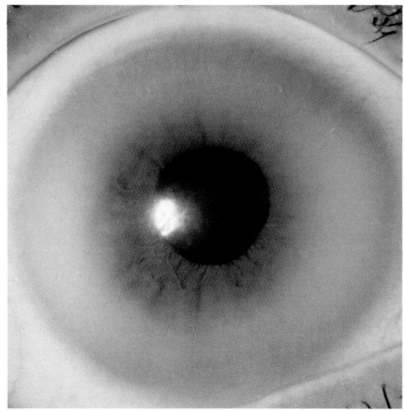

FIGURE 8-17 *Scheie's syndrome.* The deposits are fine, gray punctate opacities located throughout the corneal stroma.

FIGURE 8-18 *Scheie's syndrome.* The corneal clouding may be densest in the peripheral cornea, although the central cornea is usually affected. In this unusual case the peripheral cornea has dense clouding and the central cornea is almost clear.

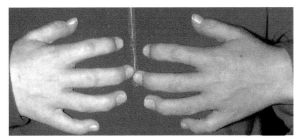

FIGURE 8-19 *Scheie's syndrome.* The hands are clawlike, and the joints are enlarged.

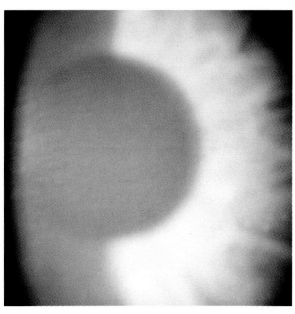

FIGURE 8-20 *Morquio's syndrome.* There is diffuse corneal clouding from keratan sulfate deposition in the corneal stroma. Morquio's syndrome is an autosomal recessive disorder of mucopolysaccharide metabolism.

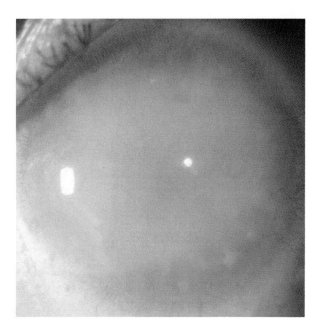

FIGURE 8-21 *Maroteaux-Lamy syndrome.* Corneal clouding is common. Dermatan sulfate accumulates in the corneal stroma. This is an autosomal recessive disorder of mucopolysaccharide metabolism.

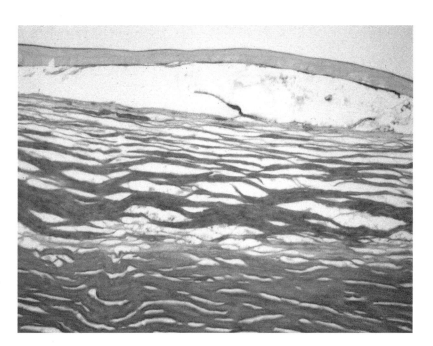

FIGURE 8-22 *Histopathology of Scheie's syndrome.* There are deposits of mucopolysaccharide throughout the corneal stroma. Mucopolysaccharide stains blue with an alcian blue stain.

Cystinosis is an autosomal recessive disorder of impaired cystine transport across lysosomal membranes. Cystine is deposited in tissues throughout the body, including the conjunctiva, cornea, and retina. Deposits of crystals in the cornea can cause severe photophobia and episodes of recurrent erosions. The infantile form is the most severe, and death usually occurs in the first decade of life from renal failure. The adolescent form manifests in the second decade of life, and renal involvement is less severe. The adult form is the mildest and has no renal involvement or retinal changes.

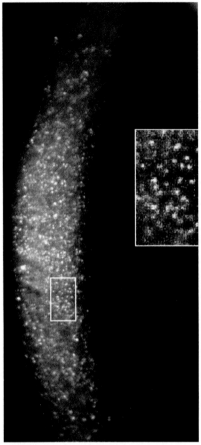

FIGURE 8-23 *Cystinosis.* The corneal crystals are polygonal, refractile, and polychromatic *(inset).*

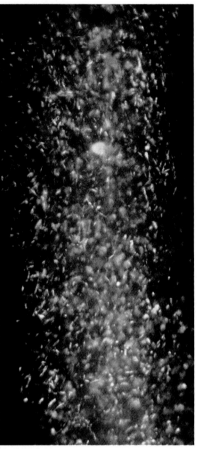

FIGURE 8-24 *Cystinosis.* High magnification of corneal crystals is seen.

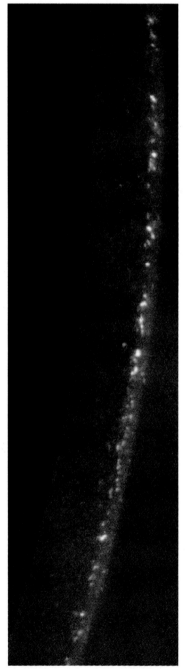

FIGURE 8-26 *Cystinosis.* In addition to corneal crystals, this patient had Fanconi's syndrome caused by cystine deposits in the kidneys.

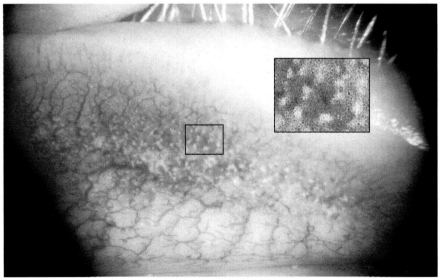

FIGURE 8-25 *Cystinosis.* Cystine crystals *(inset)* are also deposited in the conjunctiva.

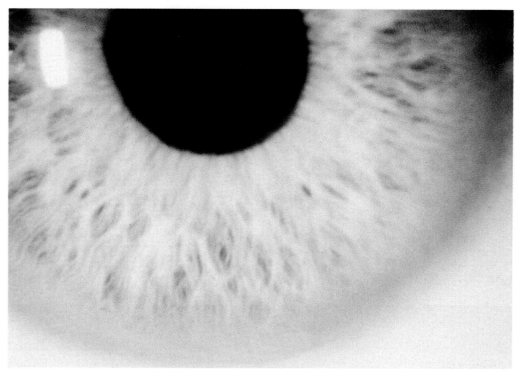

FIGURE 8-27 **Wilson's disease.** There is a defect in copper metabolism, and 95% of patients with Wilson's disease have a Kayser-Fleischer ring. Copper is deposited at the level of Descemet's membrane in the peripheral cornea. (The inferior cornea is affected first.) The ring is usually dark brown but may appear gold-yellow (as seen here) or green. There is no clear interval separating the ring from the limbus.

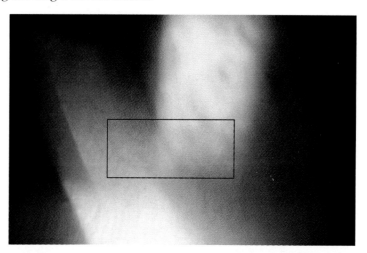

FIGURE 8-28 **Wilson's disease.** A slit beam view of a Kayser-Fleischer ring *(box)* demonstrates its deep location in Descemet's membrane.

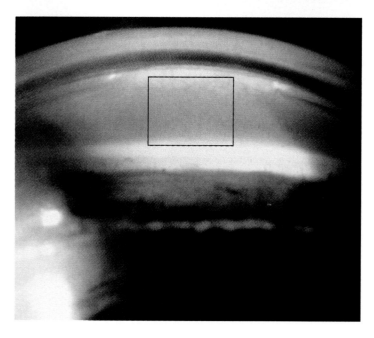

FIGURE 8-29 **Early Wilson's disease.** The copper deposition may only be appreciated with gonioscopy. In this patient, there is dark brown pigmentation extending from Schwalbe's line anteriorly *(box)*.

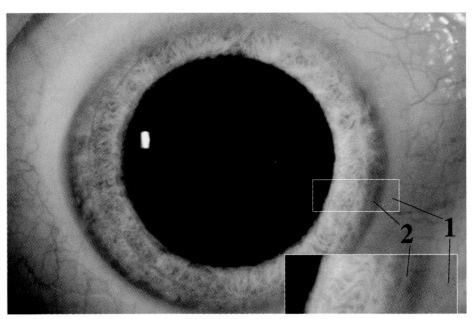

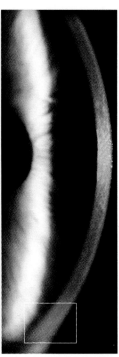

FIGURE 8-30 *Bilirubin deposits.* A Kayser-Fleischer ring should be distinguished from bilirubin deposits in the peripheral cornea. This patient with primary biliary cirrhosis has conjunctival jaundice *(1)* and peripheral yellow bilirubin deposits in the cornea *(2).*

FIGURE 8-31 *A thin slit lamp view of the same patient as in Figure 8-30.* The box shows that the bilirubin deposits are more extensive in the posterior stroma but are located throughout the stroma.

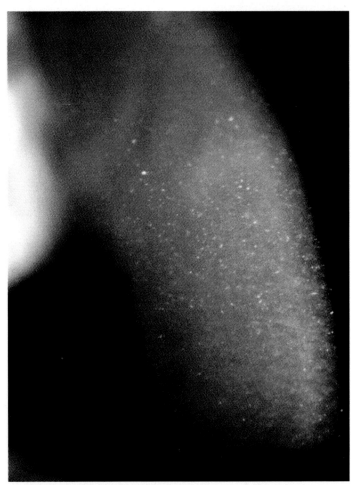

FIGURE 8-32 *Gout.* This patient has urate crystals in the corneal stroma.

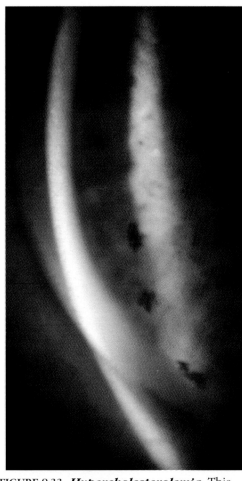

FIGURE 8-33 *Hypercholesterolemia.* This patient has arcus senilis. There is a clear area between the lipid deposits and the limbus.

Skeletal Disorders

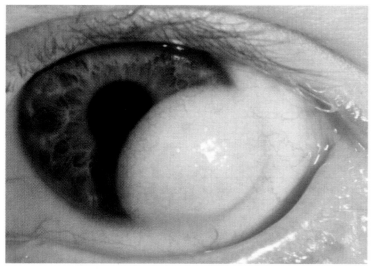

FIGURE 8-34 *Goldenhar's syndrome.* One third of patients with this syndrome (oculoauriculovertebral dysplasia) have corneal dermoids. The dermoids are usually unilateral and occur most commonly at the inferior temporal limbus.

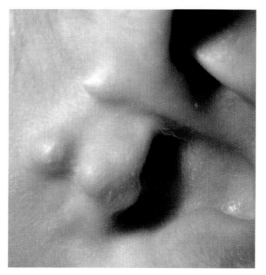

FIGURE 8-35 *Goldenhar's syndrome.* A pretragal appendage is noted.

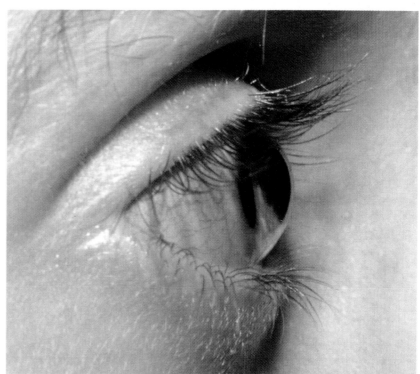

FIGURE 8-36 *Ehlers-Danlos syndrome.* This systemic disorder is characterized by poor cross-linking of collagen molecules. Systemic findings include joint hypermobility, skin hyperextensibility, easy bruising, and propensity toward organ rupture. This patient with Ehlers-Danlos syndrome type VI has keratoglobus and blue sclera. Blue sclera results from scleral thinning and increased visibility of the choroid.

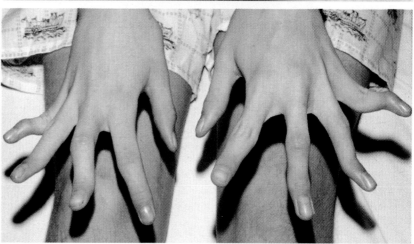

FIGURE 8-37 *Ehlers-Danlos syndrome.* Joint hypermobility is shown.

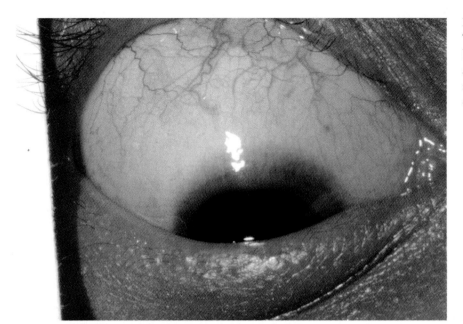

FIGURE 8-38 *Osteogenesis imperfecta.* This inherited disorder is characterized by bone fractures, deafness, and blue scleras. The blue sclera is easily appreciated when compared with the white card on the left of this figure.

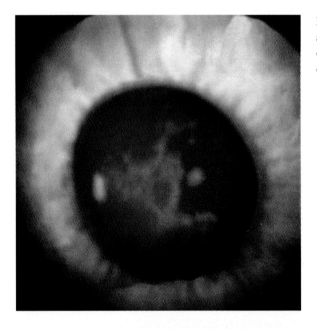

FIGURE 8-39 *Osteogenesis imperfecta.* Central corneal scarring is seen here. Other corneal abnormalities in this disease include decreased central corneal thickness, keratoconus, and megalocornea.

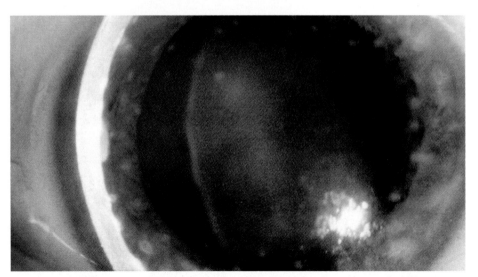

FIGURE 8-40 *Spondyloepiphyseal dysplasia tarda.* In this inherited skeletal dysplasia, multiple deep, grayish white nodular opacities may be seen in the deep peripheral corneal stroma (some project toward the anterior chamber).

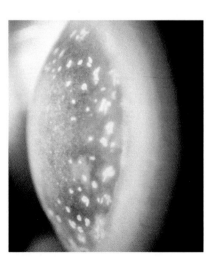

FIGURE 8-41 *Spondyloepiphyseal dysplasia tarda.* Deep peripheral opacities and fine central opacities are noted in the mid and anterior stroma.

Inflammatory Bowel Disease

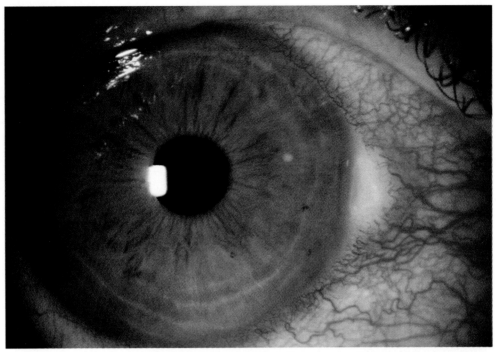

FIGURE 8-42 *Crohn's disease.* This is a chronic inflammatory disease of the gastrointestinal tract. This patient has sclerokeratitis. There is avascularity in the area of infiltration.

FIGURE 8-43 *Crohn's disease.* There is a marginal noninfected corneal ulcer. Systemic immunosuppression may be needed to control progressive ulceration.

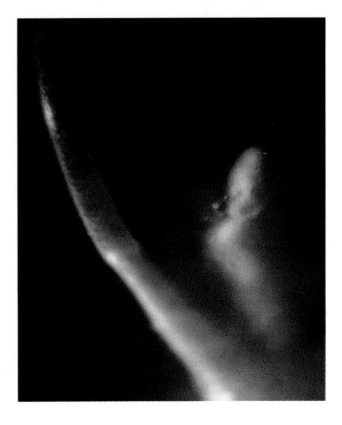

Nutritional Disorders

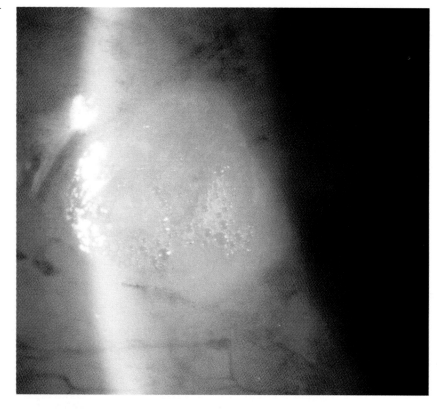

FIGURE 8-44 *Vitamin A deficiency.* Although vitamin A deficiency is rare in the United States, when it occurs, it is usually with cystic fibrosis, severe liver disease, or severe malnutrition (especially in alcoholics) or after intestinal bypass surgery. This is an example of a Bitot spot, a white-gray irregular plaque that usually occurs near the limbus in the interpalpebral region. A gas-producing bacteria, *Corynebacterium xerosis,* is responsible for the foamy appearance in this lesion.

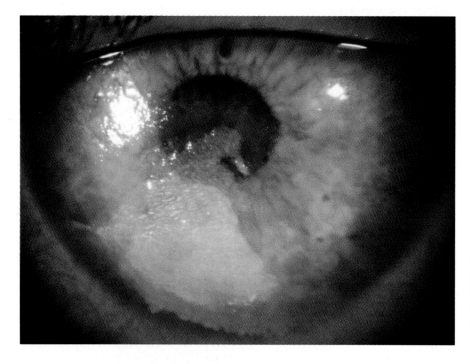

FIGURE 8-45 *Vitamin A deficiency.* This patient has marked keratinization of the inferior cornea. The corneal surface is dry, and the light reflex is irregular. Goblet cell function is impaired in this disorder, and there is a lack of mucin.

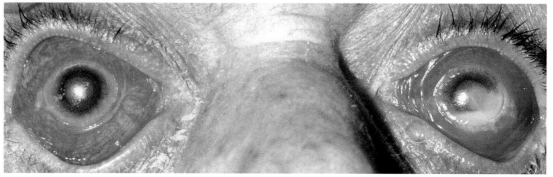

FIGURE 8-46 *Vitamin A deficiency.* In this alcoholic patient, an infected corneal ulcer has developed in the left eye. A hypopyon is present.

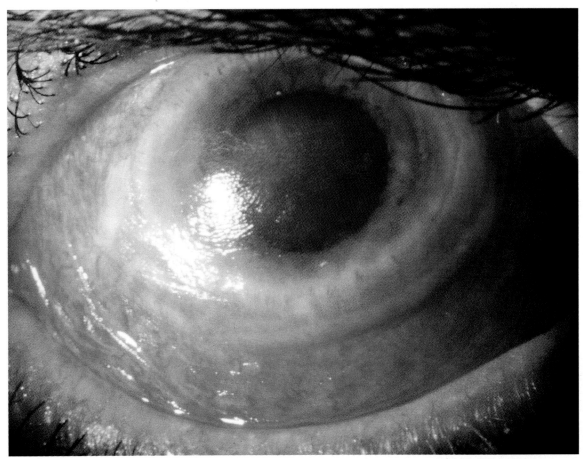

FIGURE 8-47 *The right eye of the same patient in Figure 8-46 before vitamin A treatment.*
The corneal light reflex is dulled, and the cornea and conjunctiva lack their normal luster.

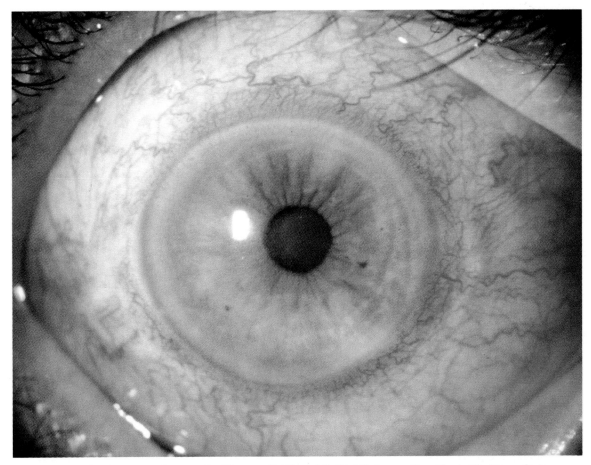

FIGURE 8-48 *Same patient as in Figures 8-46 and 8-47, 10 days after the initiation of vitamin A treatment.* The corneal light reflex is sharp, and the surface abnormalities of the conjunctiva and cornea are nearly gone.

Hematologic Disorders

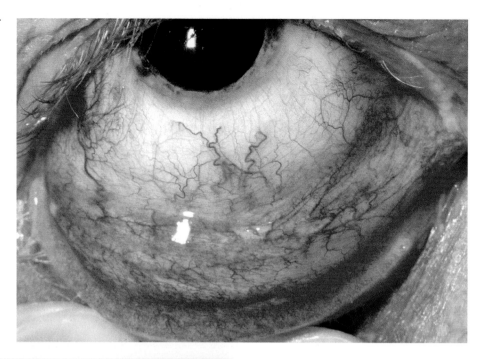

FIGURE 8-49 **Polycythemia vera.**
There is an increased red cell mass and hematocrit. Engorged blood vessels can be readily appreciated in the inferior fornix of this patient. These patients may complain of redness of the eyes, allowing the clinician the unique position of establishing the diagnosis.

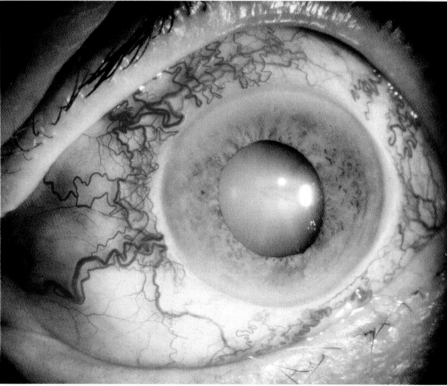

FIGURE 8-50 **Dural-cavernous fistula.**
There is a communication between the dural arteries and the cavernous sinus. The conjunctival veins in one eye become markedly enlarged and torturous, whereas the conjunctival arteries remain normal. Other signs of a dural-cavernous fistula include unilateral visual field loss, proptosis, motility disturbances, and elevated intraocular pressure.

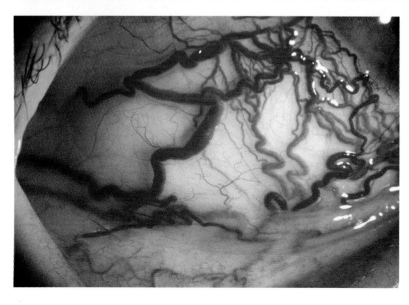

FIGURE 8-51 **Dural-cavernous fistula.** This is a higher magnification of the conjunctiva in a different patient. There is marked enlargement and tortuosity of the conjunctival veins.

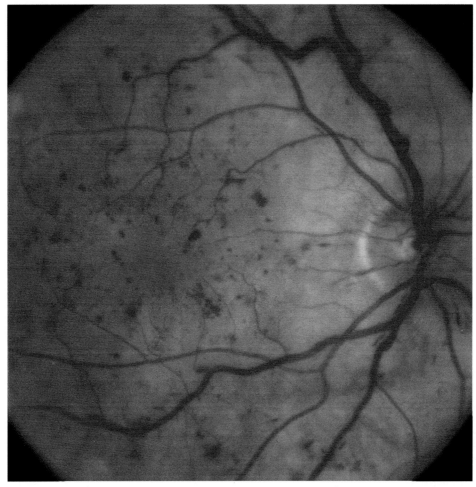

FIGURE 8-52 *Dural-cavernous fistula.* This is the retina of the same patient as in Figure 8-51. The retinal veins are enlarged, and there are scattered retinal hemorrhages from venous stasis retinopathy.

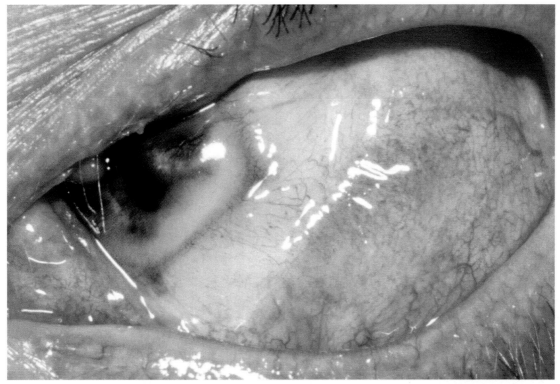

FIGURE 8-53 *Primary amyloidosis.* There is systemic deposition of abnormal proteins, which are usually composed of immunoglobulin light chains. In this patient, amyloid deposits are seen infiltrating the conjunctiva and cornea.

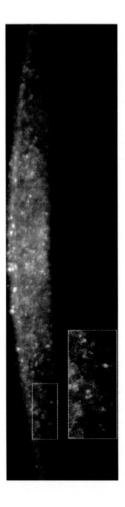

FIGURE 8-54 *Multiple myeloma.* There is systemic deposition of entire immunoglobulin molecules and an excess of light chains. Systemic findings include anemia, hypercalcemia, and osteolytic bone lesions. This patient with multiple myeloma has immunoglobulin crystals in the cornea *(inset).*

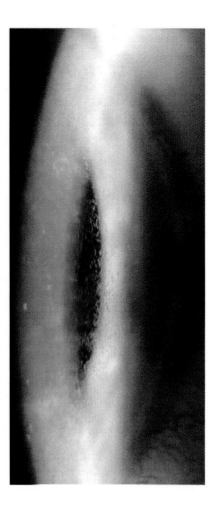

FIGURE 8-55 *Waldenström's macroglobulinemia.* There is systemic deposition of IgM. This patient demonstrates immunoglobulin deposition in the cornea. In direct illumination these deposits are white; in indirect illumination, they appear crystalline.

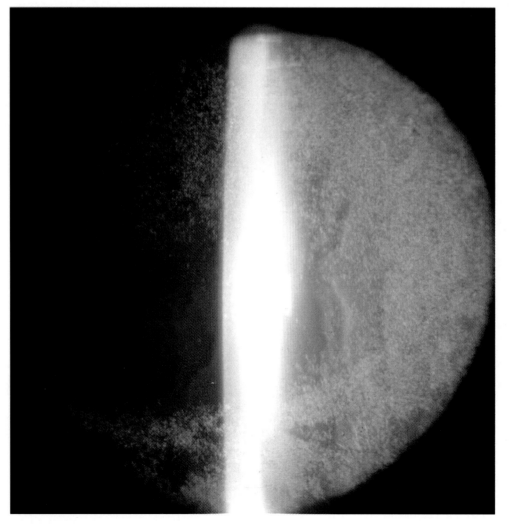

FIGURE 8-56 *Waldenström's macroglobulinemia.* In the same patient as in Figure 8-55, the red reflex demonstrates the refractile and crystalline nature of deposits.

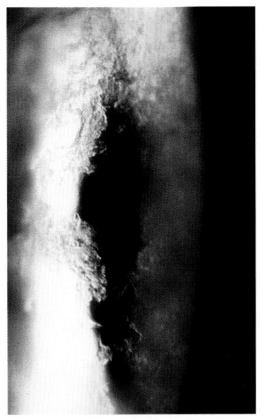

FIGURE 8-57 *Benign monoclonal gammopathy.* Immunoglobulin crystals are seen in the cornea.

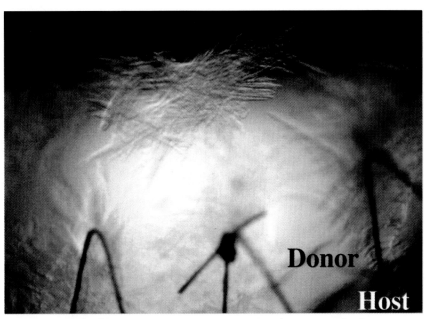

FIGURE 8-58 *Benign monoclonal gammopathy.* This patient had a recurrence of immunoglobulin crystals in a graft. Although usually a benign process, some patients develop multiple myeloma.

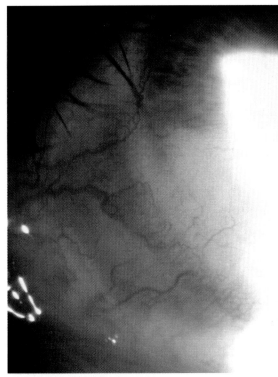

FIGURE 8-59 *Eosinophilic granuloma.* This benign tumor composed of eosinophils and histiocytes usually begins in one of the bones of the orbital rim (most commonly the frontal bone). Here the tumor has infiltrated anteriorly into the conjunctiva and cornea.

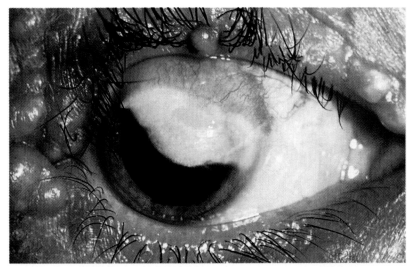

FIGURE 8-60 *Hand-Schüller-Christian disease.* A disseminated form of eosinophilic granuloma, this disease can be fatal and comprises a triad of lytic lesions in the skull, exophthalmos from orbital involvement, and diabetes insipidus. The histology is identical to that of eosinophilic granuloma. Here the tumor has extended into the subcutaneous tissue of the skin and into the conjunctiva and cornea.

Endocrine Disorders

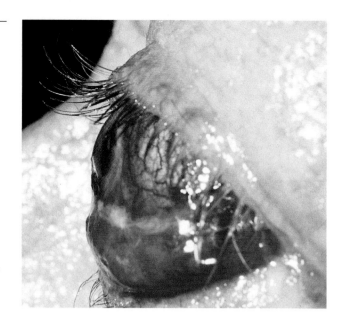

FIGURE 8-61 *Thyroid eye disease.* Infiltration of the extraocular muscles and connective tissue can result in severe proptosis and orbital inflammation.

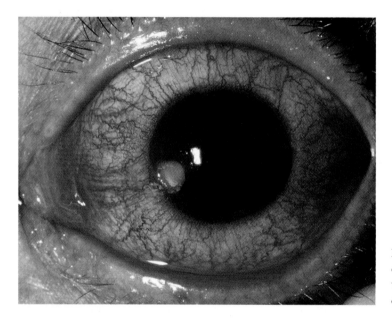

FIGURE 8-62 *Thyroid eye disease.* This patient had chronic exposure keratitis and developed an indolent ulcer. Exophthalmos and lid retraction predispose to corneal exposure.

FIGURE 8-63 *Thyroid eye disease.* There is an infected corneal ulcer with hypopyon in this patient with exposure keratitis caused by thyroid eye disease.

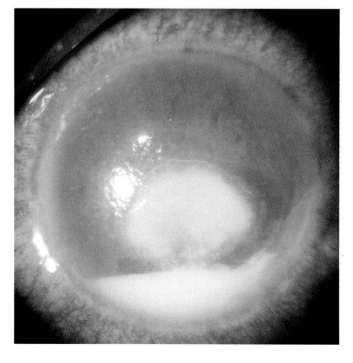

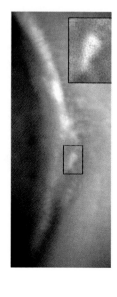

FIGURE 8-64 *Chronic renal failure.* The inset shows limbal calcium deposits in this patient.

Dermatologic Disorders

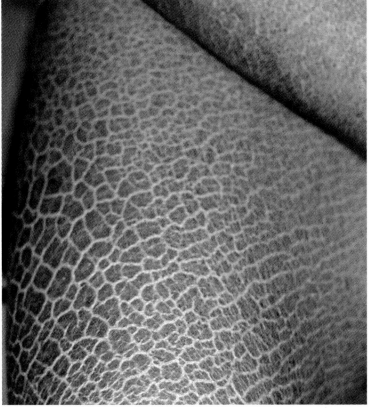

FIGURE 8-65 *X-linked ichthyosis.* There are large brown hyperkeratotic scales on the skin.

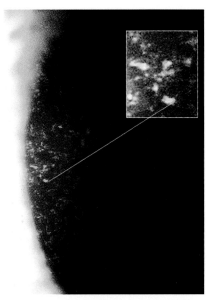

FIGURE 8-66 *X-linked ichthyosis.* There are fine white deposits just anterior to Descemet's membrane *(inset).* Other forms of ichthyosis do not have these deposits.

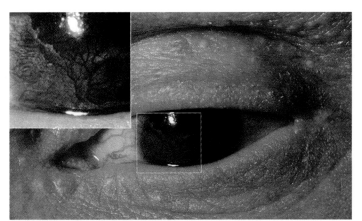

FIGURE 8-67 *Keratitis, ichthyosis, and deafness (KID) syndrome.* This rare inherited disorder may be autosomal dominant or sporadic. Hair is scant or absent, and in this case, there is an absence of the eyelashes. Corneal findings include superficial pannus *(inset),* diffuse punctate keratopathy, stromal scarring, and vascularization.

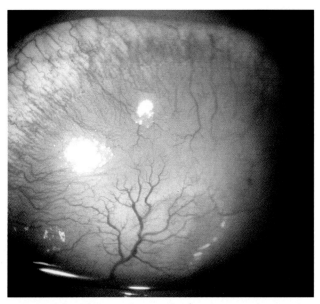

FIGURE 8-68 *KID syndrome.* In the same patient as in Figure 8-67, the cornea is scarred and vascularized.

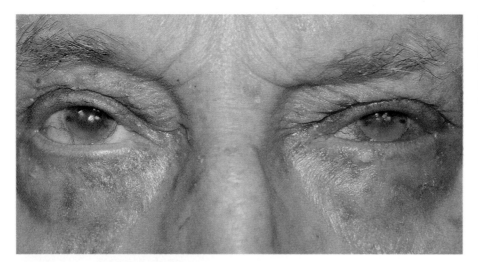

FIGURE 8-69 **Psoriasis.** This chronic skin disease is characterized by scaling papules or plaques. This patient with involvement of the skin of the eyelids has lash loss and a nonspecific conjunctivitis.

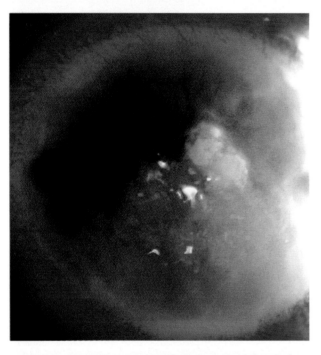

FIGURE 8-70 **Psoriasis.** An infectious corneal ulcer is seen in this patient with psoriasis of the lids. Other corneal findings include sterile ulceration, superficial vascularization, and corneal scarring.

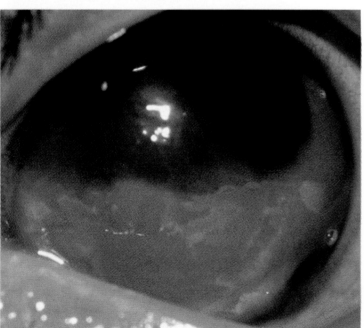

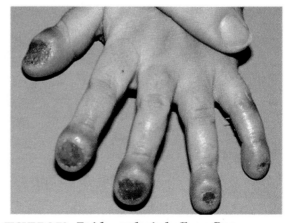

FIGURE 8-71 **Epidermolysis bullosa.** There is poor epithelial adhesion to the basement membrane. Recurrent erosion with ulceration is common.

FIGURE 8-72 **Epidermolysis bullosa.** Poor epithelial adhesion causes bullous lesions of the skin after minor trauma. The fingernails can be dystrophic, and the distal digits may be encased in a keratinized shell.

Infectious Diseases

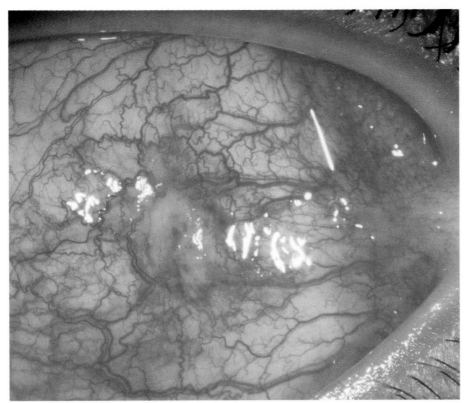

FIGURE 8-73 *Varicella (chickenpox).* This is a common viral infection of young children. The rash spreads in waves and begins as flat macules that progress to papules and vesicles. Shown is a pock in the conjunctiva.

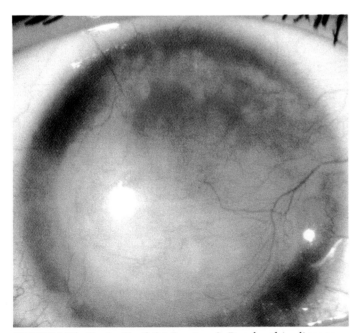

FIGURE 8-74 *Varicella (chickenpox).* Rarely, this disease is associated with interstitial keratitis. This patient has extensive corneal scarring and vascularization.

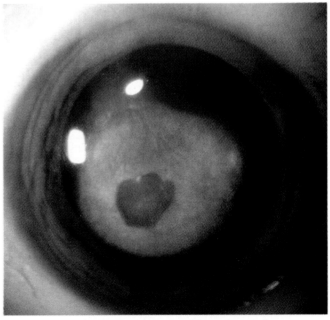

FIGURE 8-75 *Variola (smallpox).* This patient demonstrates a central corneal scar from a smallpox or variola infection. Fortunately, the variola virus has been eradicated, and complications of this type are rarely seen today.

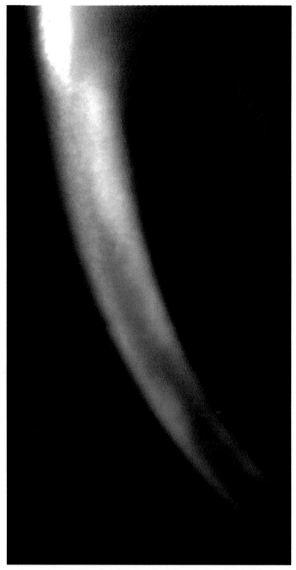

FIGURE 8-76 *Epstein-Barr virus infection.* Rarely, irregular white opacities can be found throughout the corneal stroma. These opacities can occur in patients with active mononucleosis or in the absence of systemic disease with only serologic evidence of infection. They usually respond to topical corticosteroids.

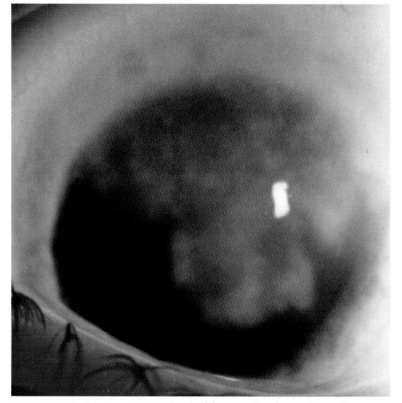

FIGURE 8-77 *Lyme disease.* Caused by a spirochete *(Borrelia burgdorferi),* Lyme disease is transmitted by ticks. In the acute infection, patients develop fever, chills, malaise, and an enlarging red rash on the thighs, buttocks, or trunk (chronicum migrans). Months later, patients may experience a relapsing migratory polyarthritis. Patients may develop an interstitial keratitis characterized by multiple corneal infiltrates with indistinct borders in all levels of the stroma. Corneal vascularization is limited, and the conjunctiva is usually uninflamed.

AIDS-Related Disorders

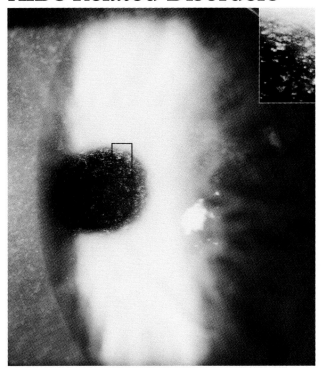

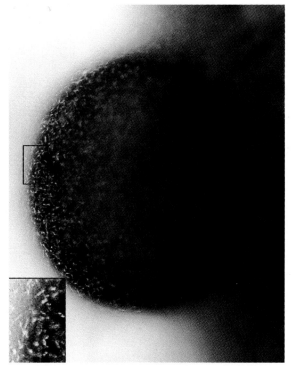

FIGURE 8-78 *Microsporidia.* In immunocompromised patients, microsporidia can cause a diffuse epithelial keratitis. There are multiple white intraepithelial infiltrates *(inset),* which represent active organisms.

FIGURE 8-79 *CMV retinitis.* Stellate keratic precipitates *(inset)* are a common finding in patients with advanced disease.

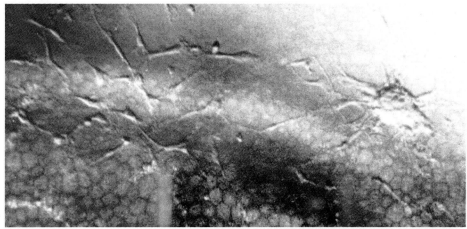

FIGURE 8-80 *CMV retinitis.* The relief mode of a specular photomicrograph shows the fine branching pattern of these stellate deposits. Histologically, they are composed of macrophages and fibrin.

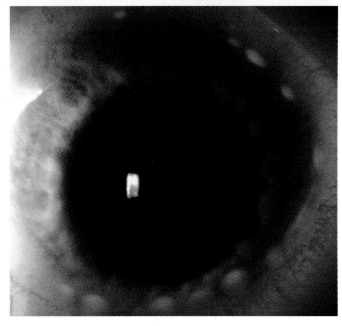

FIGURE 8-81 *Reiter's syndrome in AIDS.* There is an increased incidence of Reiter's syndrome in individuals with AIDS. In this patient with both disorders, multiple peripheral sterile corneal infiltrates can be seen.

Corneal Manifestations of Local and Systemic Therapies

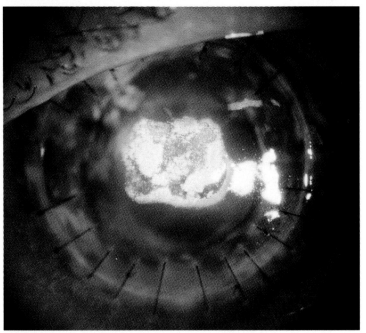

FIGURE 8-82 *Ciprofloxacin deposits.* Topical ciprofloxacin will precipitate at physiologic pH. Chalky white deposits accumulate in areas of absent epithelium.

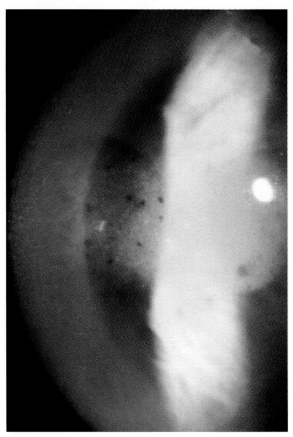

FIGURE 8-83 *Mercury deposits.* Noncalcific band keratopathy can result from mercury deposits in Bowman's layer. These are orange-brown and most commonly the result of mercury preservatives in ophthalmic drops (in this case, pilocarpine).

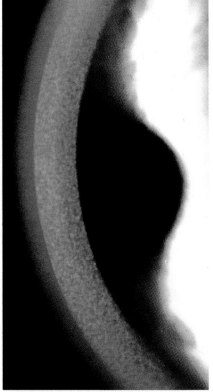

FIGURE 8-84 *Argyrosis.* This is the accumulation of silver in tissues in the body. Silver deposits in the cornea occur in the deepest portion near Descemet's membrane; they have a slate-gray appearance.

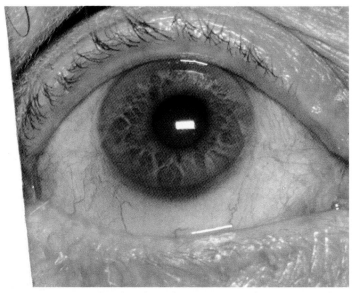

FIGURE 8-85 *Argyrosis.* Silver deposits may also occur in the conjunctiva. The conjunctiva is gray when compared with the white card on the left. Here and in Figure 8-84, the silver deposits are secondary to the topical medication Argyrol, a silver nitrate compound.

FIGURE 8-86 *Adrenochrome deposits.* These dark black deposits are commonly found in the conjunctiva of patients treated with epinephrine eyedrops for glaucoma.

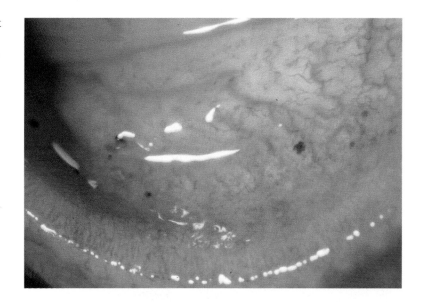

FIGURE 8-87 *Adrenochrome deposits.* These may develop on the cornea.

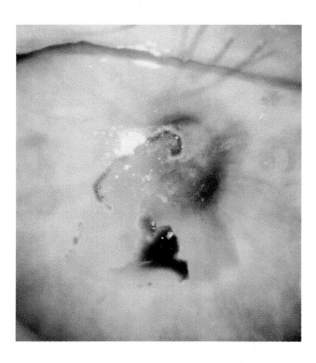

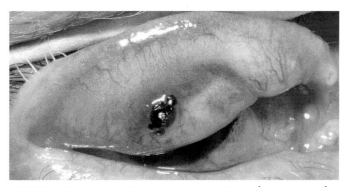

FIGURE 8-88 *Adrenochrome deposit.* Here this occurred as a concretion on the upper lid palpebral conjunctiva.

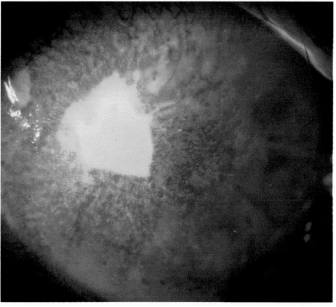

FIGURE 8-89 *Same patient as in Figure 8-88.* There is a corneal erosion resulting from mechanical irritation from this deposit.

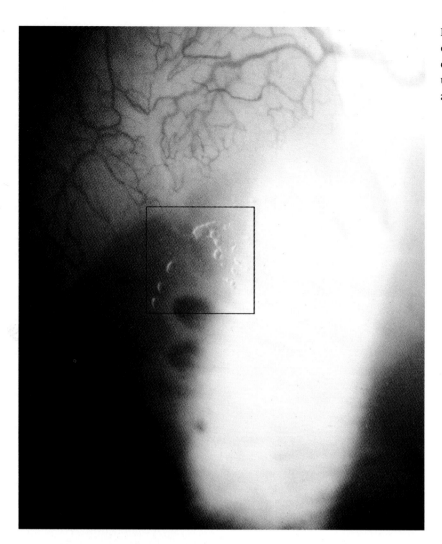

FIGURE 8-90 *Ophthalmic ointments.* These ointments can become incorporated into the epithelium, as seen here *(box).* This is very unusual and probably should not mitigate against ointment usage.

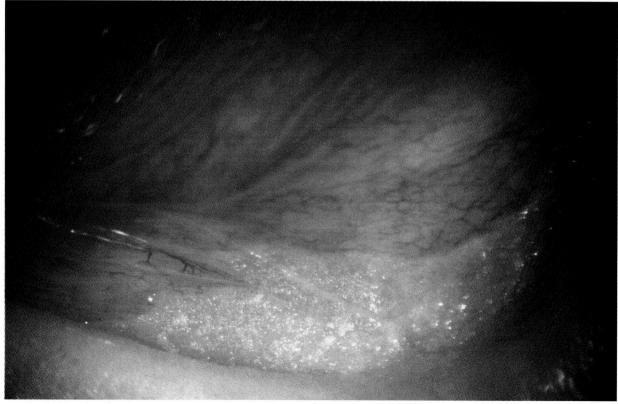

FIGURE 8-91 *Radiation therapy.* Extensive keratinization of the palpebral conjunctiva is noted after local radiation treatment for an angiosarcoma. Another example of radiation effects is seen in Figure 12-25.

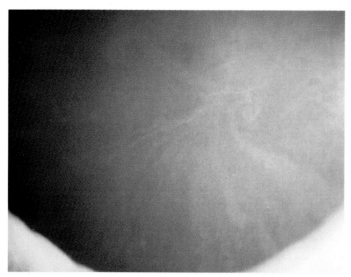

FIGURE 8-92 *Chloroquine deposits.* Whorl opacities in the corneal epithelium are termed *cornea verticillata.*

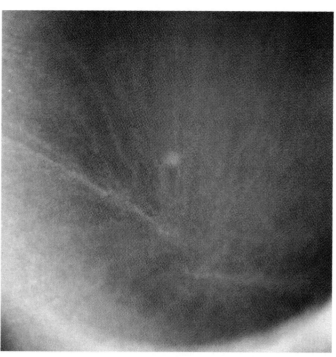

FIGURE 8-93 *Amiodarone deposits.* A cornea verticillata pattern occurred after a total cumulative dose of 56 g of amiodarone.

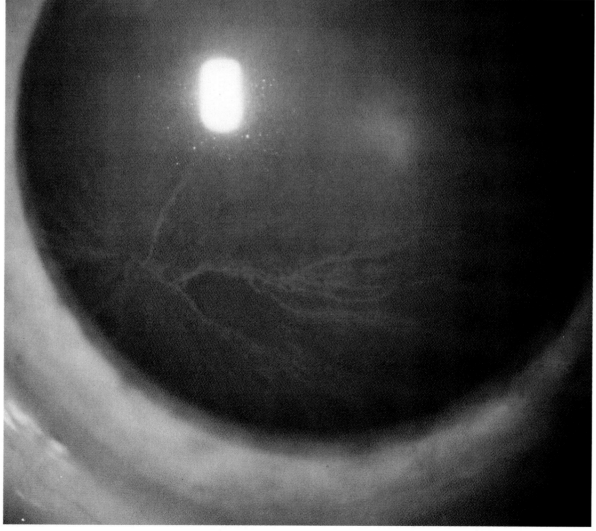

FIGURE 8-94 *Amiodarone deposits.* This example of cornea verticillata occurred after a cumulative dose of 219 g of amiodarone.

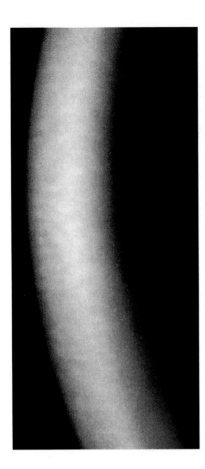

FIGURE 8-95 **_Gold accumulation in the cornea._** Termed *corneal chrysiasis,* this occurs in patients treated with both oral and intramuscular gold therapy for arthritis. The deposits are yellow-brown granules in the deep corneal stroma.

FIGURE 8-96 **_Same patient as in Figure 8-95._** There are small gold deposits in the conjunctival epithelium *(inset).*

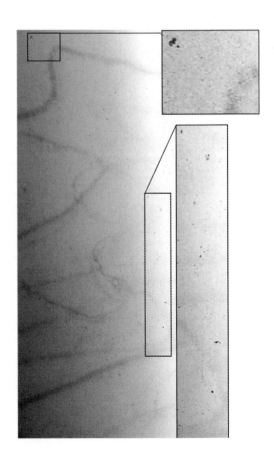

There cases highlight the anterior segment findings associated with systemic phenothiazine use. The location in the anterior lens and deep cornea suggests that these compounds (or breakdown products) enter tissue via the aqueous. Light exposure probably plays a role in the pathogenesis, since the deposits are more intense in the interpalpebral region.

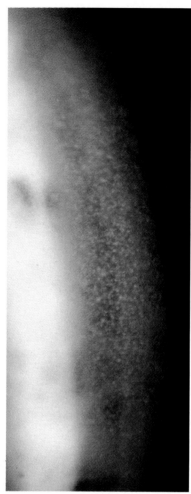

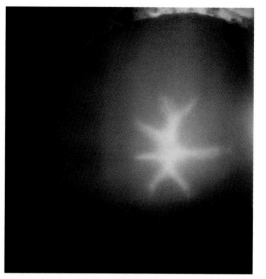

FIGURE 8-98 Stellate thorazine deposits beneath the anterior lens capsule.

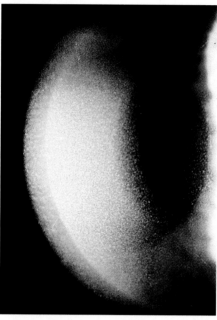

FIGURE 8-99 Heavy thorazine deposits in the posterior cornea.

FIGURE 8-97 **Thorazine deposits.** Extensive deposits are noted throughout the entire corneal stroma, although they are more numerous in the posterior stroma.

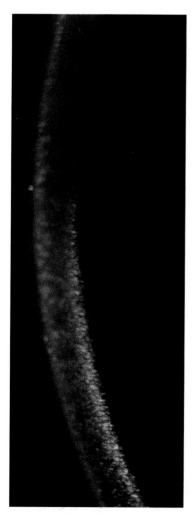

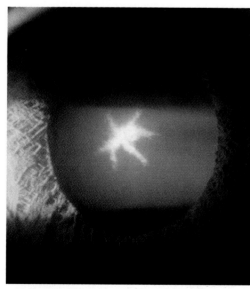

FIGURE 8-100 **Stellazine deposits.** Brown deposits in the posterior corneal stroma are primarily in the interpalpebral region.

FIGURE 8-101 Stellazine deposits beneath the anterior lens capsule.

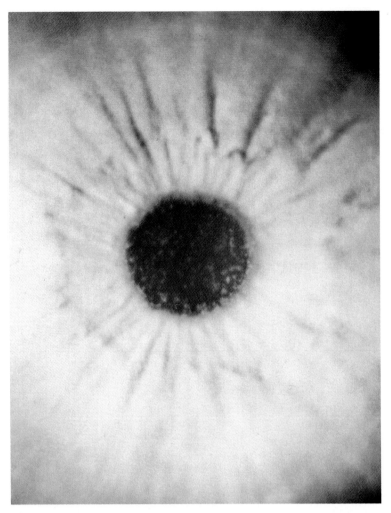

FIGURE 8-102 *Cytarabine-associated cysts.*
Cytarabine (Ara-C) is an antimetabolite used to treat systemic malignancies. Its use is associated with a keratitis characterized by multiple intraepithelial cysts and a diffuse conjunctivitis. The cysts may develop in response to altered epithelial cell metabolism. With direct illumination, the cysts are opaque. Symptoms include irritation, decreased vision, and photophobia.

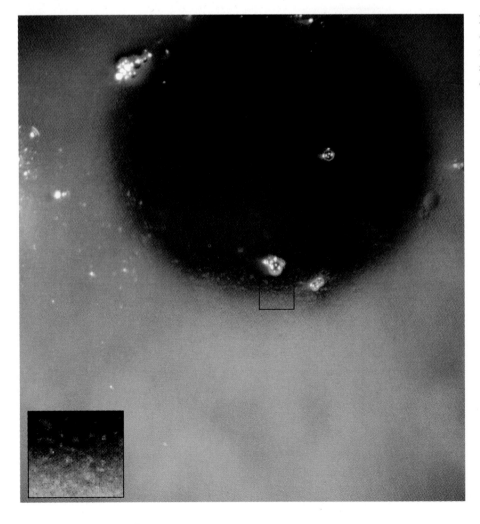

FIGURE 8-103 *Cytarabine-associated cysts.* These are seen with indirect illumination *(inset).* In addition, there are white globs of mucus on the cornea from dry eye syndrome.

CHAPTER 9

Corneal Dystrophies, Ectatic Disorders, And Degenerations

Corneal dystrophies are bilateral, inherited disorders not usually associated with any other systemic conditions. Most are autosomal dominant disorders. Patients exhibit a spectrum of pathologic conditions, so examining multiple family members may help establish the diagnosis. Degenerations, in contrast, are bilateral aging changes of the cornea and are not inherited or associated with systemic disease. Ectatic disorders are often characterized by a great reduction in vision because they alter the shape of the primary refractive element of the eye.

Anterior Membrane Dystrophies

FIGURE 9-1 *Epithelial basement membrane dystrophy (map-dot-fingerprint dystrophy).* This is the most common corneal dystrophy seen in clinical practice. The geographic figures in this disorder are caused by reduplications of basement membrane. Similar geographic reduplications of basement membrane may be seen in the area of a healed epithelial defect; therefore these changes may represent a response of the cornea to various insults. This disorder is usually bilateral and occasionally seen with an autosomal dominant pattern of inheritance. Patients are frequently asymptomatic; however, if the lesions extend into the visual axis, blurred vision and monocular diplopia may develop. Patients may also have symptoms and signs of recurrent erosion. This figure demonstrates a large, gray area with scattered, puttylike dots. The large dot seen in the inset is slightly darker superiorly, where it lies under additional basement membrane material.

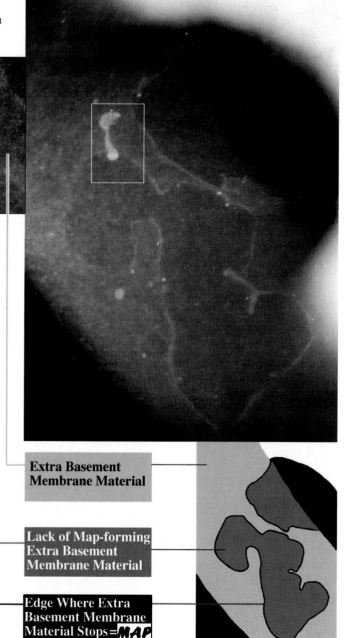

Extra Basement Membrane Material

Lack of Map-forming Extra Basement Membrane Material

Edge Where Extra Basement Membrane Material Stops=*MAP*

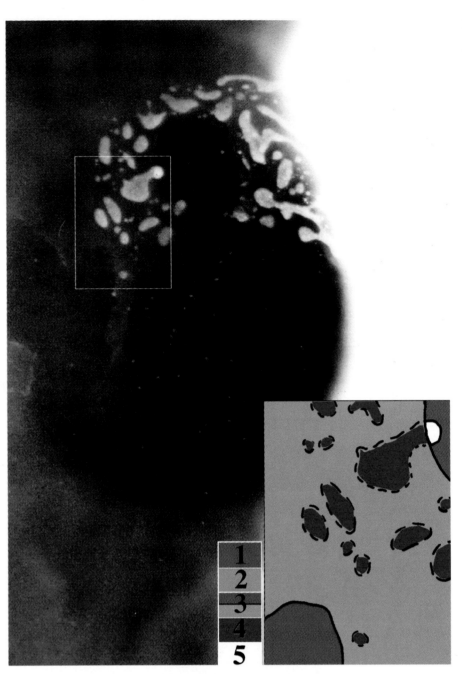

FIGURE 9-2 *Epithelial basement membrane dystrophy.* *1,* Area where extra basement membrane material is not present. *2,* Area of extra basement membrane material. *3,* Junction of *1* and *2,* the edge of which *(black line)* appears as a "map." *4,* Portion of dot beneath extra basement membrane. *5,* Portion of dot beyond extra basement membrane.

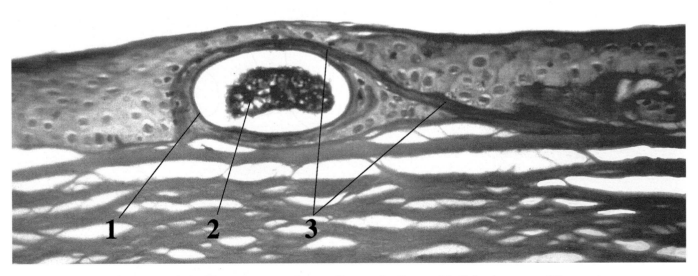

FIGURE 9-3 *Epithelial basement membrane dystrophy.* Intraepithelial microcysts *(1)* contain pyknotic nuclei and cytoplasmic debris *(2).* Extra basement membrane material *(3)* is covering cyst (dot).

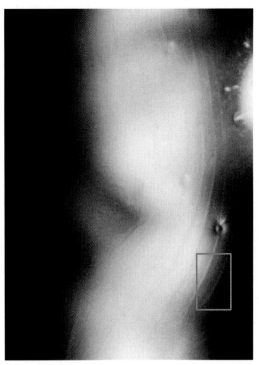

FIGURE 9-4 *Epithelial basement membrane dystrophy, fingerprint lines.* These lines *(box)* are formed when extra basement membrane material forms folds that extend into the epithelial layer.

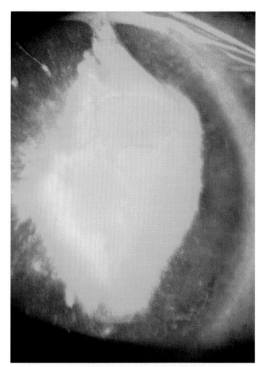

FIGURE 9-5 *Epithelial basement membrane dystrophy.* Patients occasionally develop recurrent corneal erosions.

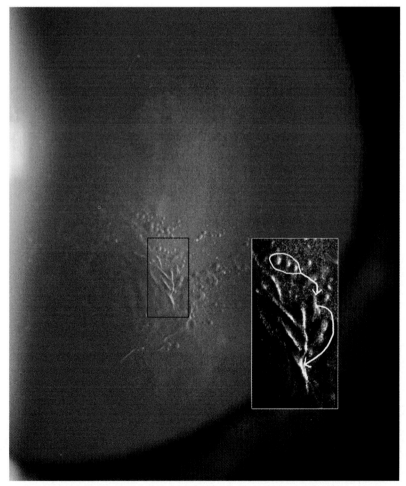

FIGURE 9-6 *Epithelial basement membrane dystrophy.* Blebs are fine, bubblelike structures that appear clear with retro-illumination. These blebs can coalesce to form groups with a linear branching pattern *(inset)*.

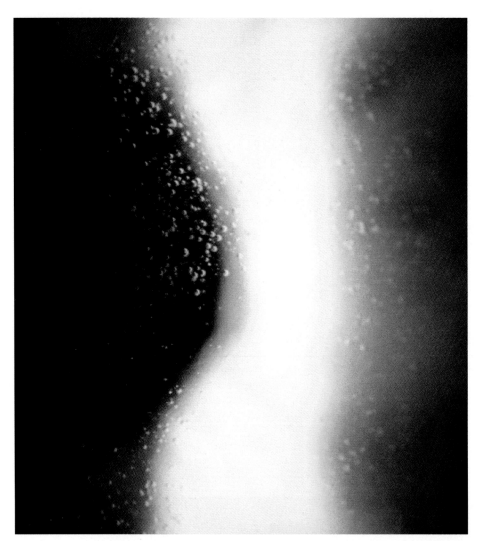

FIGURE 9-7 *Meesmann's dystrophy.* This autosomal dominant disorder is characterized by the appearance of multiple vesicular or bleblike structures within the corneal epithelium. They tend to be more numerous in the interpalpebral zone. The cysts occasionally rupture onto the ocular surface and can cause pain and decreased vision. The cysts appear as gray dots with direct illumination and as small vesicles with indirect illumination.

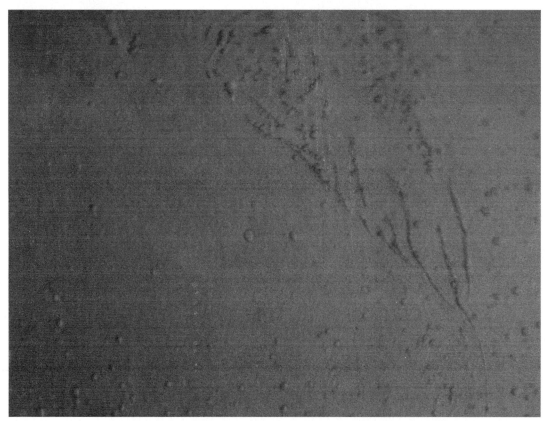

FIGURE 9-8 *Meesmann's dystrophy.* The epithelial cysts are often best appreciated with retinal retro-illumination. Here single cysts are seen, and centrally, there are linear areas where the cysts have coalesced.

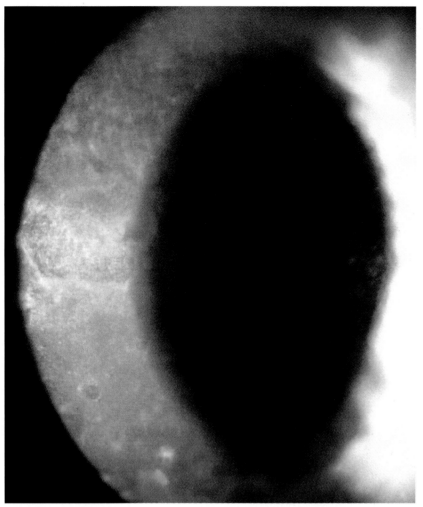

FIGURE 9-9 **Reis-Bücklers' dystrophy.** This autosomal dominant dystrophy is characterized by irregular gray-white opacities beneath the epithelium. It begins in childhood, and visual loss is progressive. Recurrent erosions occur periodically.

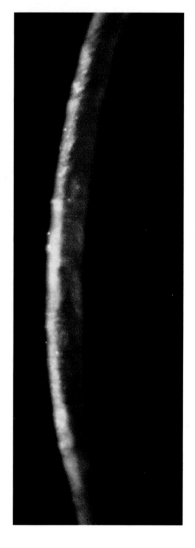

FIGURE 9-10 **Reis-Bücklers' dystrophy.** A thin slit beam view demonstrates the opacification beneath the epithelium and the irregularity of the corneal surface.

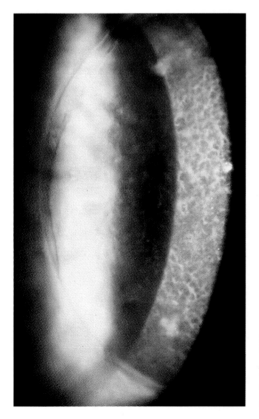

FIGURE 9-11 **Reis-Bücklers' dystrophy.** This disorder often recurs in a graft. Peripherally, there is a fine granular pattern, and centrally, the opacification is denser and the surface more irregular.

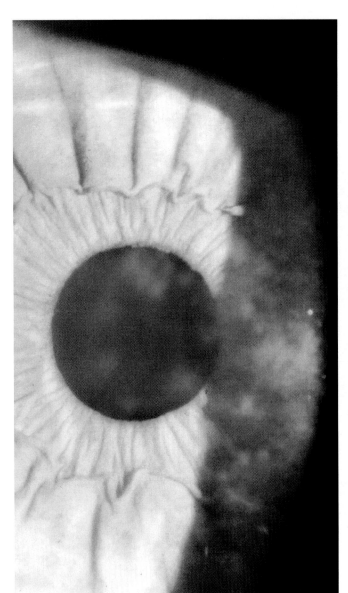

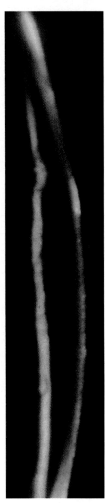

FIGURES 9-12 AND 9-13 *Subepithelial mucinous dystrophy.* This autosomal dominant disorder is characterized by subepithelial deposits of gray-white material between which there is a generalized subepithelial haze. The cornea is involved limbus to limbus. Patients experience multiple recurrent erosions, which begin in childhood. Visual loss can become significant later in life.

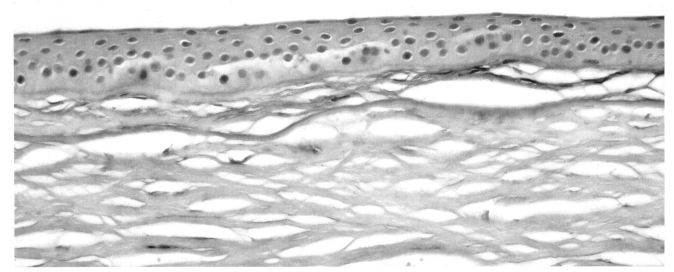

FIGURE 9-14 *Histology of subepithelial mucinous dystrophy.* The thick subepithelial layer stains with Alcian blue. The deposits are composed of chondroitin 4-sulfate and dermatan sulfate.

Stromal Dystrophies

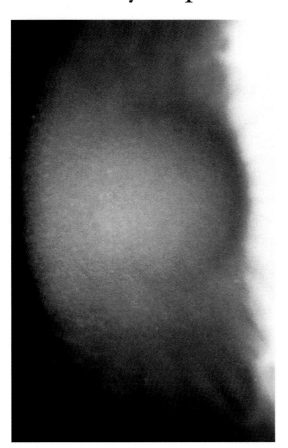

FIGURE 9-15 **_Early lattice dystrophy type I._** The corneal findings are subtle. Three findings have been described: central stromal haze (as seen here), subepithelial white spots, and filamentary lines. This is a 13-year-old girl with central stromal haze.

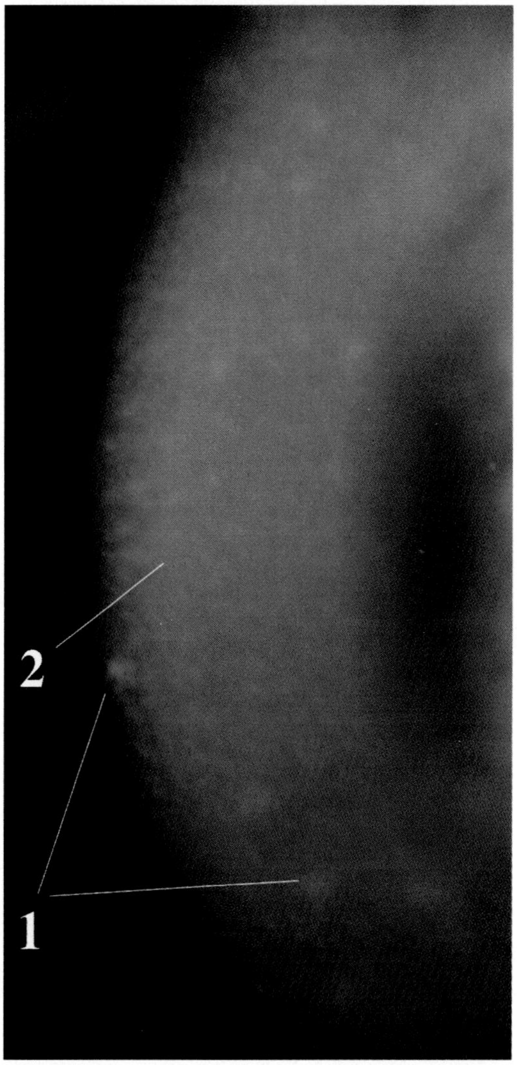

FIGURE 9-16 **_Early lattice dystrophy type I._** This 4-year-old boy has several subepithelial white spots *(1)* and central stromal haze *(2)*.

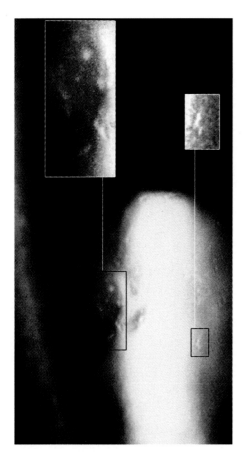

FIGURE 9-17 **_Early lattice dystrophy type I._** Refractile filamentary lines *(inset)* are seen in a 13-year-old girl.

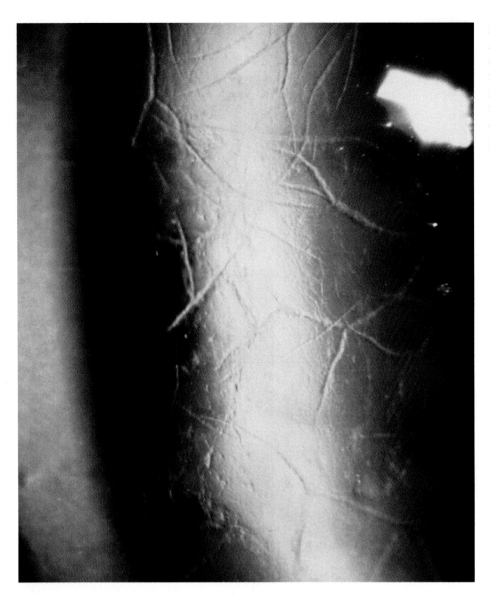

FIGURE 9-18 *Lattice dystrophy type I in an adult.* There are refractile filamentary lines with nodular dilations. The deposits are more common in the anterior stroma. Usually, there is a limbal clear zone. A fine central anterior stromal haze may be present.

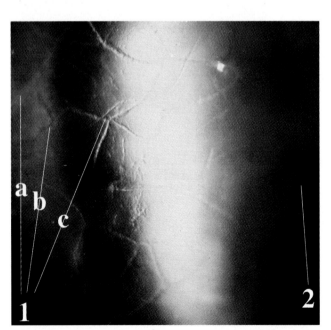

FIGURE 9-19 *Lattice dystrophy type I. 1,* Lattice lines are white (*a*) or dark (*b*) in direct light and translucent, almost crystalline in indirect light (*c*). *2,* Lattice lines do not reach the limbus except in advanced cases.

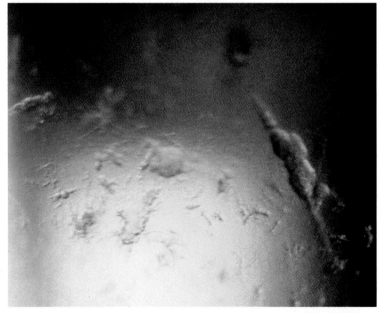

FIGURE 9-20 *Lattice dystrophy type I.* Yellow or amber refractile material can be seen in subepithelial areas in some cases. The histopathology of these areas shows elastoid degeneration.

FIGURE 9-21 *An epithelial erosion in lattice dystrophy type I.* Visual acuity may be markedly decreased in patients with epithelial involvement.

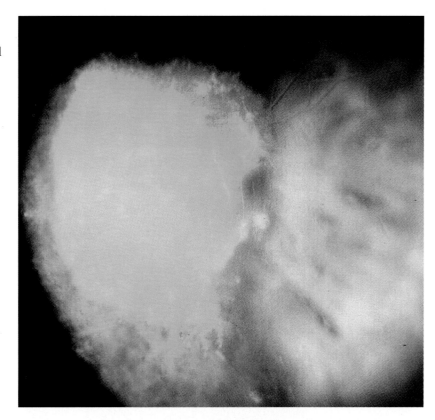

FIGURE 9-22 *Lattice dystrophy type I.* This commonly recurs in the graft, beginning in the periphery and spreading centrally. Typically there are elevated subepithelial opacities, fine lattice lines, and diffuse haze in the anterior stroma. Occasionally, adequate vision can be maintained by scraping the superficial subepithelial deposits.

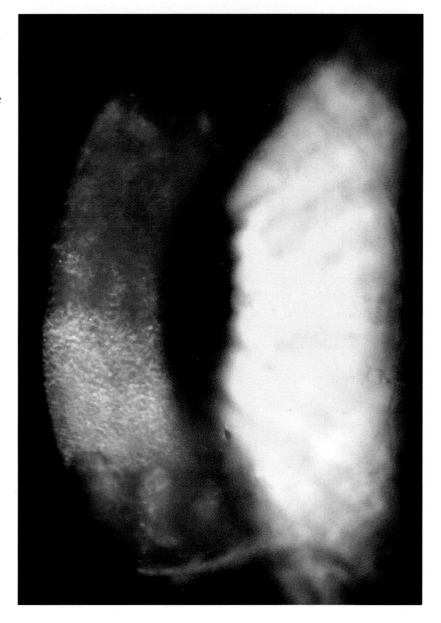

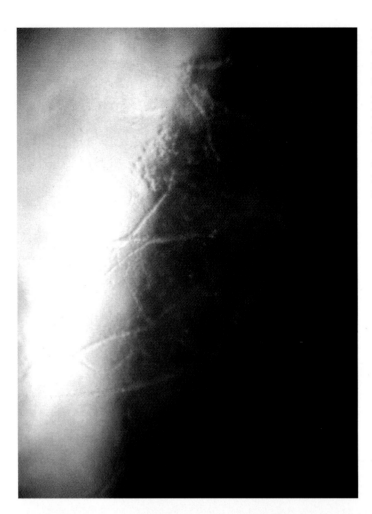

FIGURE 9-23 *Lattice dystrophy type II (Meretoja's syndrome).* There are refractile corneal deposits that differ in several respects from those seen in lattice dystrophy type I. The deposits are fewer, coarser, and most dense in the corneal midperiphery and generally extend to the limbus with a more radial orientation. The central cornea is usually spared, and the cornea is relatively clear between the lines. In contrast to lattice type I, there are systemic findings, including blepharochalasis, bilateral facial-nerve palsies, peripheral neuropathy, and systemic amyloidosis.

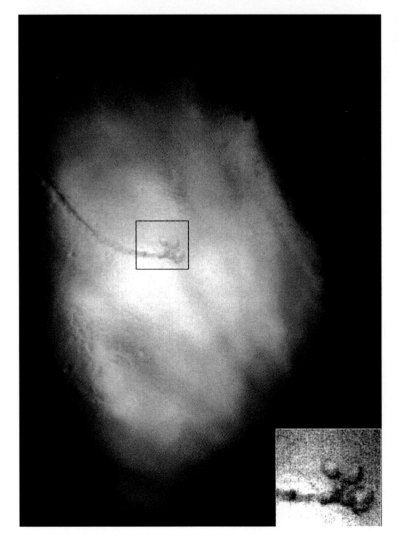

FIGURE 9-24 *Lattice dystrophy type II.* In this patient the lattice lines are coarse and there are prominent terminal bulbs *(inset).*

FIGURE 9-25 **Advanced lattice dystrophy type I.** Congo red stain reveals extracellular fusiform deposits of congophilic material *(1)* and elastoid degeneration *(2).*

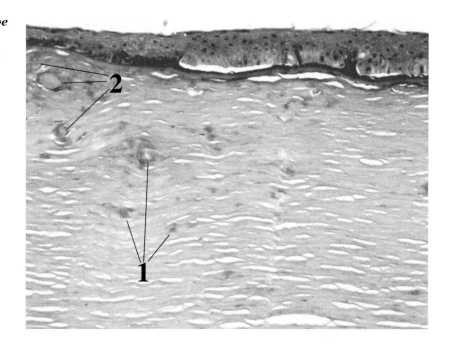

FIGURE 9-26 **Histopathology of lattice corneal dystrophy type I.** Congo red stain reveals large fusiform stromal lesion.

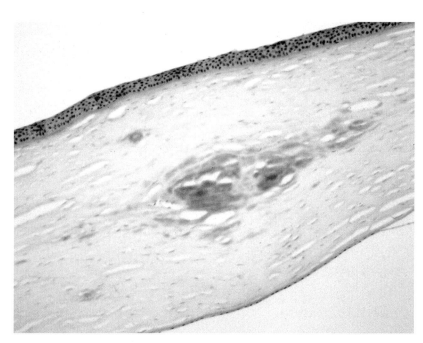

FIGURE 9-27 **Same patient as in Figure 9-26.** Birefringence of the Congo red stain is seen with polarized light.

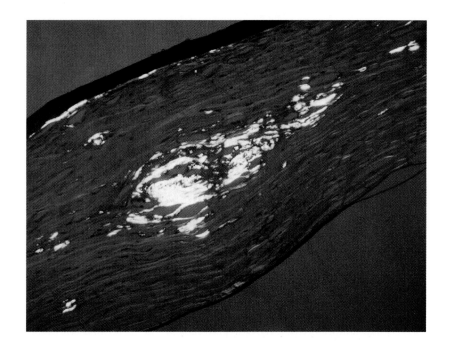

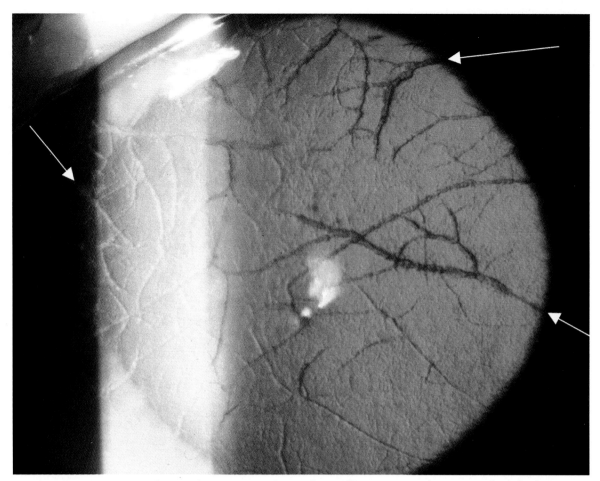

FIGURE 9-28 *Lattice dystrophy type IIIA.* Coarse lattice lines traverse the cornea from limbus to limbus *(arrows)*. This rare form of lattice dystrophy is inherited as an autosomal dominant disorder, has an adult onset, and includes frequent episodes of recurrent corneal erosions.

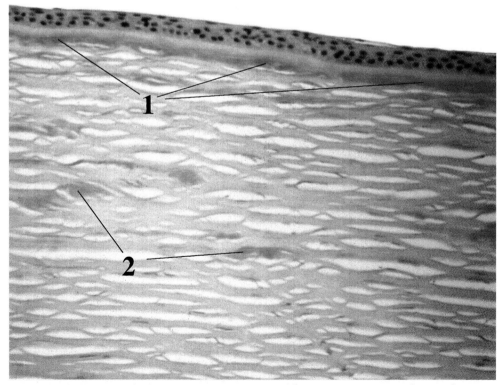

FIGURE 9-29 *Histopathology of lattice type IIIA.* There is a prominent layer of amyloid deposition just posterior to Bowman's layer *(1)* and irregular deposits in the stroma *(2)*. The amyloid deposits stain with Congo red.

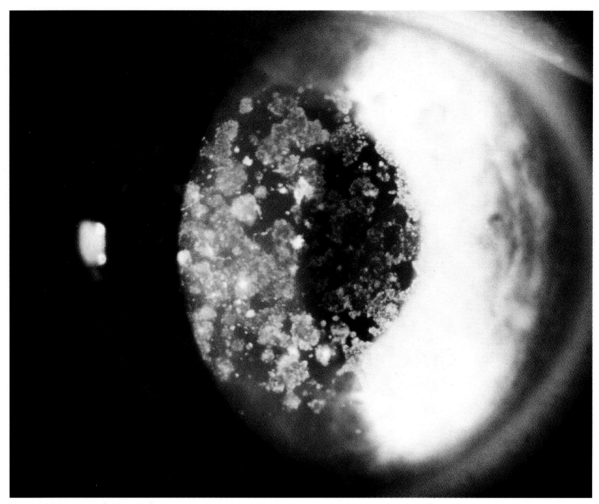

FIGURE 9-30 *Granular dystrophy.* In this autosomal dominant condition, there are numerous "bread crumb" white deposits in the corneal stroma. The deposits are concentrated centrally and in the anterior stroma. There is a peripheral clear zone of 2 to 3 mm that remains free of deposits. Visual impairment usually begins after the fifth decade of life.

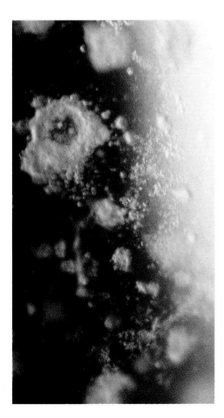

FIGURE 9-31 *Granular dystrophy.* In this high magnification view, some of the lesions are opaque with clear centers. There are small refractile deposits as well.

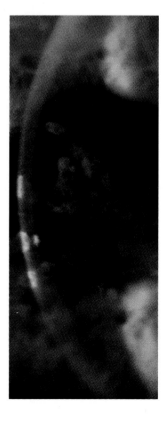

FIGURE 9-32 *A thin slit beam view of granular dystrophy.* The deposits are primarily in the anterior stroma, and the overlying epithelium is disrupted occasionally. Recurrent erosions can occur but are uncommon.

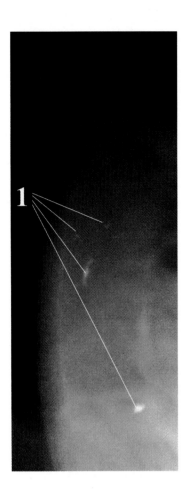

FIGURE 9-33 *Granular dystrophy in a 15-month-old child.* The earliest sign of granular dystrophy is fine dots in the superficial stroma *(1)*.

FIGURE 9-34 *Granular dystrophy in a 7½-year-old child.* As the disease progresses, there are focal white opacities with variable shapes in the anterior stroma.

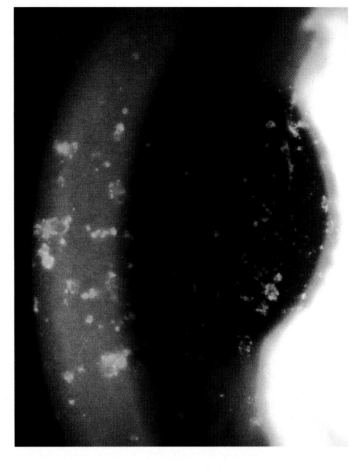

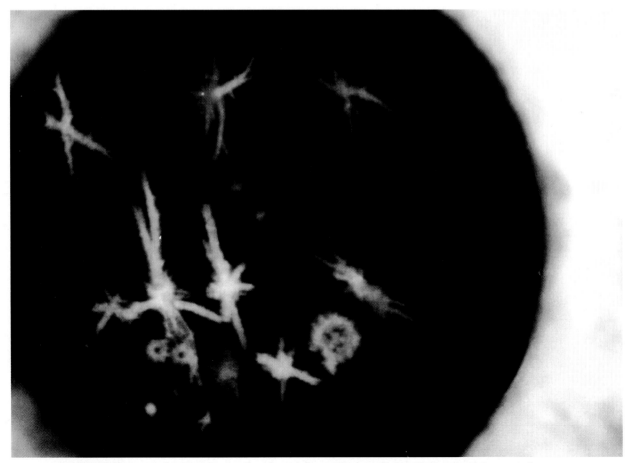

FIGURE 9-35 Unusual case of granular dystrophy with snowflake shapes in the corneal stroma.

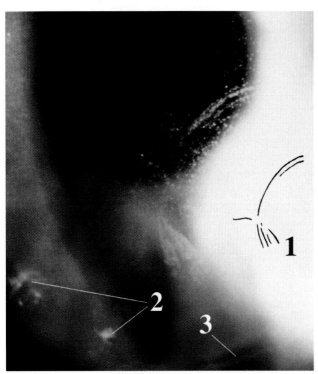

FIGURE 9-36 *Recurrence of granular dystrophy in a graft.* The most common pattern is a superficial cornea verticillata pattern *(1)*. Suture track scar *(2)* and corneal wound *(3)* are shown.

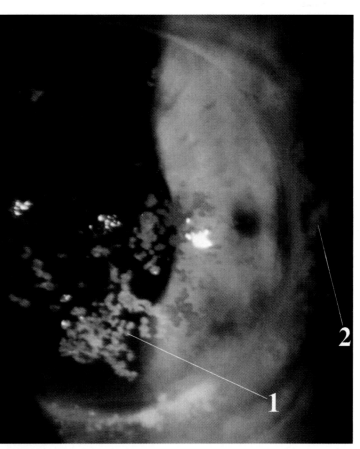

FIGURE 9-37 *Advanced recurrence of granular dystrophy in a graft.* Multiple white granular opacities are seen in the graft *(1)*. Granular deposits are also seen in the host tissue *(2)*.

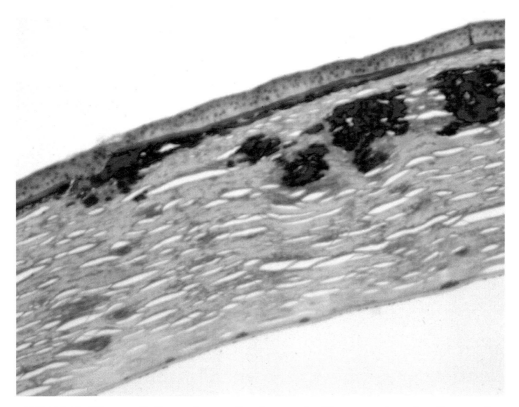

FIGURE 9-38 *Histopathology of granular dystrophy.* There are deposits of extracellular hyaline material in the corneal stroma. These deposits are primarily in the anterior stroma and have a bread crumb appearance. The hyaline material stains red with Masson's trichrome stain.

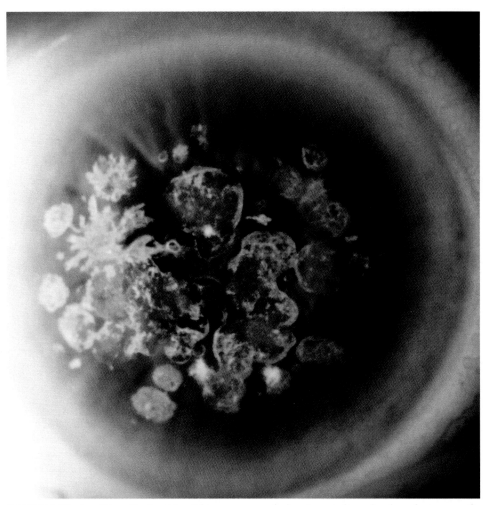

FIGURE 9-39 *Avellino dystrophy.* This autosomal dominant disorder has features of both granular and lattice dystrophy clinically and on histopathologic examination. The lattice lesions develop after the granular deposits. Recent evidence has shown that granular dystrophy, lattice dystrophy type I, and Avellino dystrophy map to a single locus on chromosome 5q.

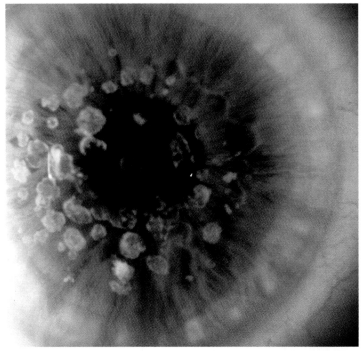

FIGURE 9-40 *Avellino dystrophy.* Another patient with Avellino dystrophy demonstrates the variable appearance characteristic of dominantly inherited disorders. These patients, like those with lattice and granular dystrophy, can have recurrent erosions.

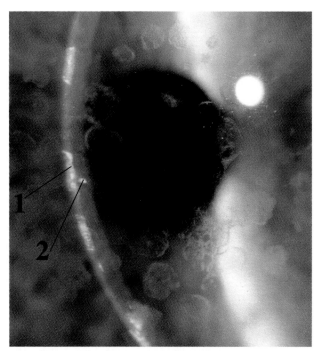

FIGURE 9-41 *Avellino dystrophy.* A typical granular deposit *(1)* appears as hyaline material on histopathologic examination. This deposit *(2)* corresponds to amyloid material on histopathologic examination.

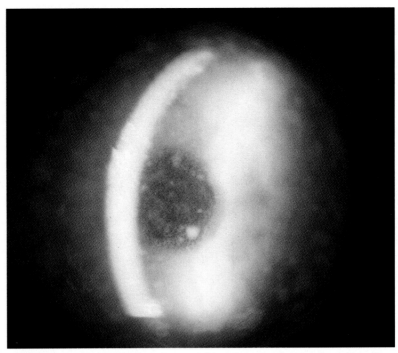

FIGURE 9-42 ***Macular dystrophy.*** This autosomal recessive disorder is characterized by a diffuse stromal haze extending limbus to limbus and throughout the corneal stroma. Multiple, irregular, gray-white nodular lesions are found within the diffuse haze. Recurrent erosions can occur, although less frequently than in lattice dystrophy. Photophobia may be out of proportion to clinical findings. Visual acuity usually is markedly decreased by the third and fourth decades of life.

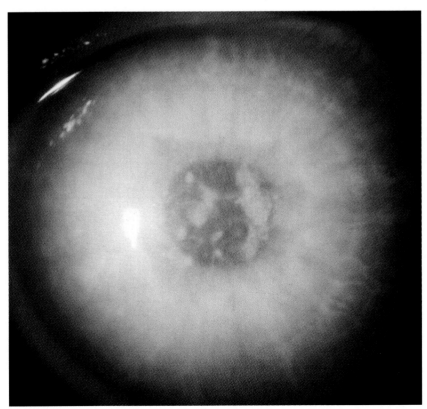

FIGURE 9-43 ***Macular dystrophy.*** The haze extends limbus to limbus.

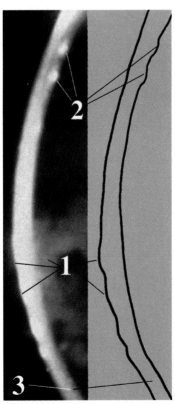

FIGURE 9-44 ***A thin slit beam view of macular dystrophy.*** The central lesions are more anterior *(1)*, and the peripheral white lesions are more posterior *(2)*. The cornea is thinner than normal *(3)*.

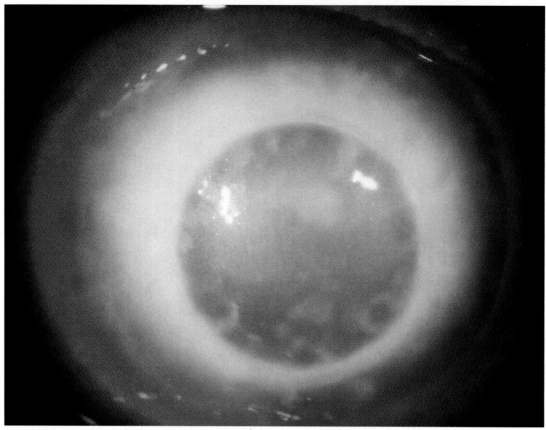

FIGURE 9-45 *Recurrence of macular dystrophy in a graft.* The graft has a generalized haze, and there are focal white nodular deposits.

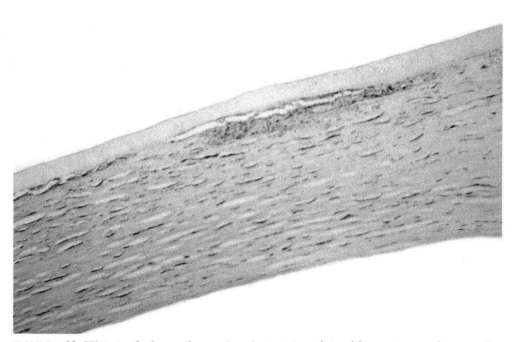

FIGURE 9-46 *Histopathology of macular dystrophy.* Alcian blue staining of extracellular and intracellular mucopolysaccharides occurs in all layers of the cornea, including the epithelium, endothelium, and Descemet's membrane.

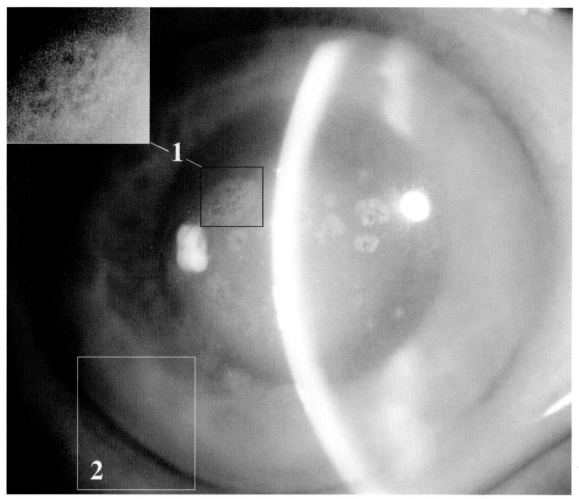

FIGURE 9-47 **Schnyder's crystalline dystrophy.** In this autosomal dominant disorder, there is central anterior stromal corneal opacity. The peripheral edge is irregular and crystalline *(1)*. The crystals are composed of cholesterol, and patients may have systemic hyperlipidemia. Arcus *(2)* is often present.

FIGURE 9-48 **The 16-year-old son of the patient in Figure 9-47.** Small white crystalline opacities are seen in the central anterior stroma.

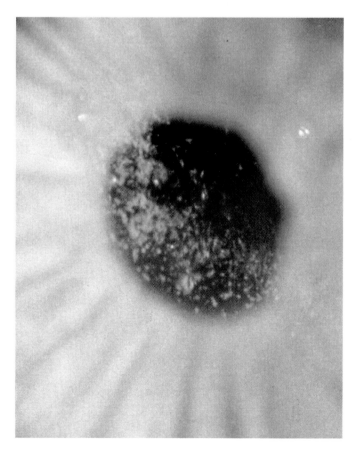

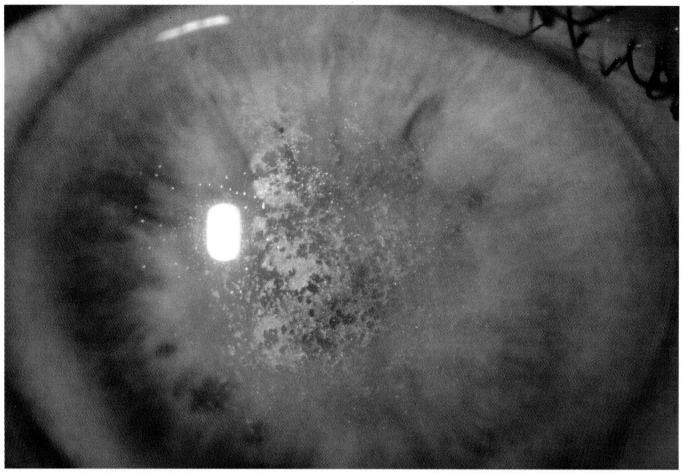

FIGURE 9-49 *Schnyder's crystalline dystrophy.* Multiple central crystalline deposits and peripheral arcus are seen.

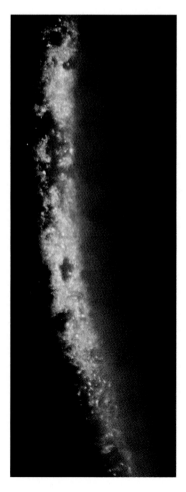

FIGURE 9-50 *A thin slit beam view of the same patient as in Figure 9-49.* There is a crystalline pattern in the anterior corneal stroma.

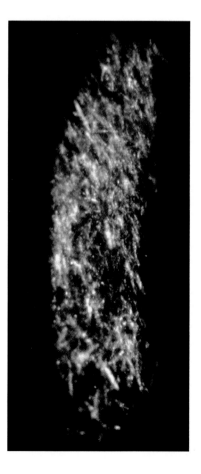

FIGURE 9-51 *Schnyder's crystalline dystrophy.* A thin slit beam view shows crystals with a spicular pattern in another patient.

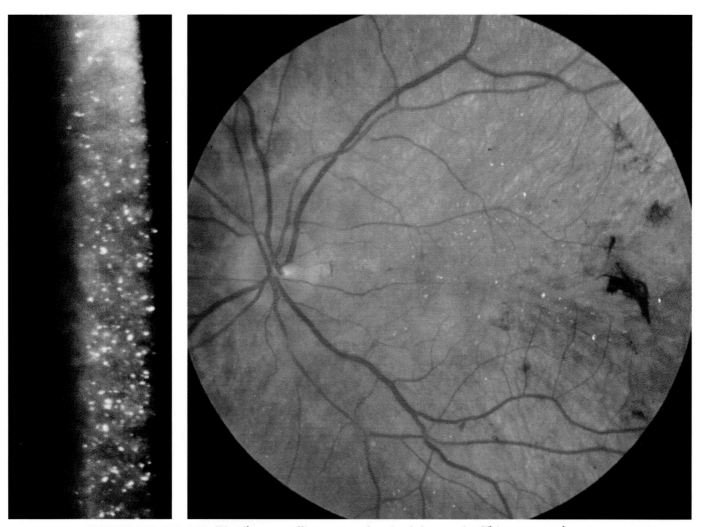

FIGURES 9-52 AND 9-53 ***Bietti's crystalline corneal-retinal dystrophy.*** This autosomal recessive disorder is characterized by crystalline deposits in the peripheral cornea (Figure 9-52,
left) and retina (Figure 9-53, ***right***). As the disease progresses, pigment changes occur within
the retina and the choriocapillaris atrophies. Patients may have symptoms of nyctalopia,
poor dark adaptation, peripheral visual field loss, and central visual acuity loss. The corneal
crystals resemble cholesterol or other lipid deposits histologically, and the disorder may represent a systemic defect in lipid metabolism.

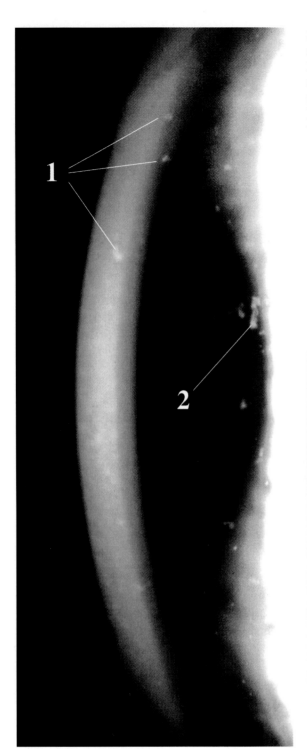

FIGURE 9-54 *Fleck dystrophy.* This autosomal dominant disorder is seen as an incidental finding. There are white, comma-shaped, stellate, circular, and wreathlike opacities at all levels of the corneal stroma. The opacities are white in direct light *(1)* and gray in indirect light *(2).* Histologically, the deposits are formed by distended keratocytes filled with complex lipids and glycosaminoglycans. Vision is not affected.

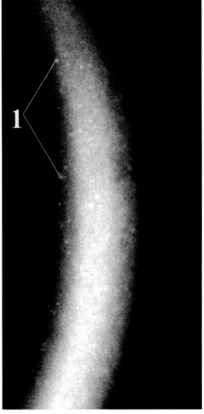

FIGURE 9-55 *Pre-Descemet's dystrophy.* There are fine white opacities in the deep stroma just anterior to Descemet's membrane *(1).*

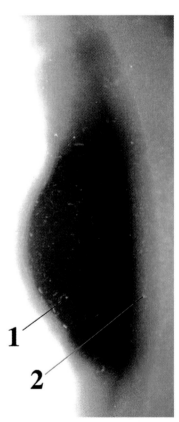

FIGURE 9-56 *Pre-Descemet's dystrophy.* This is the 30-year-old daughter of the patient in Figure 9-55. Deep white stromal opacities are seen in indirect light *(1)* and direct light *(2).*

The deep white stromal opacities in pre-Descemet's dystrophy resemble those seen in X-linked ichthyosis (see Figure 8-66). They may also resemble the deposits in cornea farinata (see Figure 9-125), although in cornea farinata the deposits are much finer.

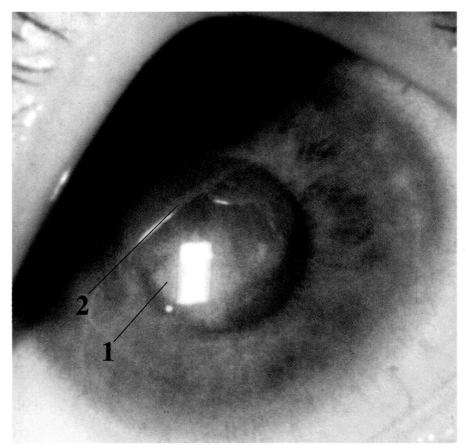

FIGURE 9-57 *Posterior amorphous stromal dystrophy in a 6-month-old infant.* There is central corneal opacification *(1)*. Reflection of the upper eyelid is seen as a white artifact *(2)*.

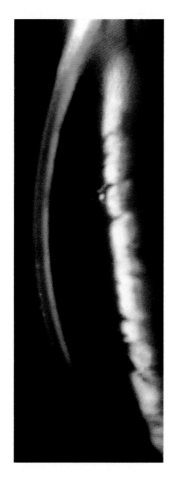

FIGURE 9-58 *Posterior amorphous stromal dystrophy.* This thin slit beam view demonstrates deep stromal opacification. The corneas in this disorder are thin, and the corneal topography is flat, leading to hyperopia. Iris anomalies may be present. The inheritance pattern is autosomal dominant. The presence of anomalies in infants and occasional iris abnormalities suggest that this may be a congenital disorder of anterior segment differentiation. Vision is not usually greatly affected but rarely can be reduced enough to require corneal transplantation.

Posterior Membrane Dystrophies

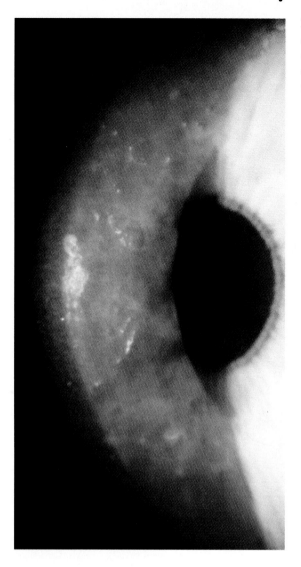

FIGURE 9-59 ***Posterior polymorphous dystrophy.*** This autosomal dominant disorder of the corneal endothelium is almost always bilateral, although it can be extremely asymmetric or unilateral. This is an example of posterior corneal vesicles, the most common finding in this disorder.

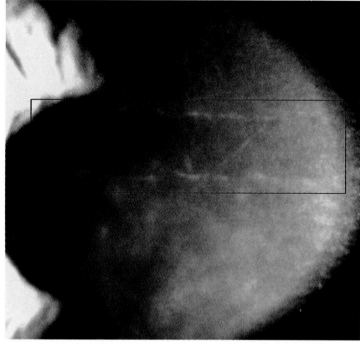

FIGURE 9-60 ***Posterior polymorphous dystrophy.*** Broad bandlike opacities can occur at the level of Descemet's membrane and the endothelium *(box)*.

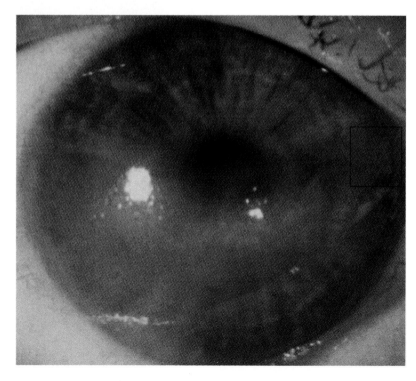

FIGURE 9-61 ***Diffuse corneal edema in a 12-year-old girl with posterior polymorphous dystrophy.*** Most patients do not develop corneal edema; however, if the edema develops, it can occur early or late in the course of the disease or even at birth. This patient also has calcific band keratopathy *(box)*.

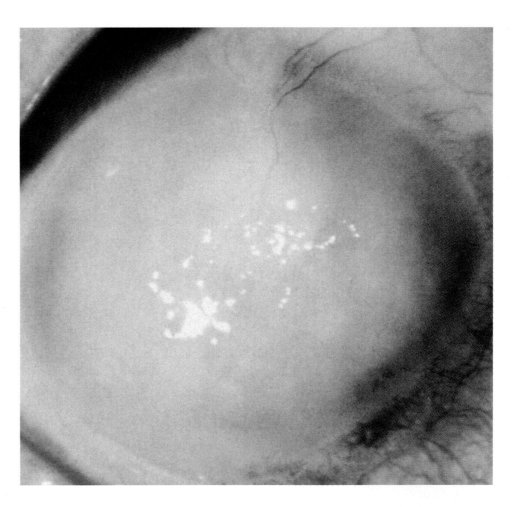

FIGURE 9-62 *Posterior polymorphous dystrophy.* This is the 74-year-old grandfather of the patient in Figure 9-61. There is extensive corneal edema, as well as calcific and lipid degeneration.

FIGURE 9-63 *Specular photomicrograph of posterior polymorphous dystrophy.* Vesicles with abnormal endothelium *(1)* are surrounded by relatively normal endothelium *(2)*.

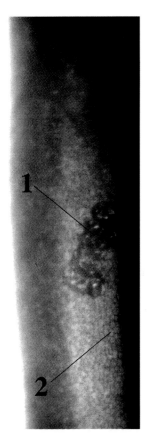

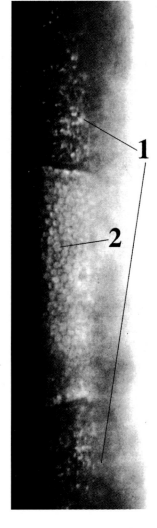

FIGURE 9-64 *Specular photomicrograph of posterior polymorphous dystrophy.* Markedly abnormal endothelium *(1)* with intervening relatively normal endothelium *(2)* is seen. There is a sharp demarcation between the normal and abnormal regions.

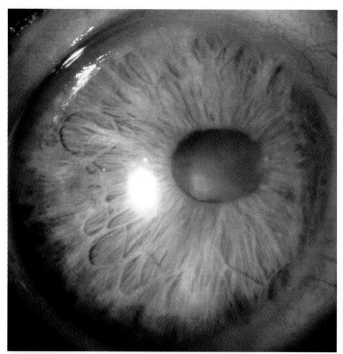

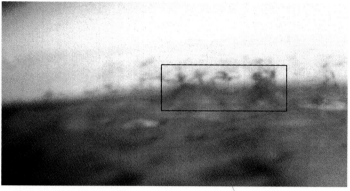

FIGURE 9-65 **Posterior polymorphous dystrophy.** The abnormal endothelium can grow across the trabecular meshwork and onto the iris. Iris traction can result in peripheral anterior synechiae and corectopia. Iris atrophy is usually not present.

FIGURE 9-66 **Posterior polymorphous dystrophy.** Peripheral anterior synechiae *(box)* is only seen with gonioscopy. The prognosis for penetrating keratoplasty in these cases is relatively good.

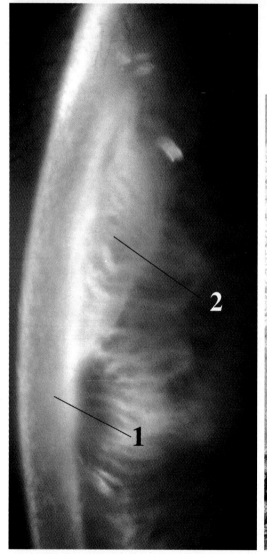

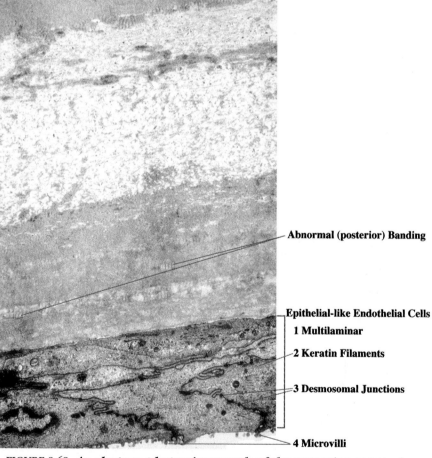

Abnormal (posterior) Banding

Epithelial-like Endothelial Cells
1 Multilaminar
2 Keratin Filaments
3 Desmosomal Junctions
4 Microvilli

FIGURE 9-67 **Posterior polymorphous dystrophy.** Corneal edema is noted *(1)*. Visible peripheral anterior synechiae are associated with a sheet of epithelial-like endothelial cells *(2)*. The prognosis for keratoplasty in these cases with easily visualized peripheral anterior synechiae is worse because of postoperative glaucoma.

FIGURE 9-68 **An electron photomicrograph of the posterior cornea in posterior polymorphous dystrophy.** Abnormal banding occurs in the posterior aspect of Descemet's membrane, and endothelial cells with epithelial-like characteristics, including a multilaminar architecture *(1)*, keratin filaments *(2)*, desmosomal junctions *(3)*, and microvilli *(4)*, are seen.

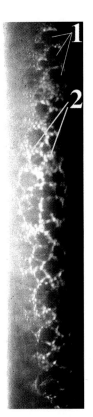

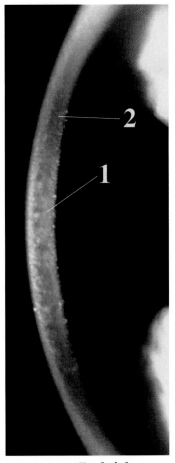

FIGURE 9-69 ***Endothelial dystrophy.*** Dark holes *(1)* in the endothelial mosaic *(2)* represent guttata.

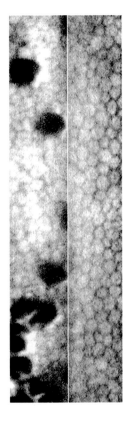

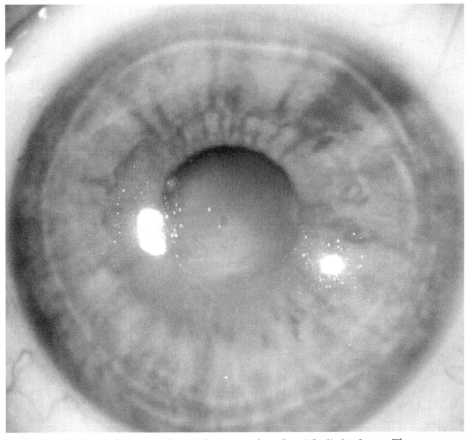

FIGURE 9-71 ***Endothelial dystrophy.*** Corneal guttata are seen with red reflex.

FIGURE 9-70 Pseudoguttata (endothelial cell edema) is seen in a patient with iritis *(left).* Normal endothelial mosaic is found in the same patient when the iritis has resolved *(right).*

FIGURE 9-72 ***Fuchs' dystrophy.*** A thicker central cornea (normally thinner) *(1)* and thinner peripheral cornea without edema *(2)* are seen.

FIGURE 9-73 ***Fuchs' dystrophy with stromal and epithelial edema.*** The term ***endothelial dystrophy*** is reserved for patients with corneal guttata and no evidence of corneal edema (see Figure 9-71).

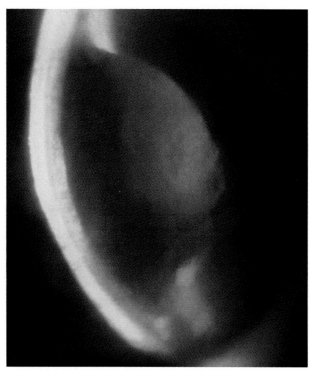

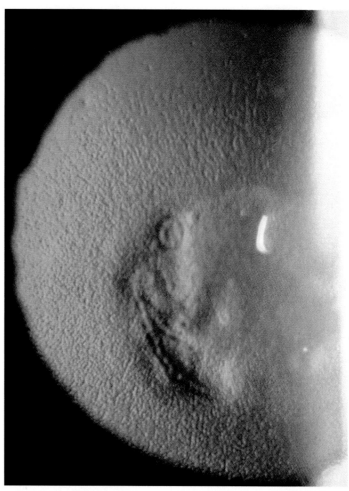

FIGURE 9-74 *Fuchs' dystrophy.* Patients with chronic corneal edema may develop subepithelial fibrosis, as seen here. At this stage, corneal sensation is often decreased.

FIGURE 9-75 *Red reflex of Fuchs' dystrophy.* Peripherally, there are numerous guttata, and centrally, there is localized corneal edema with bullae.

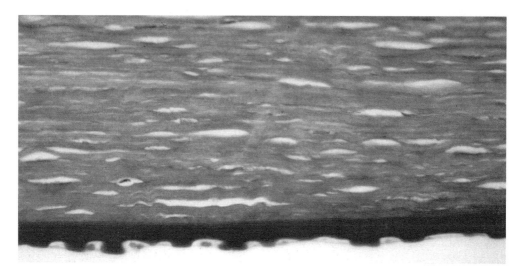

FIGURE 9-76 *Histopathology of the posterior cornea in Fuchs' dystrophy.* Seen is the thickened Descemet's membrane with nodular excrescences (cornea guttata). Endothelial cells are sparse.

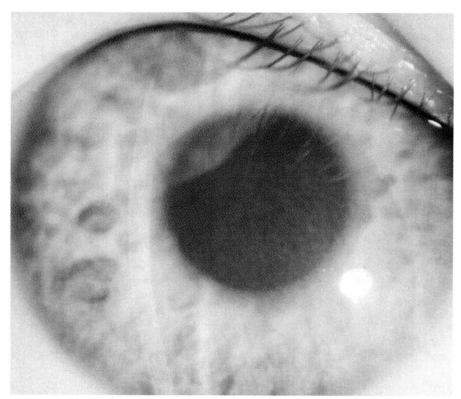

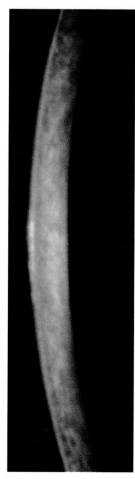

FIGURE 9-77 *Congenital hereditary endothelial dystrophy.* In this condition, diffuse stromal edema is present at birth or develops in the first decade of life, and there is no evidence of cornea guttata.

FIGURE 9-78 *Congenital hereditary endothelial dystrophy.* A thin slit beam view of the patient in Figure 9-77 shows diffuse stromal edema. The central cornea is thicker than the peripheral cornea.

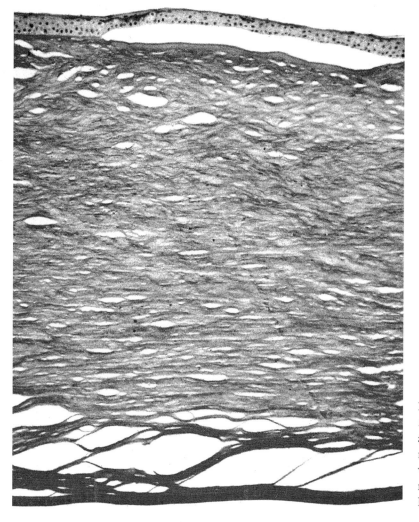

FIGURE 9-79 *Histopathology of congenital hereditary endothelial dystrophy.* There is an absence of endothelial cells, and Descemet's membrane is thickened. There is corneal edema, with loss of the artifactual stromal clefting and random orientation of collagen lamellae. Epithelial bullae are present.

Noninflammatory Ectatic Disorders

Keratoconus is a noninflammatory progressive thinning of the cornea. The cornea assumes a cone shape. Keratoconus is usually bilateral but often asymmetric. Most cases are sporadic, but in approximately 10% of patients, there is a positive family history.

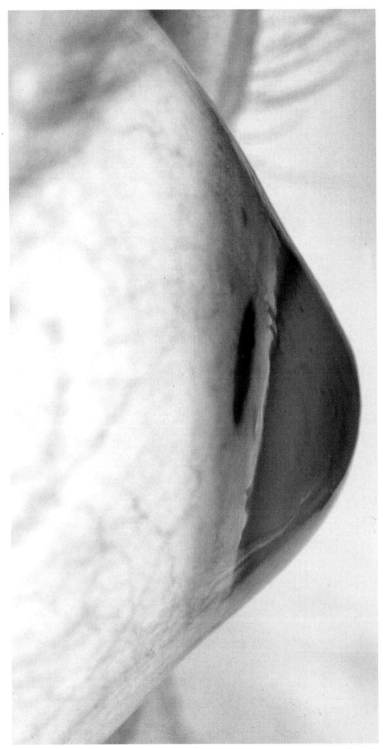

FIGURE 9-80 **Keratoconus.** The thinning is most pronounced at the apex of the cone, which is usually inferior to the visual axis. As the thinning progresses, patients develop increasing degrees of irregular myopic astigmatism. In this case, the angle structures can be directly visualized because of the extreme protrusion of the cornea.

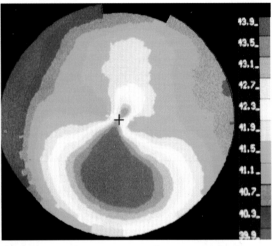

FIGURE 9-81 **Computerized topography in early keratoconus.** The corneal curvature is 43.90 diopters inferior to fixation.

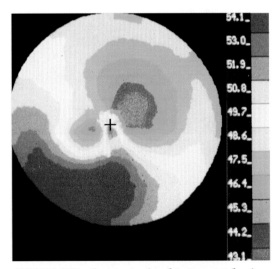

FIGURE 9-82 **Computerized topography in advanced keratoconus.** The corneal curvature is 54.10 diopters inferior to fixation.

FIGURE 9-83 **Keratoconus.** In this case the observer is shining a penlight from the right, resulting in a triangle of light on the left portion of the iris. The triangle is formed from focused light from the cone. This is known as **Rizutti's sign.**

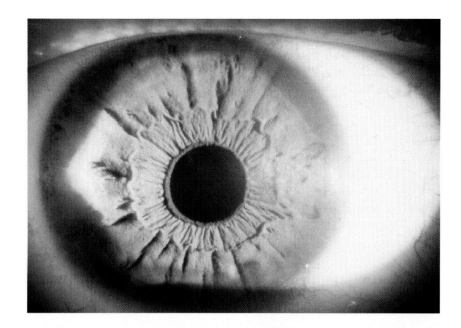

FIGURE 9-84 **Keratoconus.** Munson's sign is a late finding. When the patient looks down, the lower lid protrudes conically.

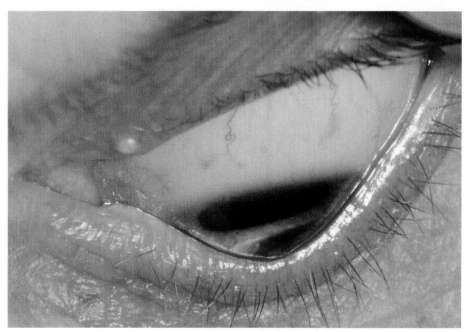

FIGURE 9-85 **Keratoconus.** The central red reflex is irregular because of the steepness of the cone and irregular astigmatism. Dynamic retinoscopy results in a scissoring reflex.

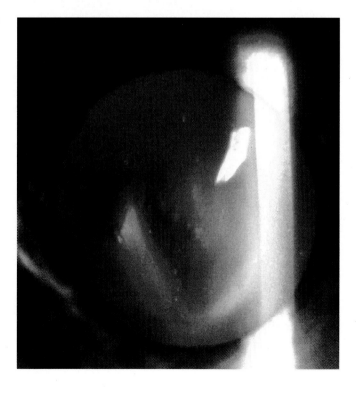

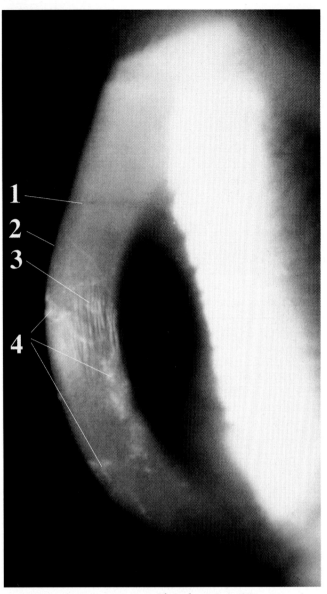

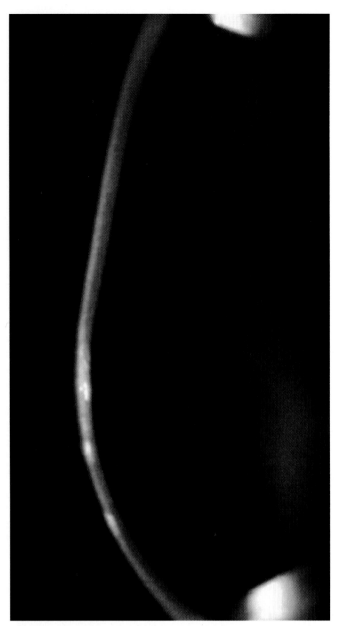

FIGURE 9-86 *Keratoconus.* Fleischer ring *(1)*, protrusion of the cone *(2)*, Vogt's striae *(3)*, and anterior stromal scarring *(4)* are shown.

FIGURE 9-87 *A thin slit beam view of keratoconus.* The cornea is thinnest at the region of maximal protrusion.

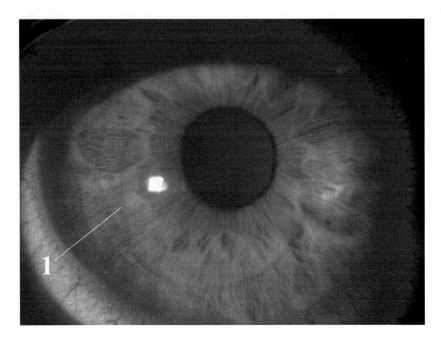

FIGURE 9-88 *Keratoconus.* A Fleischer ring *(1)* is composed of iron in the corneal epithelium. The ring configuration is produced by an irregular distribution of tears at the base of the cone and resultant iron deposition. It is easier to see the iron line with the cobalt blue light.

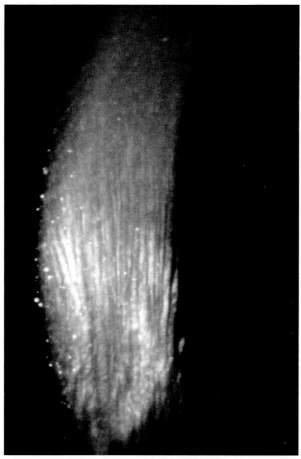

FIGURE 9-89 *Keratoconus.* Vogt's striae are stress lines in the posterior cornea stroma and occur near the apex of the cone.

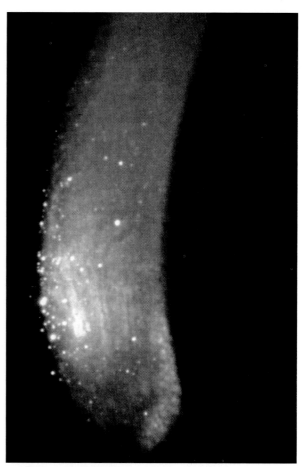

FIGURE 9-90 *Keratoconus.* When digital pressure is applied to the globe, Vogt's striae disappear.

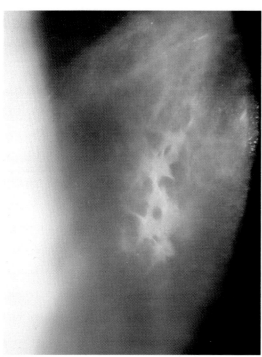

FIGURE 9-91 *Keratoconus.* Breaks in Bowman's membrane result in anterior stromal scarring.

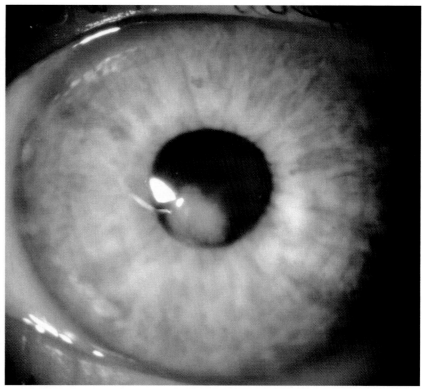

FIGURE 9-92 *Keratoconus.* Occasionally, an elevated subepithelial nodule occurs from chronic rubbing of a contact lens on the apex of the cone. These nodules can usually be scraped from the surface of the cornea.

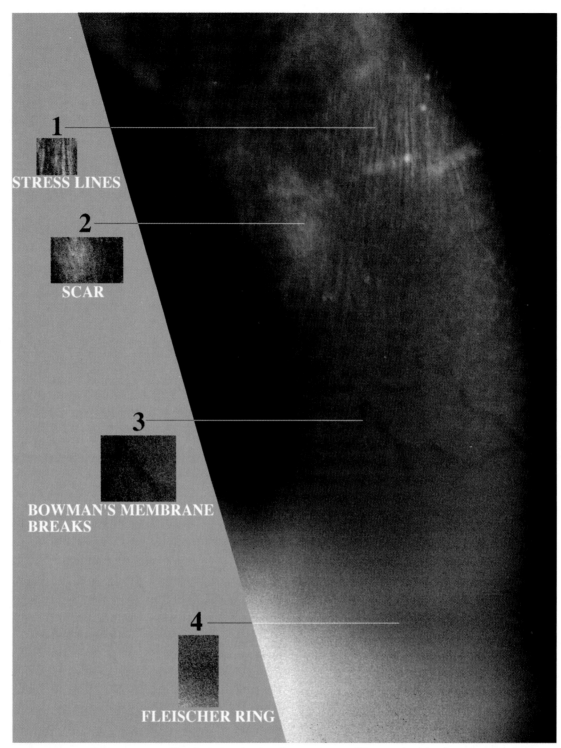

FIGURE 9-93 *Keratoconus.* Vogt's striae in the deep stroma *(1)*, scarring in the anterior stroma from old breaks in Bowman's membrane *(2)*, fresh breaks in Bowman's membrane with clear areas between breaks *(3)*, and iron deposition in the epithelium (Fleischer ring) *(4)* are shown.

FIGURE 9-94 *Keratoconus.* Corneal hydrops occurs when there is an acute break in Descemet's membrane. The cornea is edematous, and patients complain of pain and sudden decreased vision.

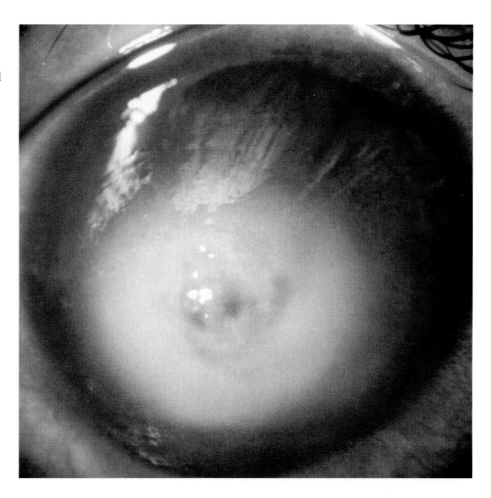

FIGURE 9-95 *Keratoconus.* This is a thin slit beam view of hydrops. The cornea is markedly edematous. With time, the edema resolves and stromal scarring occurs. Rarely, the visual acuity can improve if the scar flattens the cone.

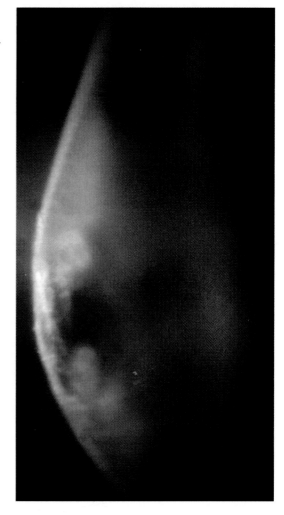

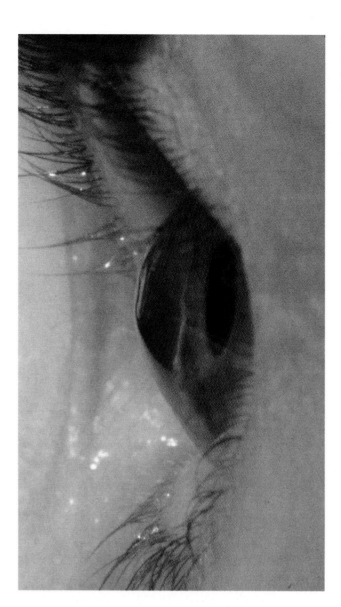

FIGURE 9-96 ***Keratoconus in a patient with Leber's congenital amaurosis.*** The cone is more central and superior in this case. Patients with Leber's congenital amaurosis frequently rub their eyes (the oculodigital sign), and this may predispose the development of keratoconus.

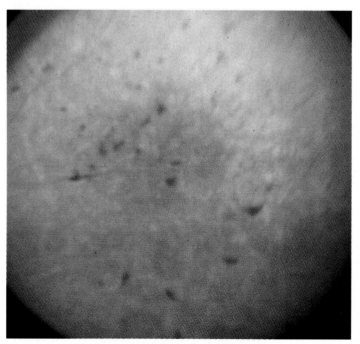

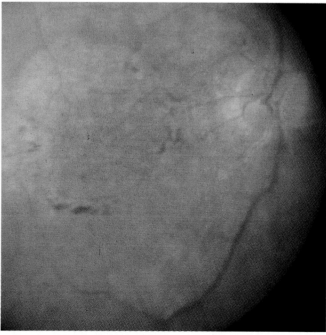

FIGURES 9-97 AND 9-98 ***Keratoconus in a patient with Leber's congenital amaurosis.*** The peripheral retina (Figure 9-97, *left*) and central retina (Figure 9-98, *right*) in the same patient as in Figure 9-96 are shown. There is a diffuse pigmentary retinopathy. Both pictures are slightly out of focus because of the difficulty in focusing the image through an irregularly shaped cornea.

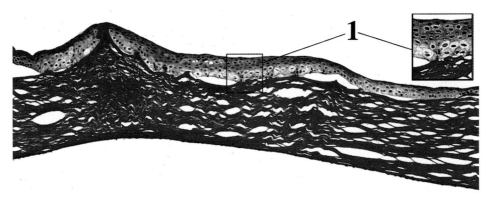

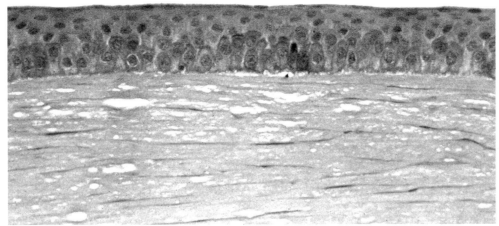

FIGURE 9-99 *Keratoconus.* There is an irregular thickness of the epithelium and a rupture of Bowman's membrane with epithelial stromal apposition *(1)*. The stroma is thinner in the central portion (cone) of the specimen. The endothelium is normal.

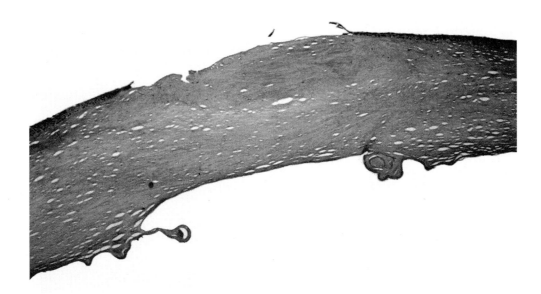

FIGURE 9-100 *Keratoconus.* Prussian blue stains iron deposits in the epithelium, especially the basal cells. The loss of Bowman's membrane is demonstrated.

FIGURE 9-101 *Keratoconus.* Corneal hydrops and the break in Descemet's membrane with scrolled edges are shown. There is scarring in the central stroma, and a large epithelial defect is present.

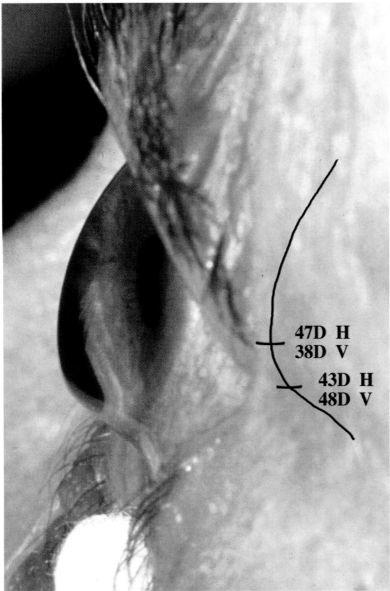

FIGURE 9-102 ***Pellucid marginal degeneration.*** This is an inferior thinning of the cornea that usually extends from 4 to 8 o'clock. The thinning is 1 to 2 mm wide and located 1 to 2 mm from the inferior limbus. It is not associated with vascularization. It typically begins between the ages of 20 and 40, and the progression may be slow. Unlike keratoconus, there is no Fleischer ring or Vogt's striae. Centrally, there is against-the-rule astigmatism (in this example, 47 diopters horizontally, 38 diopters vertically), and inferiorly, there is with-the-rule astigmatism (in this example, 43 diopters horizontally, 48 diopters vertically).

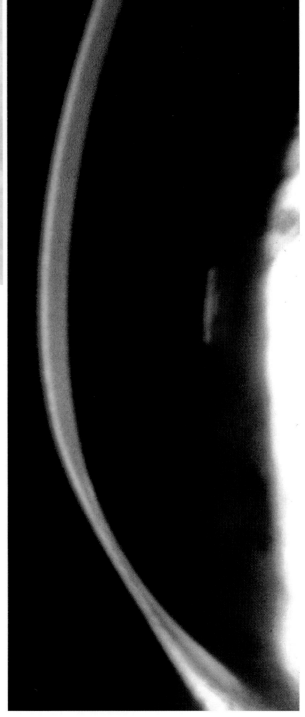

FIGURE 9-103 ***A thin slit beam view of pellucid marginal degeneration.*** There is marked thinning of the cornea inferiorly, well below the area of maximal corneal protrusion. In contrast, the thinning in keratoconus is in the area of maximal corneal protrusion (see Figure 9-87).

FIGURE 9-104 *Corneal scarring in a patient with pellucid marginal degeneration after an episode of acute hydrops.* There is peripheral vascularization of the cornea in reaction to the hydrops *(box).*

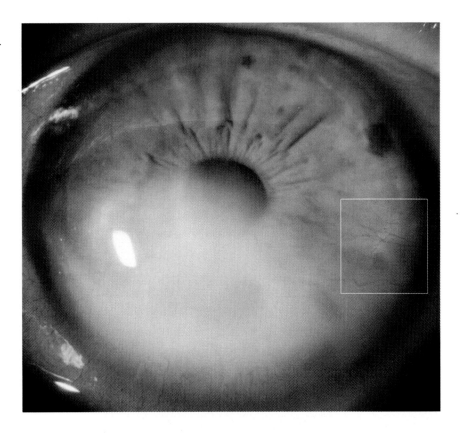

FIGURE 9-105 *Photokeratoscopy of pellucid marginal degeneration.* Typically, the central mire has an egg shape. Centrally, the horizontal rings are closer together than the vertical rings, which indicates corneal steepening in the horizontal axis (against-the-rule astigmatism). Inferiorly *(inset),* the vertical rings become close together, indicating a shift in steepening to the vertical axis (with-the-rule astigmatism).

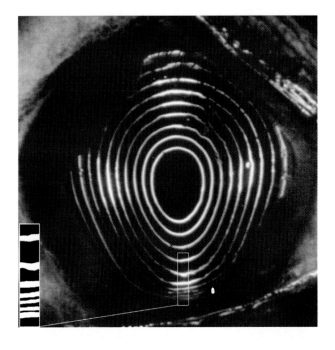

FIGURE 9-106 *Computerized topography of pellucid marginal degeneration.* Centrally, there is corneal steepening in the horizontal meridian (against-the-rule astigmatism). The shift to with-the-rule astigmatism inferiorly cannot be seen in this photograph, since the corneal imaging system does not image the far peripheral cornea.

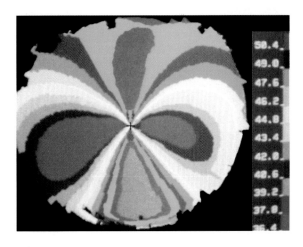

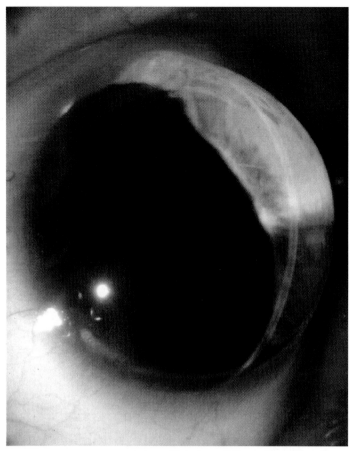

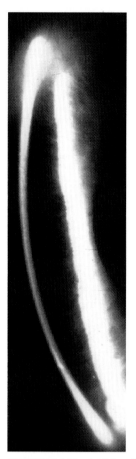

FIGURE 9-107 **Keratoglobus.** This is a diffuse thinning of the cornea to ⅓ to ⅕ normal thickness. In this case the thinning is more pronounced in the periphery, as seen in the inferior portion of the slit beam. It is noted in early life, and progression is minimal.

FIGURE 9-108 **A thin slit beam view of keratoglobus.** The cornea is diffusely thin.

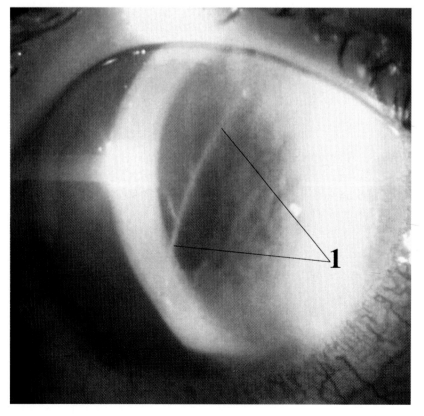

FIGURE 9-109 **Acute hydrops in keratoglobus.** In this case, Descemet's membrane is detached *(1)*. Keratoglobus has been associated with Leber's congenital amaurosis and Ehlers-Danlos syndrome type VI. Some families with both keratoglobus and keratoconus have been reported.

Secondary Ectasias

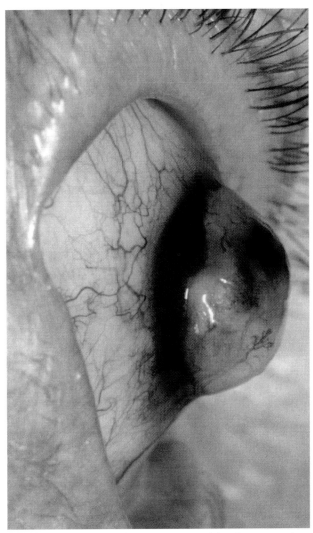

FIGURE 9-110 Corneal ectasia caused by long-standing glaucoma and chronic corneal inflammation with thinning.

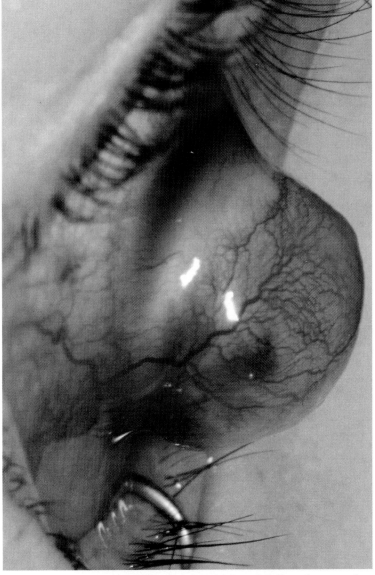

FIGURE 9-111 *Corneal ectasia caused by a childhood corneal infection of unknown etiology.* In both Figures 9-110 and 9-111, the corneas are scarred and vascularized, distinguishing them from keratoconus, pellucid marginal degeneration, and keratoglobus.

Iridocorneal Endothelial Syndrome

The iridocorneal endothelial syndrome (ICE syndrome) is not inherited and almost always unilateral, occurs more often in females, and has its onset between the ages of 30 and 50. ICE is an acronym for iris-nevus syndrome (Cogan-Reese), Chandler's syndrome, and essential iris atrophy.

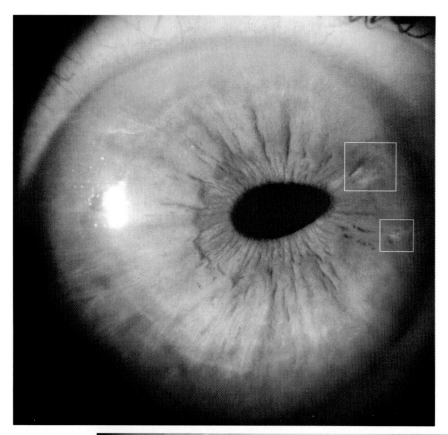

FIGURE 9-112 *Chandler's syndrome.* Areas of iris atrophy are highlighted in the two boxes. The pupil is drawn toward the areas of iris atrophy. The histopathology of this disorder shows abnormal endothelial cells that migrate across the trabecular meshwork and onto the iris. This abnormal endothelial cell proliferation can cause corneal edema, peripheral anterior synechiae with glaucoma, and traction and atrophy of the iris.

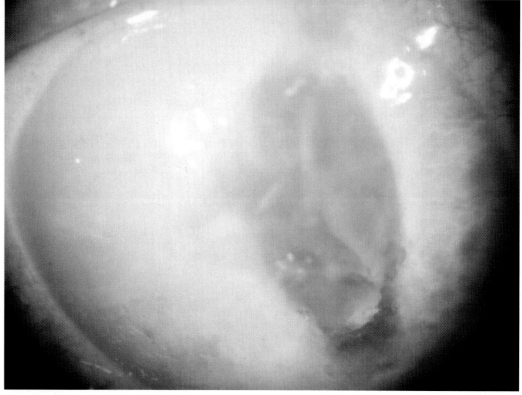

FIGURE 9-113 *Chandler's syndrome.* This advanced case has extensive corneal edema. The pupil is irregular, and there is ectropion uvea.

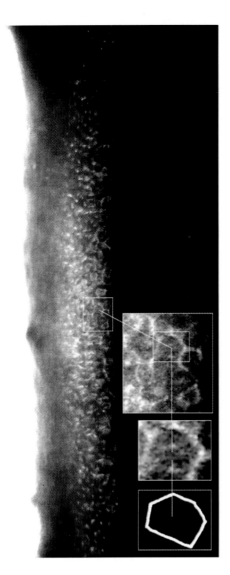

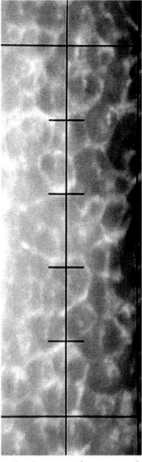

FIGURE 9-114 ***Specular photomicroscopy, low magnification, of Chandler's syndrome.*** The endothelial cells are markedly abnormal. Insets show progressively more magnified views and a schematic of endothelial cells. The dark areas between cells are not cornea guttata but represent undulations in the endothelial surface, with some areas in focus and some out of focus.

FIGURE 9-115 Specular photomicroscopy, high magnification, of Chandler's syndrome.

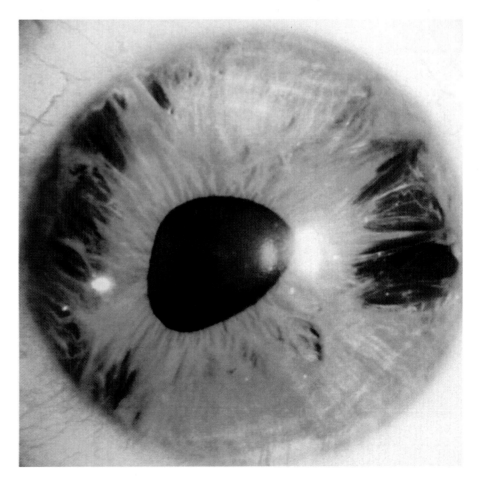

FIGURE 9-116 ***Essential iris atrophy.*** The peripheral iris is atrophic, and there are areas of absent tissue. The pupil is drawn toward the areas of maximal iris atrophy.

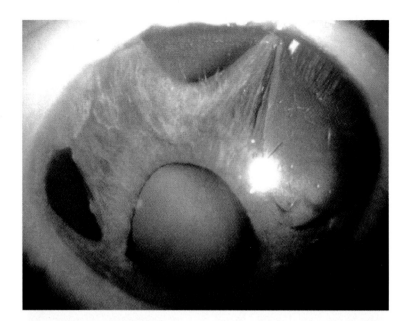

FIGURE 9-117 *Essential iris atrophy, advanced case.* Large portions of the iris are atrophic or absent. Ectropion uvea is present inferiorly.

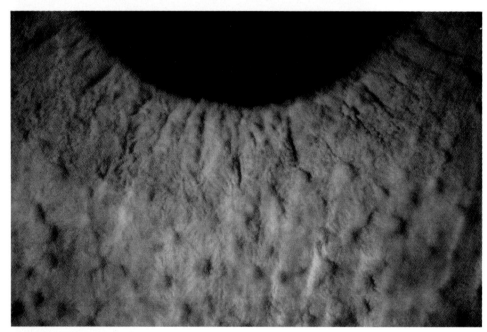

FIGURE 9-118 *Iris-nevus (Cogan-Reese) syndrome.* There are multiple fine brown nodules on the iris surface.

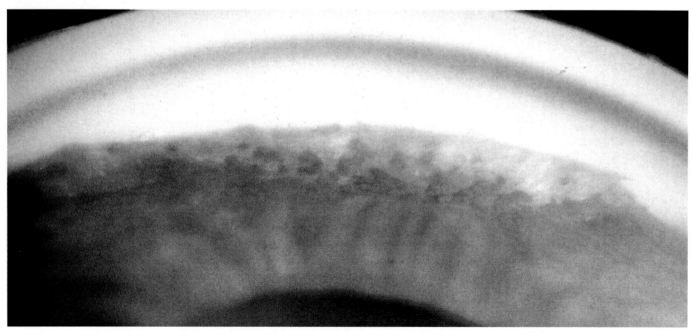

FIGURE 9-119 *Gonioscopy view of iris-nevus (Cogan-Reese) syndrome.* Multiple brown iris nodules are seen on the peripheral iris. There is a broad band of peripheral anterior synechiae.

Conjunctival and Corneal Degenerations

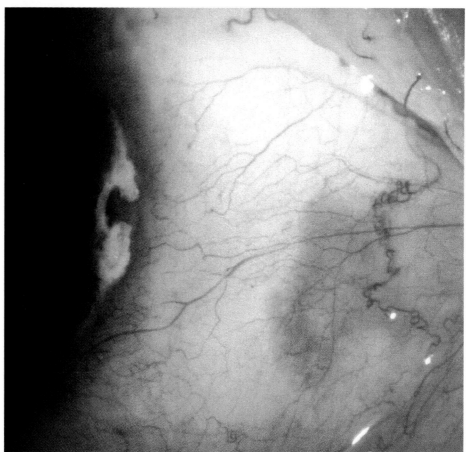

FIGURE 9-120 **Vogt's limbal girdle type I.** This is actually a mild form of limbal calcific band keratopathy. It is usually irregular and slightly elevated and may contain small "Swiss cheese" holes. This patient also has a calcified scleral plaque.

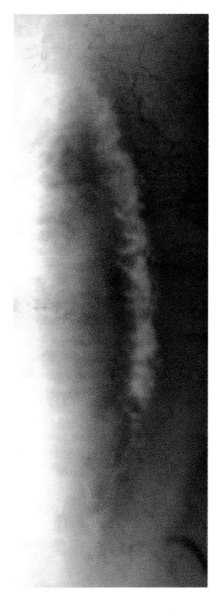

FIGURE 9-121 **Vogt's limbal girdle type II.** Similar to the lesion in Figure 9-120, this occurs in the interpalpebral zone. There is a vertical chalklike band of material in the superficial cornea. Several conical protrusions point toward the pupil. Histologically, this is a region of elastoid degeneration. This lesion is often associated with pinguecula.

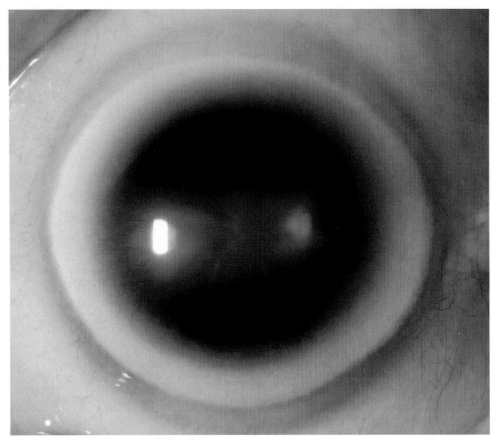

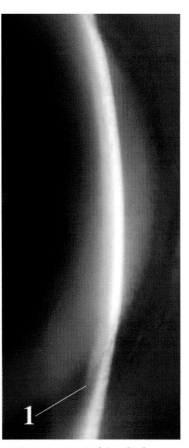

FIGURE 9-122 *Advanced arcus senilis.* This lesion is composed of lipid, and there is a characteristic clear zone between the limbus and outer edge of the lesion. The central edge of the lesion has an irregular border as compared with the peripheral edge.

FIGURE 9-123 *A thin slit beam view of arcus senilis.* Posteriorly, there is a peripheral wedge of lipid *(1)*.

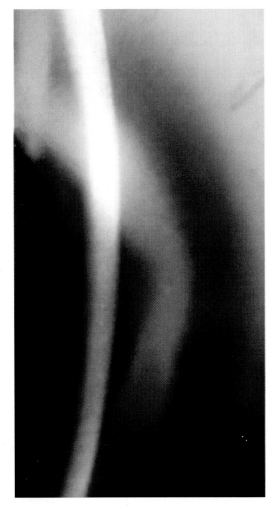

FIGURE 9-124 *Arcus juvenilis.* Peripheral lipid deposition in a young patient often signifies a systemic lipid abnormality. Serum lipid profiles should be obtained.

FIGURE 9-125 *Cornea farinata.* This represents an accumulation of fine, white, dustlike particles in the deep corneal stroma. In this case, they are best seen in retro-illumination to the left of the pupillary margin. The deposits are bilateral and not visually significant. They should not be mistaken for cornea guttata (see Figure 9-71). The term *cornea farinata* is derived from the word *farina*, which means "flour."

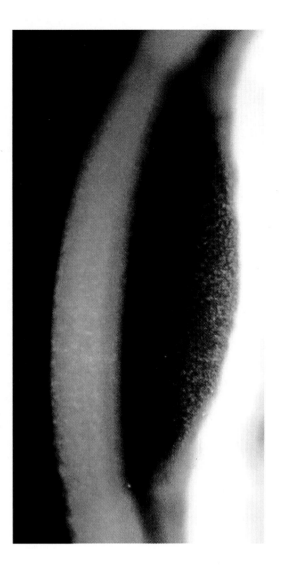

FIGURE 9-126 *Glass striae (1).* These are vertical striations in the deep corneal stroma or Descemet's membrane. They are seen in older patients and tend to be more common in patients with diabetes. They are best seen on retro-illumination and appear as fine twisted strands, some of which have a double-walled configuration. This patient also has cortical spoking from a cataract *(2).*

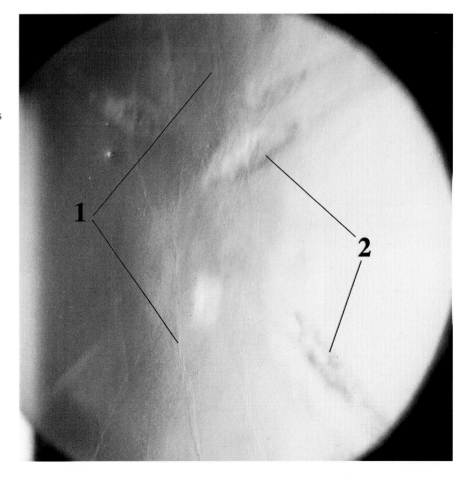

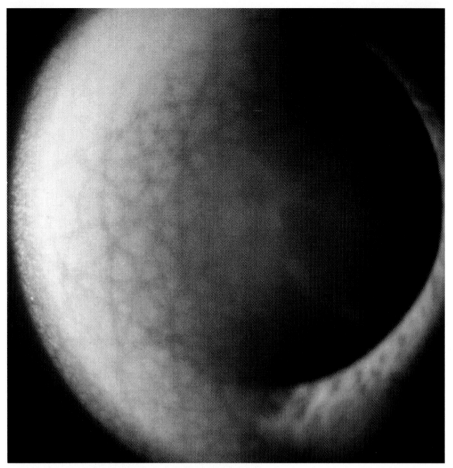

FIGURE 9-127 ***Posterior crocodile shagreen.*** There are polygonal opacities in the deep corneal stroma separated by relative clear areas. The disorder is bilateral, seen late in life, and not visually significant. Electron microscopy of one case showed an irregular arrangement of the collagen lamellae. There is no heritable pattern, but it is clinically identical to central cloudy dystrophy of François, which occurs in an autosomal dominant pattern.

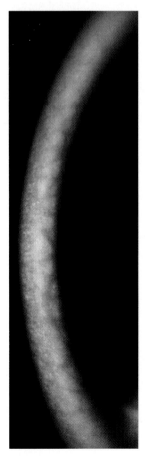

FIGURE 9-128 Thin slit beam of posterior crocodile shagreen.

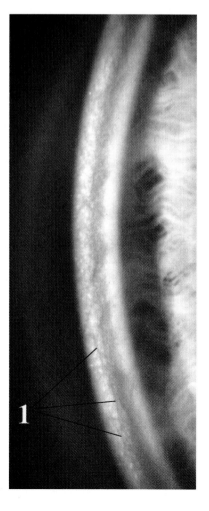

FIGURE 9-129 Thin slit beam of posterior crocodile shagreen highlighting the clear areas (*1*) between the areas of polygonal opacification.

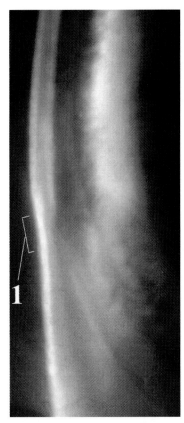

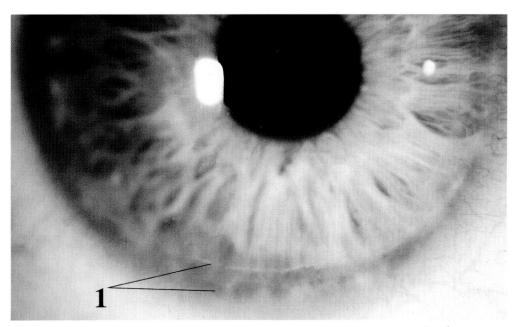

FIGURE 9-131 ***Furrow degeneration, diffuse illumination (1).*** Occasionally, fine superficial vessels extend into the area of thinning, but this is not associated with acute inflammation.

FIGURE 9-130 ***Furrow degeneration.*** This is a peripheral thinning of the cornea *(1)* near the limbus.

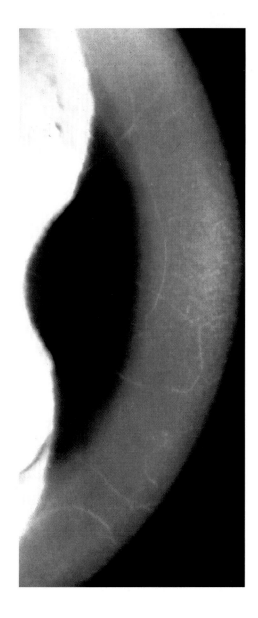

FIGURE 9-132 ***Prominent corneal nerves.*** These appear as fine, branching white lines that originate at the limbus in the mid to anterior stroma. They can be associated with multiple endocrine neoplasia type IIB, leprosy, Refsum's syndrome, neurofibromatosis, and keratoconus.

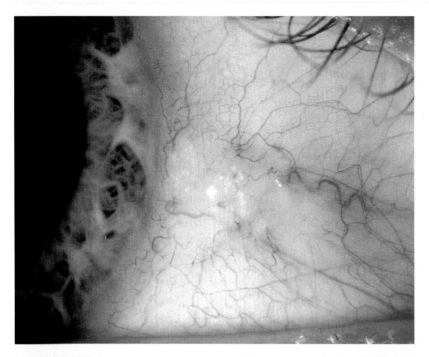

FIGURE 9-133 *Pinguecula.* These elevated, fleshy conjunctival masses are located in the interpalpebral region, most commonly on the nasal side. They are yellow or light brown. They are associated with chronic actinic exposure, repeated trauma, and dry and windy conditions. Histologically, they are composed of abnormal collagen bundles with staining characteristics similar to elastic tissue. The condition is termed *elastotic degeneration,* but the tissue is not actually composed of elastin.

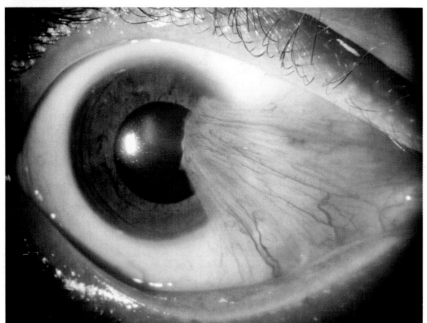

FIGURE 9-134 *A pterygium.* These fibrovascular growths extend from the conjunctiva onto the cornea. They are almost always preceded by pinguecula and, like pinguecula, are associated with chronic actinic exposure, trauma, and dry and windy conditions. There is destruction of Bowman's membrane in the cornea, and for this reason, there is residual corneal scarring when these growths are removed. The histopathology, like pinguecula, shows elastotic degeneration.

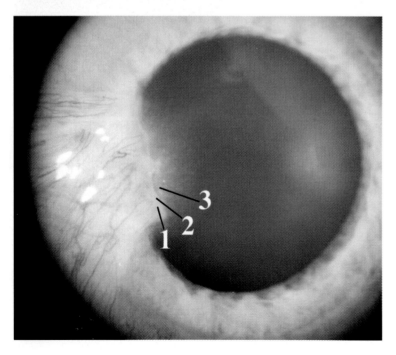

FIGURE 9-135 *A pterygium.* The head of the pterygium has a thick white scar *(1)* that is avascular *(2).* There is an iron line (Stocker line) in the epithelium *(3),* which results from an irregular tear distribution adjacent to the raised edge of the pterygium.

Iron lines appear as faint brown deposits in the corneal epithelium. Sometimes they are best seen with the cobalt blue light. Iron deposits occur in areas of irregular tear distribution. Histologically, the iron is seen in the epithelium, especially the basal layer.

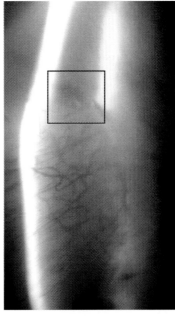

FIGURE 9-136 Pterygium with a Stocker line *(box)*.

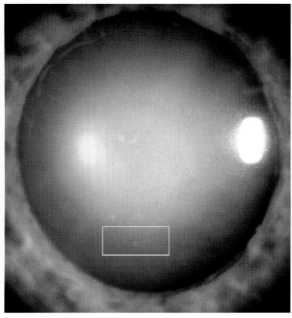

FIGURE 9-137 Hudson-Stähli line at the junction of the upper two thirds and lower one third of the cornea *(box)*.

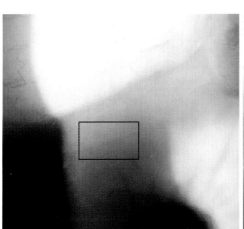

FIGURE 9-138 Filtering bleb with Ferry line *(box)*, white light.

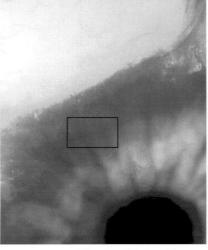

FIGURE 9-139 Filtering bleb with Ferry line *(box)*, blue light.

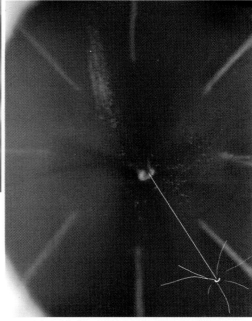

FIGURE 9-140 Iron lines associated with radial keratotomy.

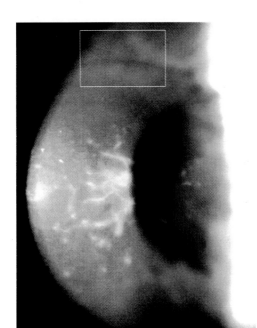

FIGURE 9-141 Iron in keratoconus (Fleischer ring) *(box)*.

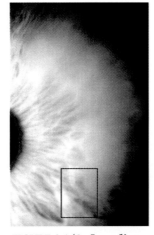

FIGURE 9-142 ***Iron lines can be seen in many corneal conditions.*** This case shows Salzmann's nodular degeneration *(box)*.

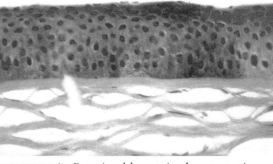

FIGURE 9-143 Prussian blue stain demonstrating iron in the epithelium *(box)*.

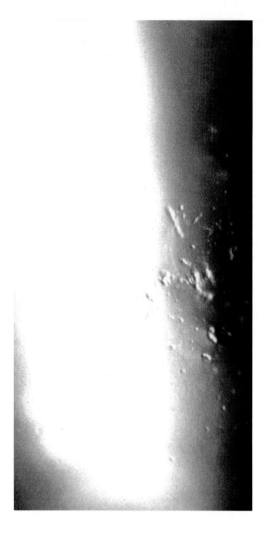

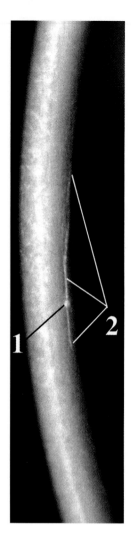

FIGURE 9-144 *Polymorphic amyloid degeneration.* This age-related change of the cornea is usually bilateral and does not affect vision. In the deep corneal stroma, there are small polygonal gray-white opacities and lines that are refractile with indirect illumination. The opacities themselves appear similar to those seen in lattice dystrophy; however, they are usually less extensive, are located in the deepest level of the stroma, and are not associated with any of the sequelae of lattice dystrophy. These deposits are not associated with any systemic disorder of amyloid deposition.

FIGURE 9-145 *Polymorphic amyloid degeneration.* An amyloid deposit *(1)* and Descemet's fold caused by pressure from the deposit *(2)* are shown.

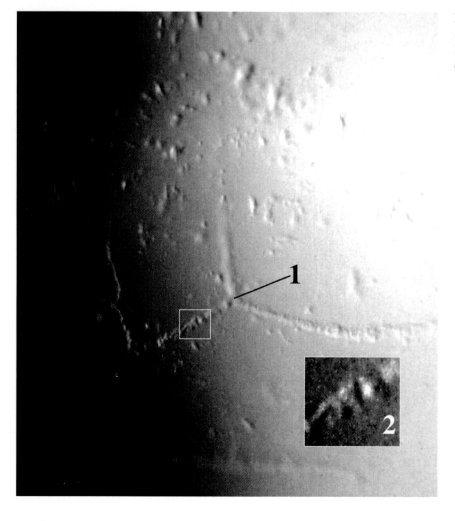

FIGURE 9-146 *Polymorphic amyloid degeneration.* This can appear similar to lattice dystrophy with branching lines *(1)* composed of smaller nodules *(inset [2])*.

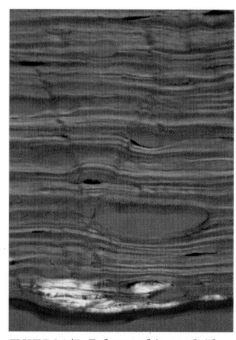

FIGURE 9-147 *Polymorphic amyloid degeneration.* Fusiform extracellular amyloid material is seen in the very deep stroma (birefringence of Congo red stain).

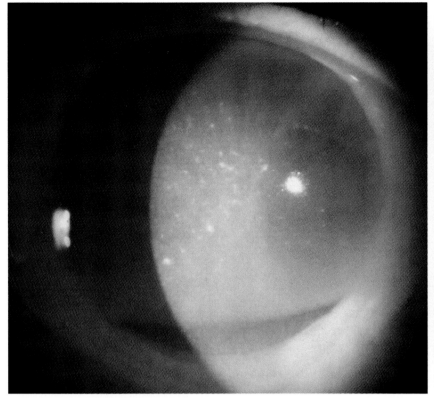

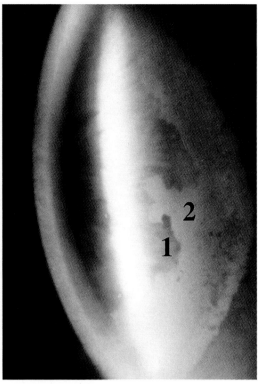

FIGURE 9-148 **_Calcific band keratopathy._** Characteristically this occurs in the interpalpebral region. Calcium deposits in this region result from localized elevations of pH favoring calcium precipitation and increased evaporation, which increases the local concentration of calcium. This condition may be idiopathic but is usually associated with localized ocular inflammatory processes or systemic hypercalcemia.

FIGURE 9-149 **_Same patient as in Figure 9-148 after chelation with EDTA._** The area where calcium was removed is shown *(1)*. Calcium remnants are seen in the peripheral cornea *(2)*. The small holes represent areas where corneal nerves penetrate through Bowman's layer to the superficial epithelium.

FIGURE 9-150 **_Calcific degeneration._** Calcium deposition in the cornea is associated with chronic vascularization or inflammation. Histopathologically, the calcium may be associated with a fibrovascular pannus or may occur deep in the corneal stroma, as opposed to calcific band keratopathy in which the calcium deposition is confined to the region of Bowman's membrane (see Figure 9-152). In this case the calcific degeneration was associated with chronic inflammation from interstitial keratitis.

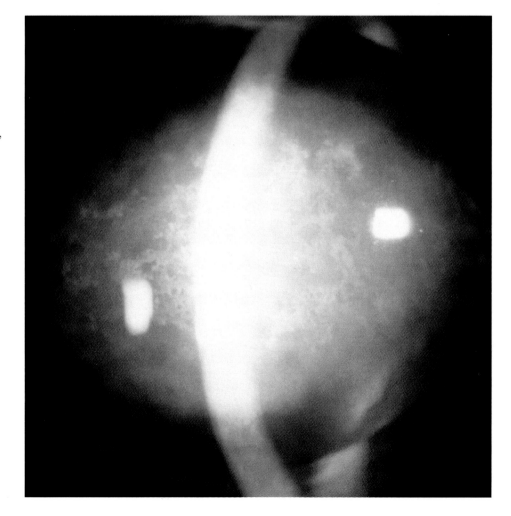

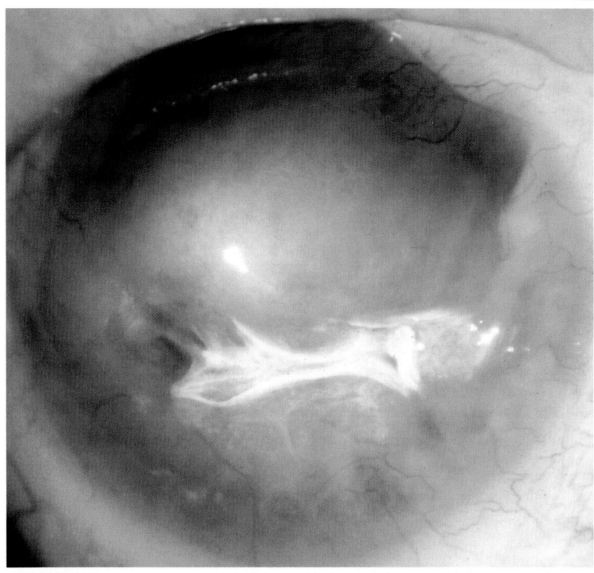

FIGURE 9-151 *Calcific degeneration.* This patient had severe glaucoma and chronic corneal edema from aphakic bullous keratopathy. The histopathology showed calcium associated with a fibrovascular pannus.

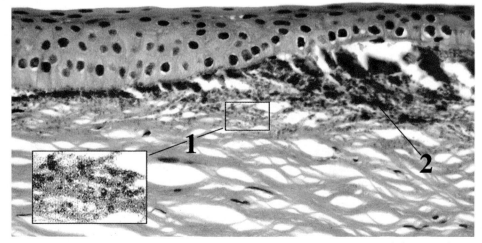

FIGURE 9-152 *Histopathology of calcific band keratopathy.* Basophilic stippling from calcium diffusely replaces Bowman's membrane *(1)* with larger pieces of calcium *(2)* in localized accumulations.

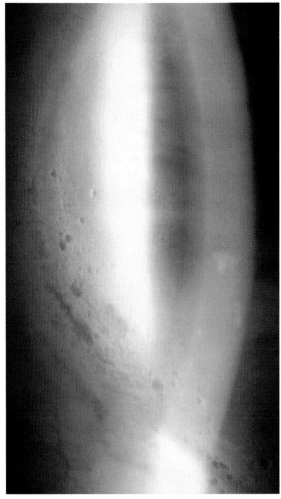

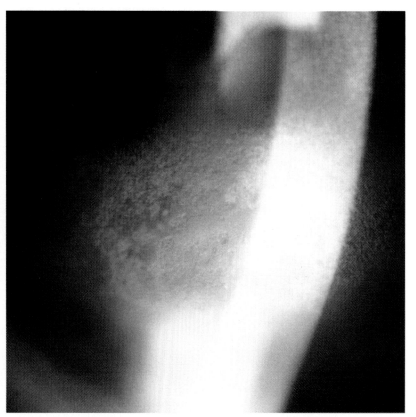

FIGURE 9-154 *Spheroidal degeneration, advanced.* The brownish-yellow deposits are more confluent and are located in the central cornea in this case. Spheroidal degeneration characteristically occurs in the interpalpebral zones and is associated with chronic actinic exposure and dry and windy conditions. Similar to band keratopathy, it may also be associated with chronic localized ocular inflammation.

FIGURE 9-153 *Spheroidal degeneration, mild.* There are multiple golden-brown spherules in the superficial cornea.

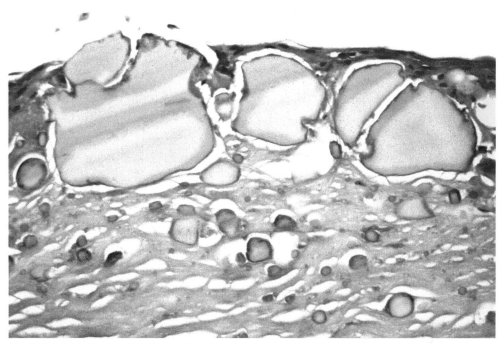

FIGURE 9-155 *Histopathology of spheroidal degeneration.* Extracellular deposits of globular, faintly basophilic material are noted in the superficial stroma and Bowman's layer. The globules are irregularly shaped with well-demarcated borders. It is similar to calcific band keratopathy except that the deposits are more homogenous and not stippled.

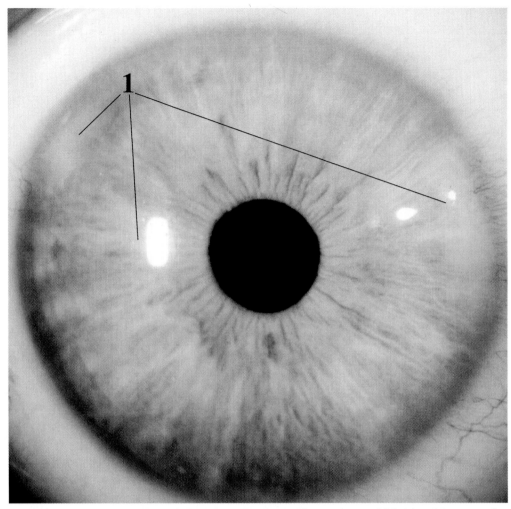

FIGURE 9-156 *Salzmann's nodular degenerations.* These elevated bluish-white superficial nodules *(1)* are more common in females and most commonly occur in the fifth decade of life or later. The condition may be associated with localized corneal inflammation. Histopathology shows subepithelial hyaline nodules that replace Bowman's layer.

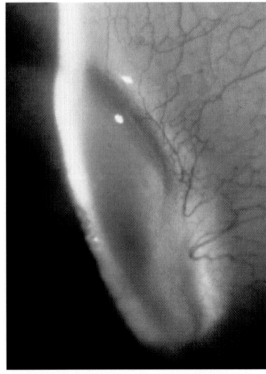

FIGURE 9-157 Peripheral Salzmann's nodule showing characteristic elevation.

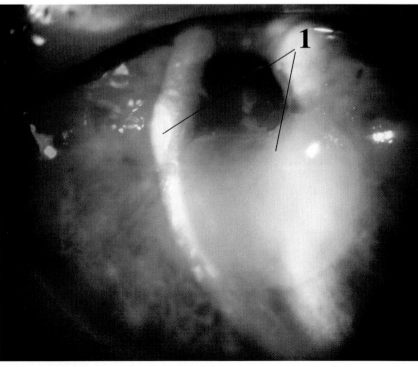

FIGURE 9-158 Salzmann's nodules *(1)* near the visual axis.

FIGURE 9-159 *Terrien's marginal degeneration.* This slowly progressive marginal thinning of the cornea is more common in males and can occur in all age groups, including children. In contrast to other causes of marginal corneal thinning such as Mooren's ulcer, there is no pain, there are very minor or no episodes of acute inflammation, and the corneal epithelium remains intact. The thinning usually begins superiorly *(1)*, and it is associated with a fine line of lipid deposition *(2)* at the edge of fine superficial vessels *(3)*.

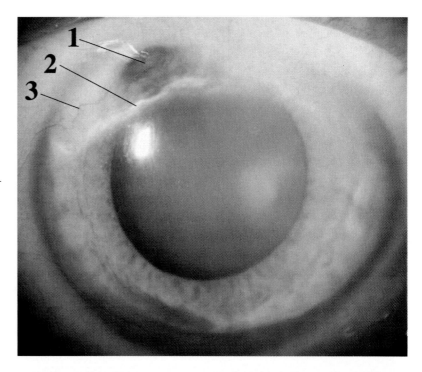

FIGURE 9-160 *Terrien's marginal degeneration.* With time, the thinning spreads circumferentially, as seen in this example. The cornea becomes extremely thin *(1)* and may bulge anteriorly. There is lipid deposition *(2)* and superficial vascularization *(3)*.

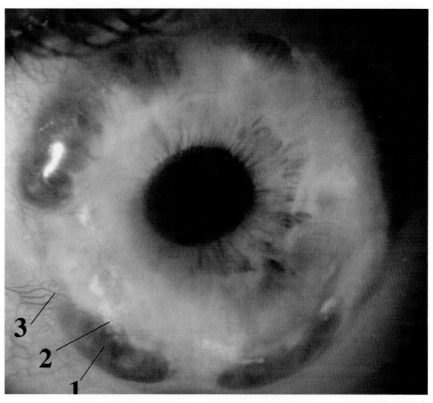

FIGURE 9-161 *A thin slit beam view of Terrien's marginal degeneration.* The cornea is extremely thin *(1)* and bulges anteriorly. The epithelium overlying the thin cornea is intact. Minor ocular trauma may result in ocular perforation. Lipid deposition *(2)* and superficial vascularization *(3)* are also seen.

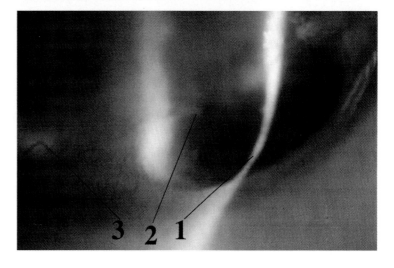

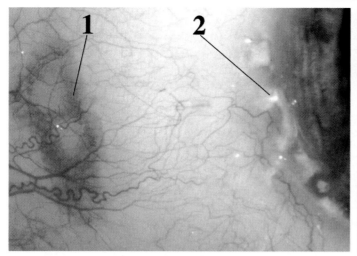

FIGURE 9-162 *Calcified scleral plaques.* Occasionally, calcified plaques *(1)* are seen in older patients. This patient also has Vogt's limbic girdle type I *(2)*, which represents mild calcific band keratopathy (see Figure 9-120).

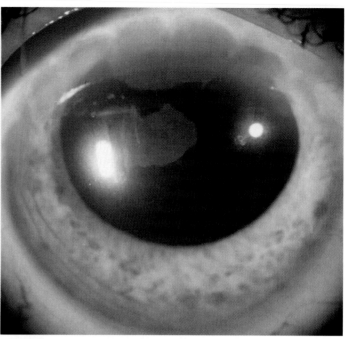

FIGURE 9-163 *Posterior proliferative endothelial pigmentation in a patient after cataract surgery.* These membranes may grow and change shape with time.

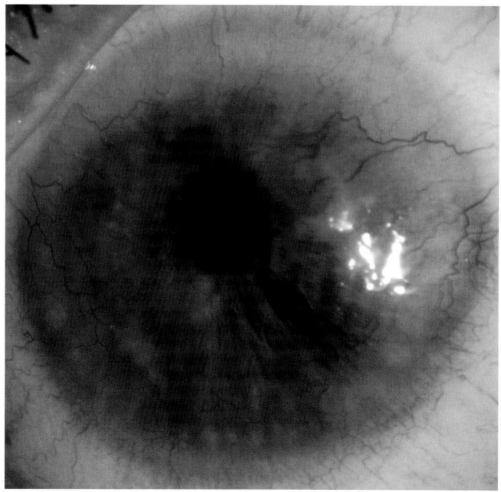

FIGURE 9-164 *Aniridia.* This congenital disorder is associated with glaucoma, cataracts, ectopia lentis, and foveal hypoplasia. These patients may have superficial corneal vascularization and severe corneal scarring. Penetrating keratoplasty is often complicated by poor epithelial healing, recurrence of superficial vascularization, and scarring in the graft. The term *aniridia* is a misnomer, since all of these patients have some iris tissue present (sometimes only histologically) and in some cases the iris may be only mildly abnormal (as seen here).

Corneal Infections

There are four basic classes of organisms responsible for infectious keratitis: bacterial, viral, fungal, and parasitic. Whenever possible, the exact diagnosis should be established by direct examination of corneal material and/or culture techniques. However, the clinical appearance of some of these disorders can establish a definitive diagnosis (e.g., herpes simplex epithelial keratitis) or guide treatment until the exact diagnosis is known.

Bacterial Infections

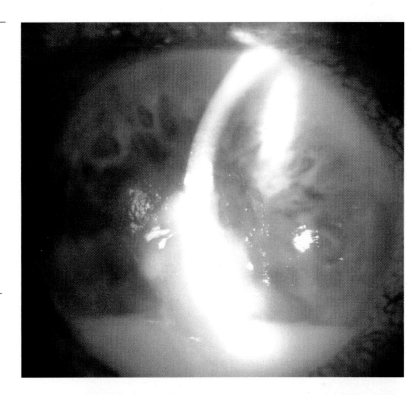

FIGURE 10-1 *Acute bacterial keratitis.* This infection is associated with symptoms of pain, redness, and decreased vision. Here there is a central corneal ulcer caused by *Staphylococcus aureus* and an anterior chamber reaction severe enough to produce a hypopyon.

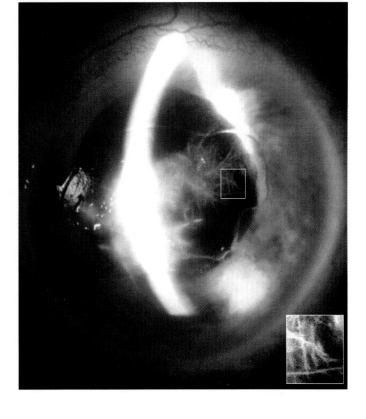

FIGURE 10-2 *Infectious crystalline keratopathy.* This is a descriptive term for a keratitis that has a crystalline appearance in the stroma *(inset).* The most common bacterial organisms implicated are the *Streptococcus viridans* group (specifically, nutritionally variant streptococci). In this case the causative organism was *S. faecalis.* Fungal keratitis and calcium deposits can have a similar appearance. The crystalline appearance results from the pattern of the organism within the corneal stroma and a lack of any host inflammatory response. (An abundance of white cells would obscure the pattern.) The nutritionally variant streptococci may be difficult to culture on routine media, and the clinical response to antibiotics may not correlate with in vitro sensitivities. Infectious crystalline keratopathy occurs more commonly in patients with corneal grafts (see Figure 18-26).

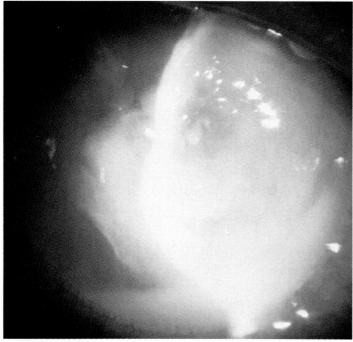

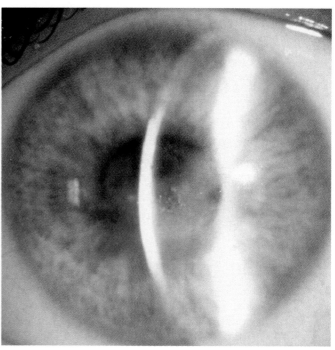

FIGURE 10-3 *Pseudomonas keratitis in a soft contact lens wearer.* There is extensive tissue destruction and a layered hypopyon.

FIGURE 10-4 *Same patient as in Figure 10-3.* The ulcer has resolved after treatment with fortified antibiotics, and there is corneal scarring.

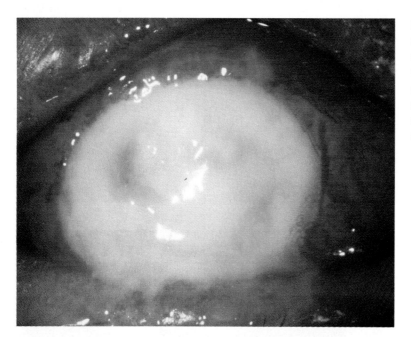

FIGURE 10-5 *Severe bacterial keratitis with infectious scleritis caused by Pseudomonas organisms.* Pseudomonas infections can be associated with a large degree of tissue destruction because of enzymes and exotoxins released from the organism and a vigorous host inflammatory response. The prognosis with scleral extension is extremely poor.

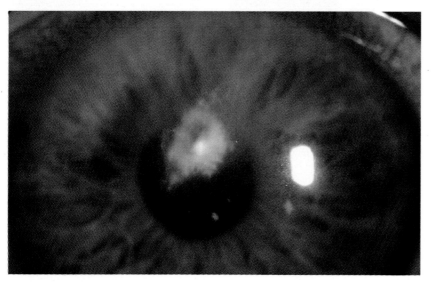

FIGURE 10-6 *Mycobacterium fortuitum keratitis.* These infections usually arise after trauma or surgical intervention. This indolent infection may progress slowly over several weeks, and there is a minimal host inflammatory response.

Herpes Simplex Keratitis

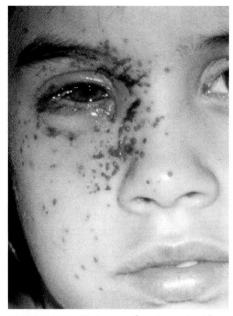

FIGURE 10-7 ***Primary herpes simplex infection of the facial skin.*** There are multiple vesicular lesions, some of which are crusted over. A blepharoconjunctivitis is present in the right eye.

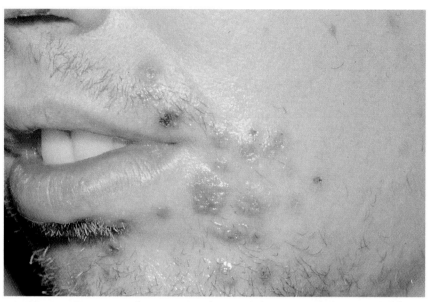

FIGURE 10-8 ***Recurrent herpes simplex vesicles around the mouth.*** These lesions are usually painless and resolve in 2 to 3 weeks without scarring.

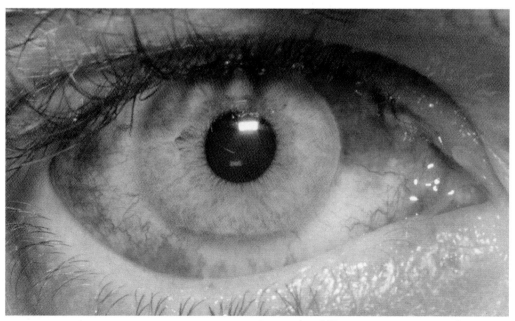

FIGURE 10-9 ***Same patient as in Figure 10-8.*** Note the diffuse conjunctivitis. With primary herpes infections, there may be a follicular response and preauricular adenopathy.

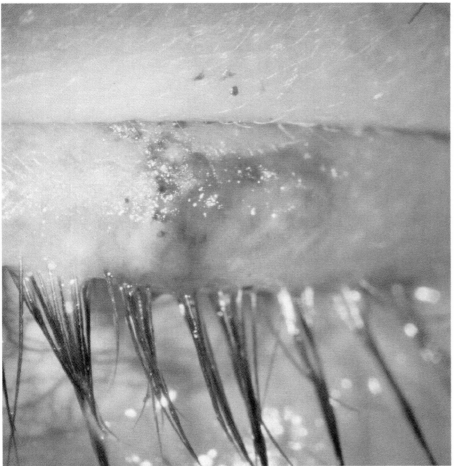

FIGURE 10-10 *A magnified view of herpes blepharitis.* An ulcerative lesion is present on the skin.

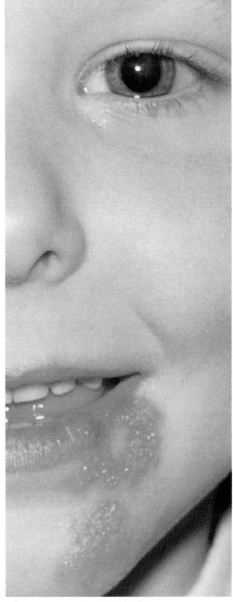

FIGURE 10-11 *Herpes simplex infection of the skin with a conjunctivitis.* A corneal scar is present from previous infections.

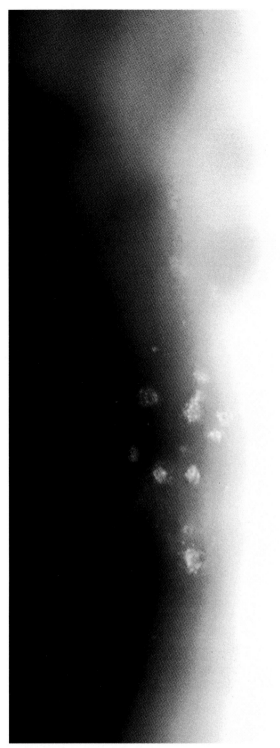

FIGURE 10-12 **Earliest stage of epithelial keratitis.** Small punctate vesicular lesions can be seen in the epithelium. These coalesce into plaques that eventually enlarge to form dendrites. It is rare to see this early stage.

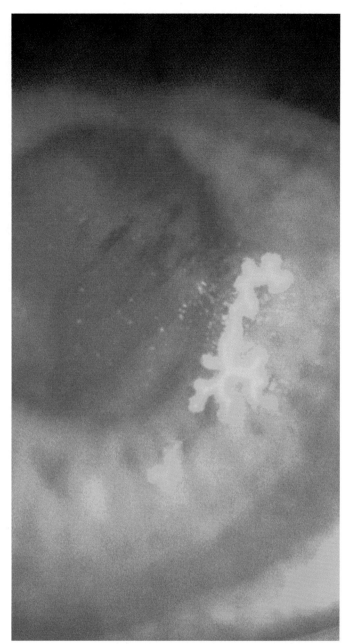

FIGURE 10-13 **Same patient as in Figure 10-12, 1 week later with a typical dendrite.** The epithelial defect stains with fluorescein. The peripheral cells lining the dendrite are often raised and contain active virus. These cells stain with rose bengal. When the dendrite resolves, scarring occurs.

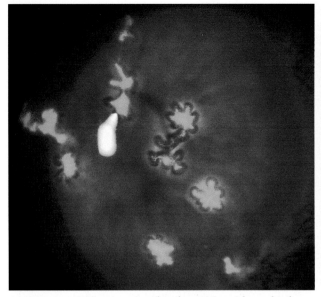

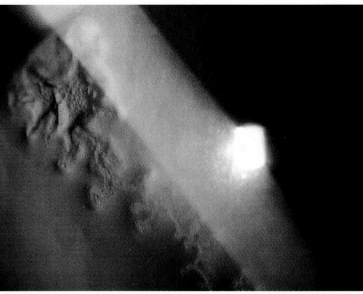

FIGURE 10-14 Herpes simplex keratitis with multiple epithelial dendrites.

FIGURE 10-15 *Herpes simplex keratitis.* The opened portion of the dendrite is seen in the upper left (geographic ulcer); the remaining closed portion (dendritic ulcer) is also seen. Notable is that herpes "bites" deeper than the epithelium.

FIGURE 10-16 *Herpes simplex keratitis with a large geographic ulcer.* These ulcers take longer to heal than dendritic ulcers.

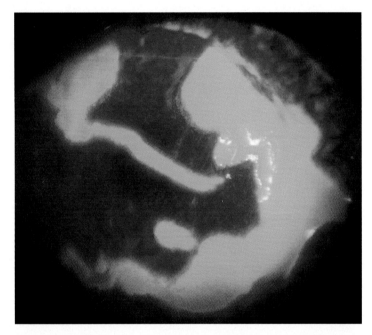

FIGURE 10-17 Herpes simplex conjunctival ulcers.

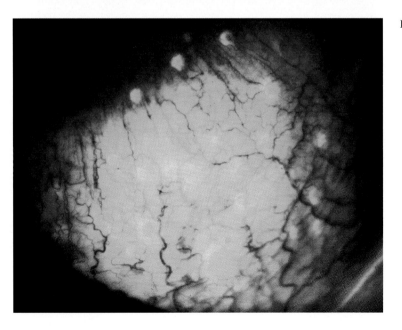

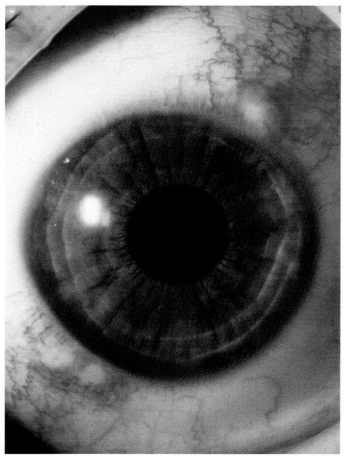

FIGURE 10-18 Herpes simplex with multiple conjunctival phlyctenules.

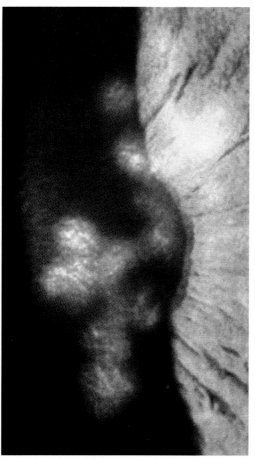

FIGURE 10-19 *Anterior stromal scars.* "Footprints" in a pattern of herpetic ulceration indicate previous herpetic infection.

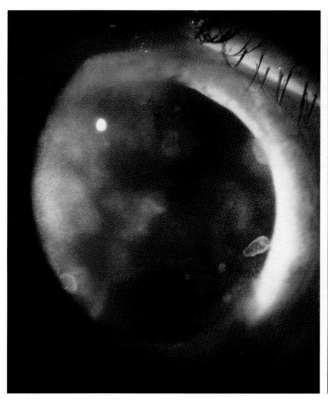

FIGURE 10-20 Herpes simplex scars with typical ground glass appearance.

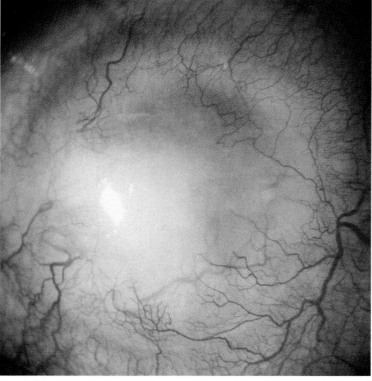

FIGURE 10-21 *Herpes simplex.* Advanced scarring and vascularization are seen.

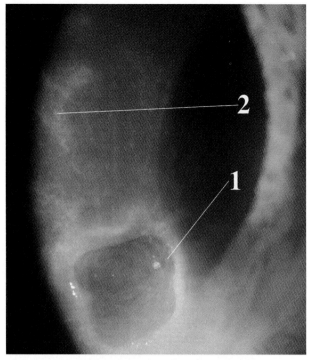

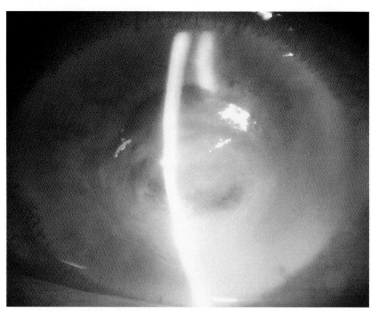

FIGURE 10-22 *Neurotrophic (metaherpetic) ulcer (1).* These ulcers are usually round, oblong, or square and have a characteristic broad, rolled-up epithelial edge. Anterior stromal scarring—evidence of a previous infection from herpes simplex virus—is seen *(2).*

FIGURE 10-23 *Neurotrophic herpes ulcer.* These ulcers occur in eyes with long-standing herpetic disease and are caused by corneal anesthesia rather than active viral infection. Typically, these ulcers are in the lower half of the cornea.

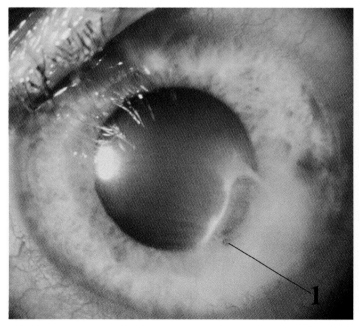

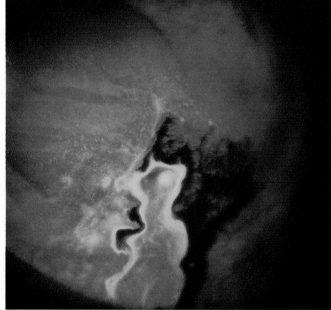

FIGURE 10-24 Herpes simplex keratitis with corneal perforation *(1).*

FIGURE 10-25 *Same patient as in Figure 10-24.* The perforation site is Seidel positive.

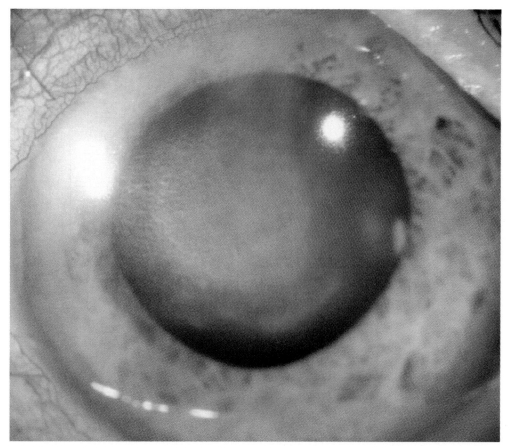

FIGURE 10-26 *Herpes simplex disciform keratitis.* There is a circular area of corneal edema. Although not seen here, keratic precipitates may be seen on the corneal endothelium, and there may be a low-grade iritis. The intraocular pressure is often elevated.

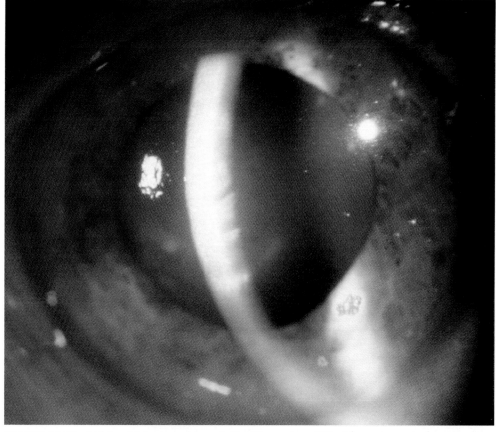

FIGURE 10-27 *A thin slit beam view of disciform keratitis.* There is central corneal edema.

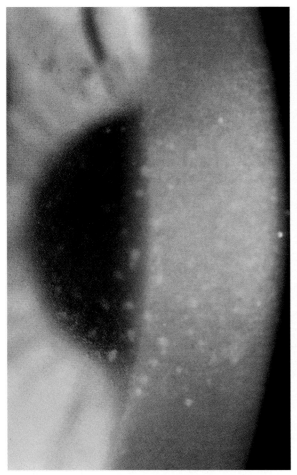

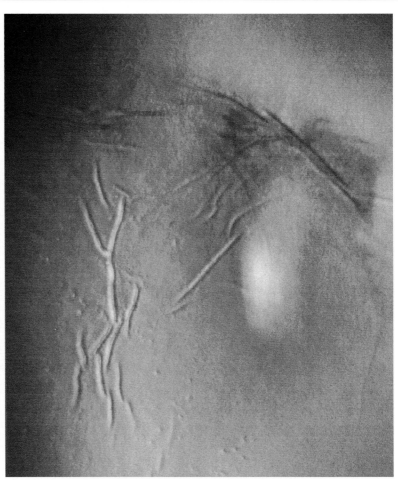

FIGURE 10-28 *Herpes simplex keratouveitis.* In contrast to disciform keratitis, there is diffuse corneal edema and the uveitis is more pronounced. A hypopyon may occur.

FIGURE 10-29 *Herpes simplex.* Areas of Descemet's proliferation are evident.

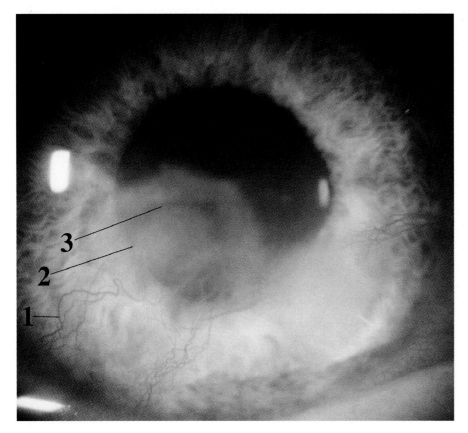

FIGURE 10-30 *Herpes simplex interstitial keratitis.* This is characterized by stromal infiltration and vascularization with an intact epithelium. Here there is vascularization *(1)* and scarring *(2)* of the corneal stroma, with an iron line *(3)* in the epithelium.

FIGURE 10-31 Herpes simplex keratitis with peripheral inflammatory disease.

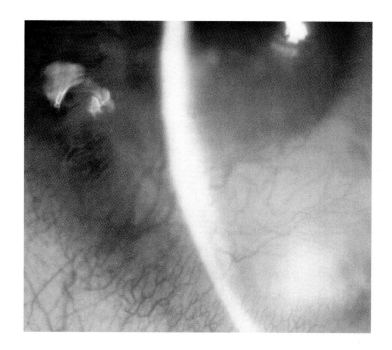

FIGURE 10-32 *Chronic keratouveitis caused by herpes simplex.* Keratic precipitates are seen centrally, and there is diffuse corneal haze with stromal vascularization.

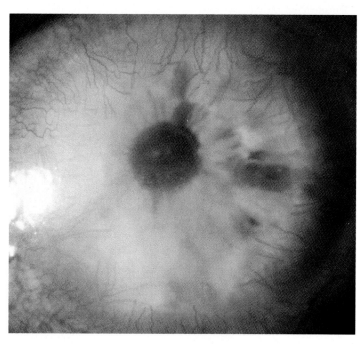

FIGURE 10-33 *Necrotizing herpes simplex keratitis.* Necrotizing infections are characterized by ulceration with tissue loss. This is one of the most serious forms of keratitis because tissue loss can lead to perforation. It is not known whether this form of keratitis results from active viral infection of the stroma or an immunologic reaction to viral antigens.

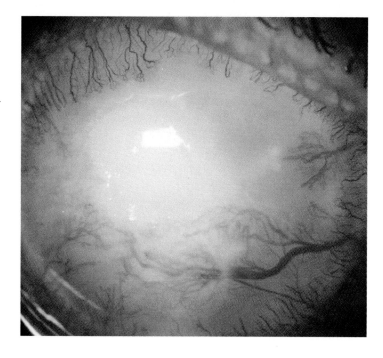

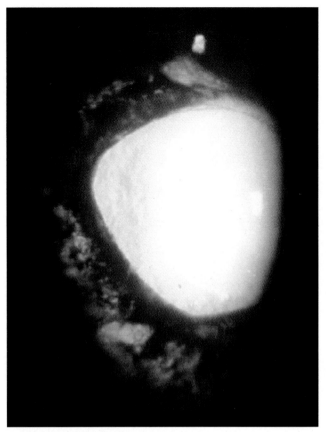

FIGURE 10-34 Diffuse iris atrophy caused by recurrent herpes simplex keratouveitis.

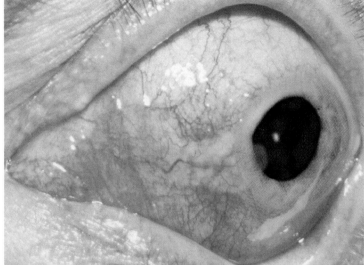

FIGURE 10-35 *Herpes simplex scleritis.* There is diffuse injection of the conjunctiva and deep episcleral vessels, and the inflammation extends into the sclera. This condition is characterized by severe pain and is often difficult to treat.

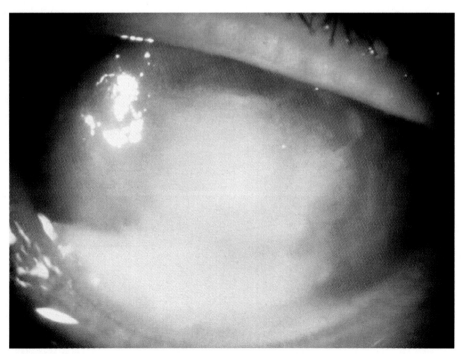

FIGURE 10-36 *Chronic herpes simplex keratitis with secondary bacterial infection.* Eyes with this disorder are more susceptible to secondary infection. Here there is an extensive corneal ulcer caused by *Moraxella* organisms.

Herpes Zoster Keratitis

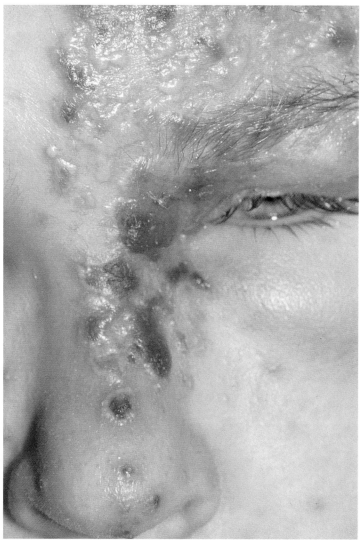

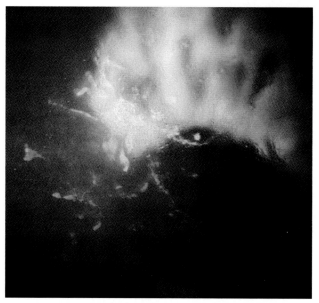

FIGURE 10-38 *Epithelial dendrites from herpes zoster infection.* In contrast to the dendrites seen in herpes simplex infection, these lesions are elevated and appear as mucous plaques stuck on the epithelium. In addition, these dendrites are coarser and do not have the terminal bulbs seen in herpes simplex.

FIGURE 10-37 *Herpes zoster keratitis.* This patient has vesicular and crusted lesions from herpes zoster infection in the distribution of the first division of the fifth cranial nerve. If the tip of the nose is involved (as in this case), it is likely that there is ocular involvement, since both regions are supplied by the nasociliary nerve (Hutchinson's sign).

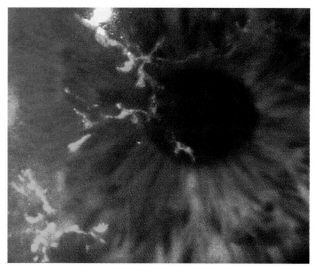

FIGURE 10-39 *Herpes zoster dendrites.* These stain weakly with fluorescein.

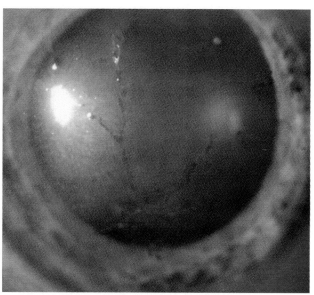

FIGURE 10-40 *Herpes zoster dendrites.* These stain well with rose bengal.

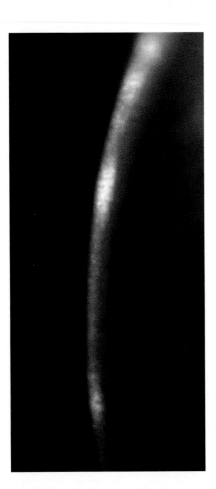

FIGURE 10-41 *Subepithelial infiltrates in herpes zoster ophthalmicus.* These infiltrates probably represent an immunologic reaction to viral proteins. Similar to the subepithelial infiltrates in epidemic keratoconjunctivitis, these occur 10 to 14 days after the onset of active disease and respond to treatment with topical corticosteroids. They can recur many months to years after active infection.

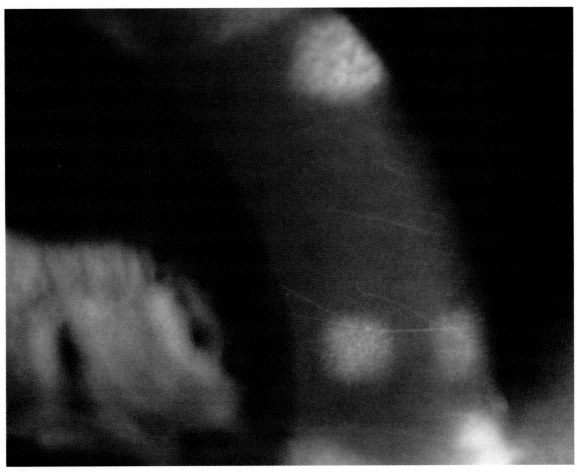

FIGURE 10-42 Multiple subepithelial infiltrates along the path of prominent corneal nerves.

FIGURE 10-43 _Herpes zoster._
Some patients develop a stromal infiltrate. This patient has an infiltrate near the limbus.

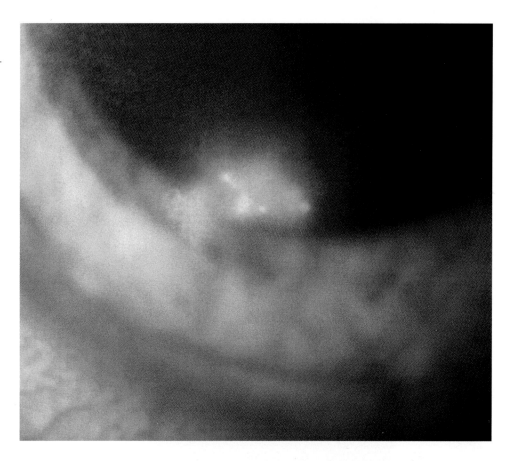

FIGURE 10-44 _Large keratic precipitates in herpes zoster uveitis._ This uveitis may begin with the initial herpes attack and can persist or recur for years after the initial episode. At least half the patients with zoster uveitis have elevated pressure, which in some cases can lead to severe glaucoma. Patients may need to be maintained on low-dose topical corticosteroids chronically to prevent reactivation.

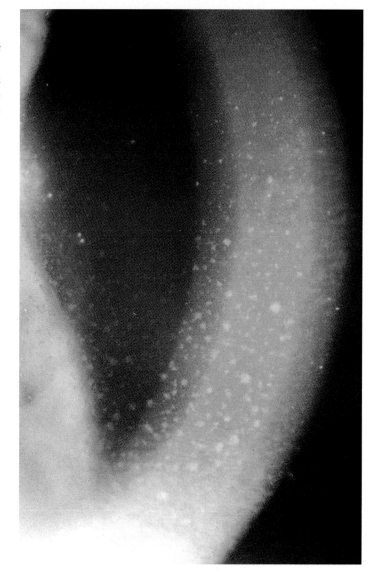

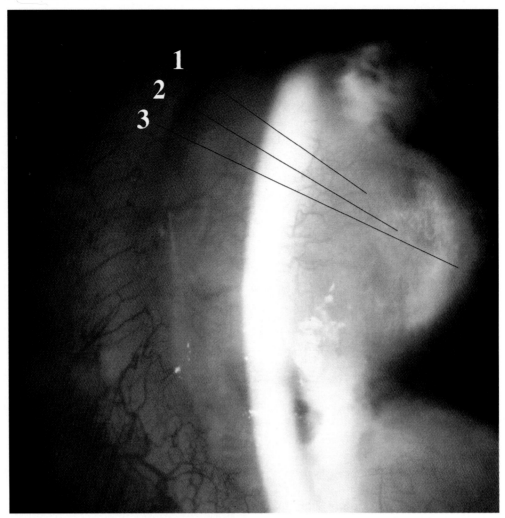

FIGURE 10-45 *Herpes zoster keratitis in a right eye.* Although not limited to previous herpes zoster infection, the findings in this patient should alert the examiner to that possibility. There is a combination of temporal location, vascularization *(1)*, scarring *(2)*, and lipid deposit *(3)*.

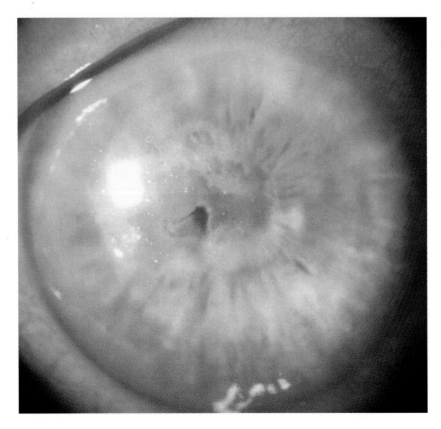

FIGURE 10-46 *Diffuse corneal scarring from herpes zoster ophthalmicus.* Scarring may result from inflammatory disease of the corneal stroma or chronic surface problems. (This eye has a small central epithelial defect.) Surface problems may be caused by many factors, including corneal anesthesia, dry eye, lagophthalmos, entropion, and ectropion.

FIGURE 10-47 *Herpes zoster ophthalmicus with a neurotrophic ulcer.* The lesion is characteristically oval; has broad, gray epithelial edges; and is usually located in the lower half of the cornea. If untreated, these lesions often progress to perforation. Treatment includes increasing corneal lubrication and coverage of the lesion with a tarsorrhaphy or, in extreme cases, a conjunctival flap. Topical corticosteroids are not indicated.

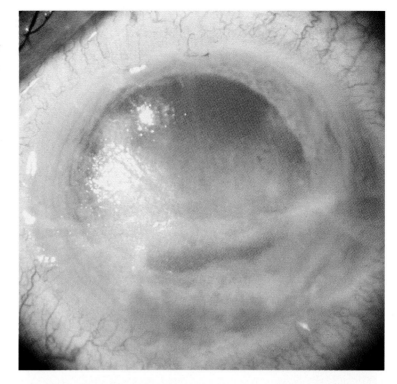

FIGURE 10-48 *Herpes zoster ophthalmicus with an indolent corneal ulcer.* The ulcer is shallow, with fairly discrete edges and a dense, very level base. Predisposing factors include corneal anesthesia, dry eye, and lid abnormalities.

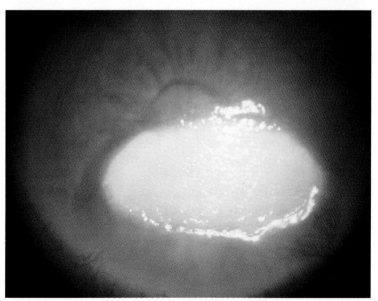

FIGURE 10-49 *Neurotrophic ulcer after a herpes zoster infection.* This patient has a hypopyon, and although this was not infectious, it is prudent to obtain routine cultures and treat with antibiotics until the diagnosis is certain.

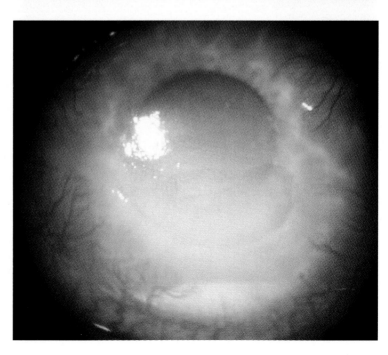

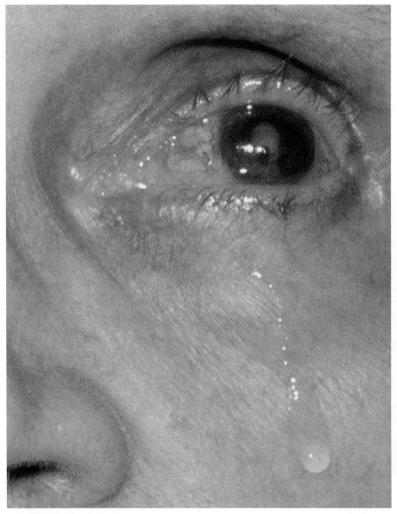

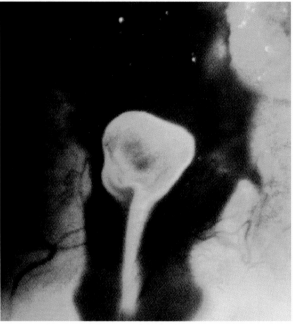

FIGURE 10-50 *Corneal perforation from a chronic herpes zoster neurotrophic ulcer.* There is an aqueous tear on the patient's cheek.

FIGURE 10-51 *Same patient as in Figure 10-50.* The perforation site is Seidel positive.

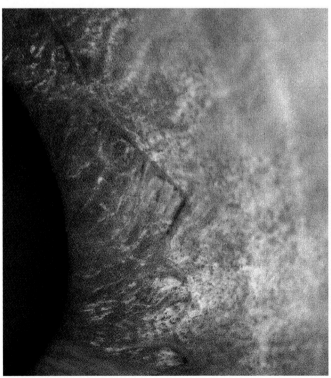

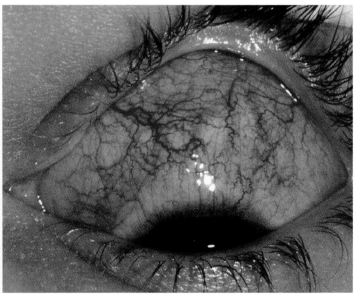

FIGURE 10-53 *Herpes zoster scleritis 2 weeks after the initial episode of herpes zoster infection.* This process was localized to the superior sclera. Similar to other forms of scleritis, it is extremely painful.

FIGURE 10-52 *Sectoral iris atrophy in herpes zoster.* This finding is attributed to a localized vasculitis.

Fungal Keratitis

FIGURE 10-54 *Fungal keratitis.* Infection with filamentous fungi is usually associated with outdoor trauma, particularly from vegetable matter. This is a case of an *Aspergillus* corneal ulcer. There is a ring infiltrate, and the edges of the infiltrate have a feathery appearance.

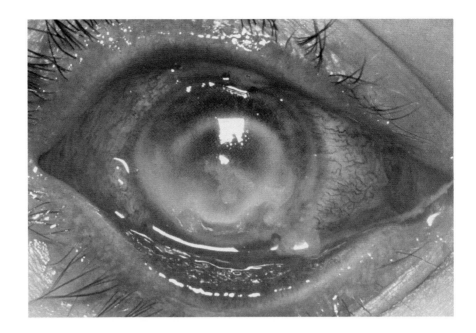

FIGURE 10-55 *Fungal keratitis.* This is a higher magnification of the infiltrate in an *Aspergillus* corneal ulcer. The edges are nondistinct and have filamentary extensions.

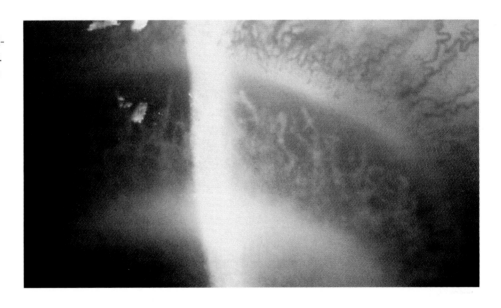

FIGURE 10-56 *Fusarium infection of the cornea.* There is a dense stromal infiltrate with indistinct margins.

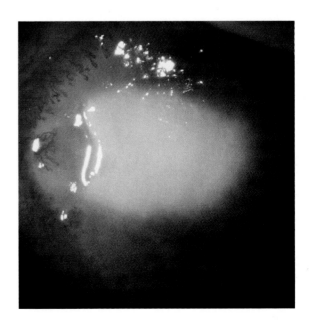

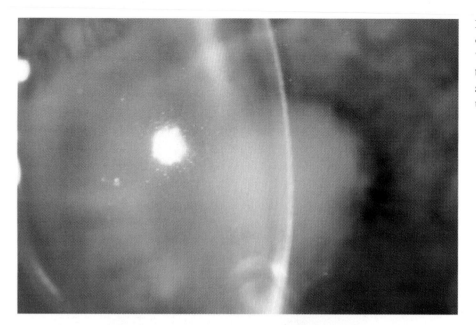

FIGURE 10-57 *Candida keratitis.* This case resulted in an anterior chamber "puff ball." The patient had been treated for several weeks with intensive topical corticosteroids for an unexplained keratitis.

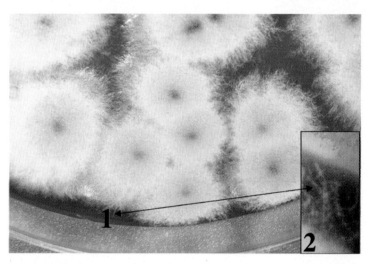

FIGURE 10-58 *Filamentous growth on blood agar from a case of Fusarium keratitis.* The growth on the agar plate *(1)* is similar to that on the cornea *(2)* in the patient in Figure 10-55.

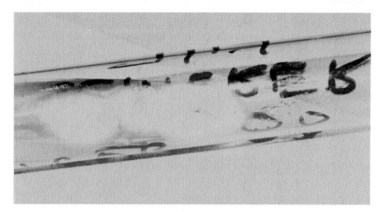

FIGURE 10-59 *Aspergillus* growth on Sabouraud's agar.

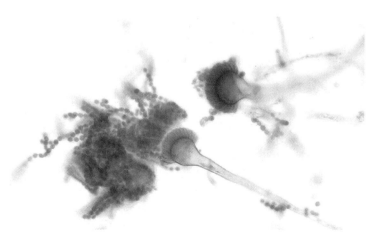

FIGURE 10-60 *Aspergillus infection, shown by lactophenol cotton blue stain.* Septate hyphae with phialides are seen on top of swollen vesicles. The phialides produce chains of round conidia spores.

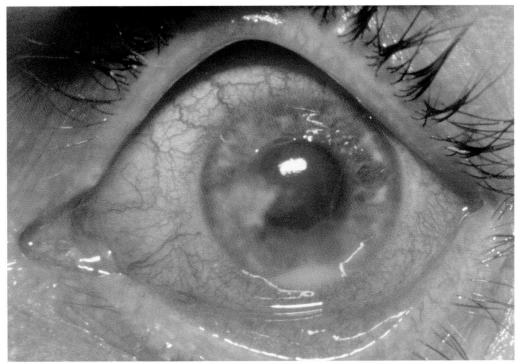

FIGURE 10-61 *Fungal keratitis.* This deep ulcer with hypopyon was caused by *Cephalosporium* infection. It did not respond to medical treatment.

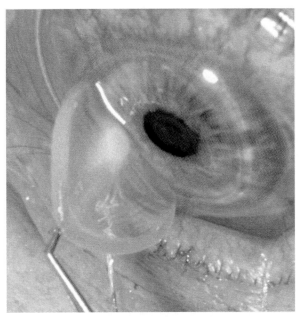

FIGURE 10-62 *Same patient as in Figure 10-61 during penetrating keratoplasty.* The deep infiltrate can be seen on the posterior cornea. There is fibrin overlying the lens.

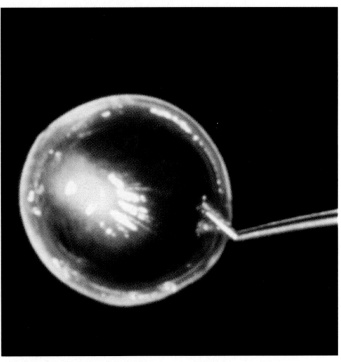

FIGURE 10-63 *Same patient as in Figures 10-61 and 10-62.* The excised host button with fungal infiltrate is shown.

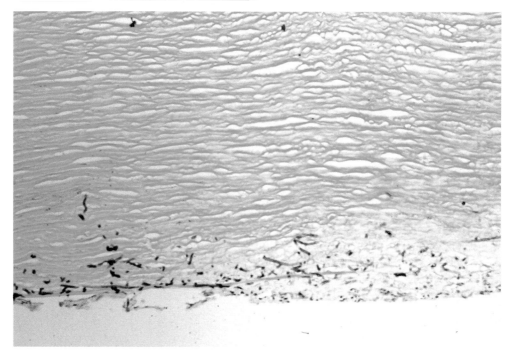

FIGURE 10-64 *Histopathology of fungal keratitis in same patient as in Figures 10-61 to 10-63.* Hyphae with right-angled branching pattern are seen penetrating the deep posterior cornea.

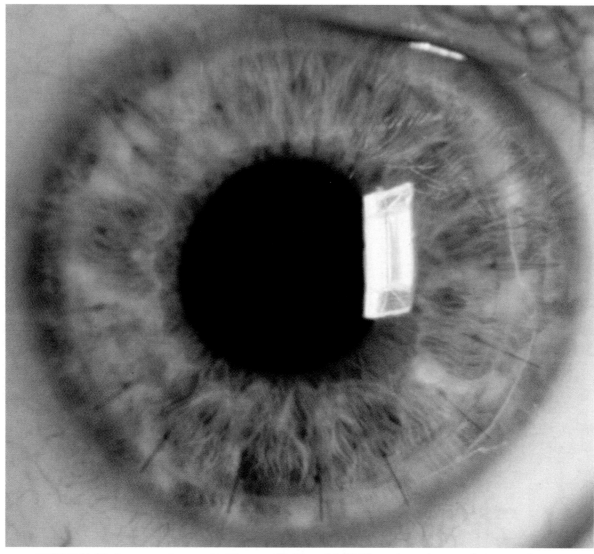

FIGURE 10-65 *Same patient as in Figures 10-61 to 10-64.* There is a clear graft 1 year after penetrating keratoplasty.

Acanthamoeba Keratitis

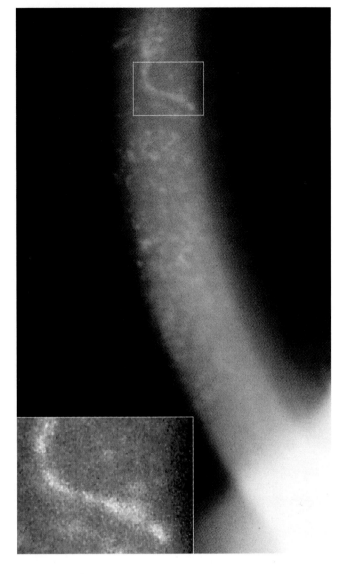

FIGURE 10-66 ***Acanthamoeba keratitis.*** This occurs most commonly in the setting of contact lens wearers who use tap water in their care regimen; however, it can occur with non-contact lens–related trauma. This patient was diagnosed with *Acanthamoeba* keratitis 2 weeks after the onset of symptoms. In the earliest stages, there is a diffuse epitheliopathy with multiple intraepithelial linear infiltrates *(inset).* These linear infiltrates often form dendritic patterns. At this stage, *Acanthamoeba* keratitis is often misdiagnosed as herpes simplex keratitis. Similar to herpes simplex keratitis, it may have a waxing and waning course and may respond favorably to topical corticosteroids. The diagnosis of *Acanthamoeba* keratitis must be made early, as in this patient, since the prognosis is markedly improved with early detection.

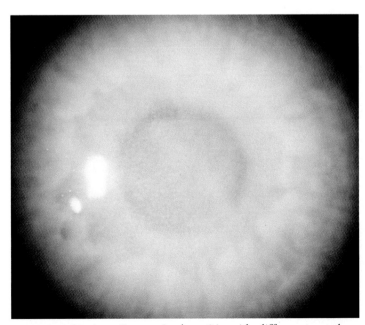

FIGURE 10-67 *Acanthamoeba* keratitis with diffuse stromal infiltration.

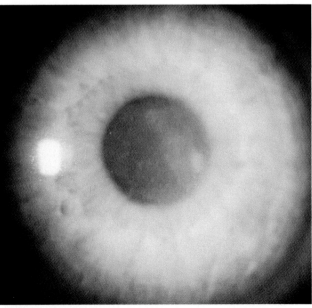

FIGURE 10-68 ***Same patient as in Figure 10-67.*** This is the appearance of the eye after 5 months of treatment.

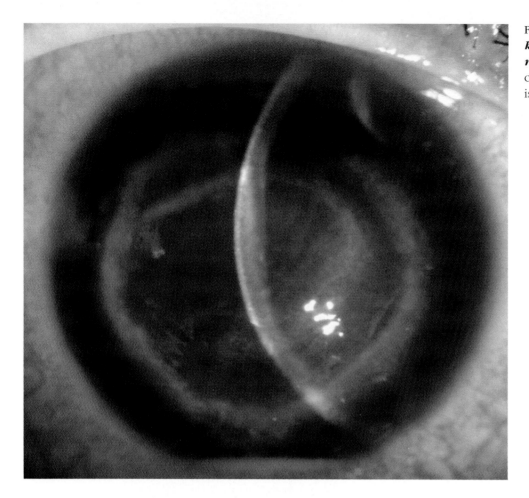

FIGURE 10-69 *Acanthamoeba keratitis with a characteristic ring infiltrate.* The central cornea is edematous, and there is a layered hypopyon.

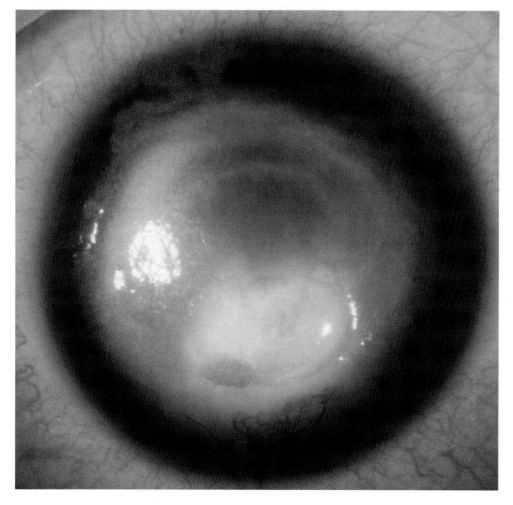

FIGURE 10-70 *Same patient as in Figure 10-69.* The disease progressed despite 4 months of treatment. This patient eventually needed a penetrating keratoplasty.

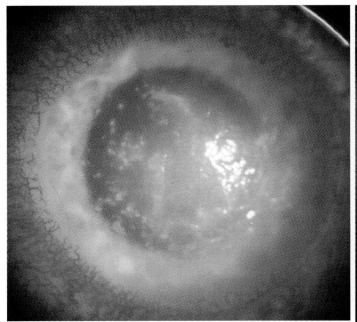

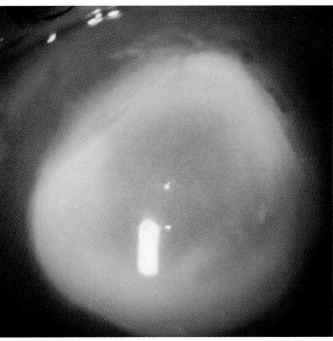

FIGURE 10-71 *Diffuse Acanthamoeba keratitis with scleritis.* Severe pain usually occurs with both scleritis and keratitis. Early epithelial involvement does not produce severe pain.

FIGURE 10-72 *Severe case of Acanthamoeba keratitis, unresponsive to treatment.* This case was complicated by topical anesthetic abuse.

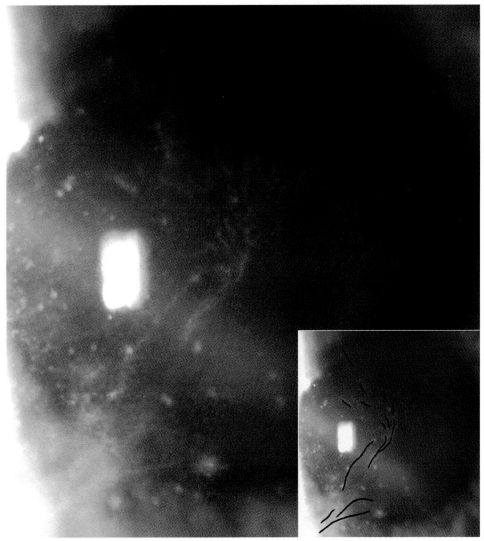

FIGURE 10-73 *Acanthamoeba keratitis with radial neuritis.* This finding may precede advanced stromal keratitis and is highly suggestive of *Acanthamoeba* infection. It usually begins centrally and progresses peripherally toward the limbus. The inset is a minification of the entire figure. The black lines were drawn to emphasize the pattern of infiltration.

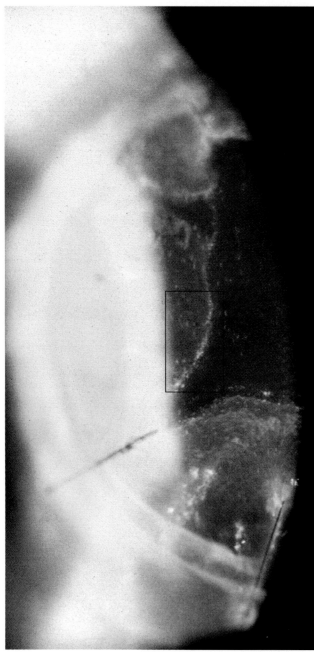

FIGURE 10-74 *Acanthamoeba keratitis.* This patient presented with irregular epithelial lines *(box)* 6 months after penetrating keratoplasty for *Acanthamoeba* infection. Initially these lines were felt to be an epithelial rejection; however, when they failed to respond to topical corticosteroids, a scraping confirmed the diagnosis of recurrent *Acanthamoeba* infection in the graft.

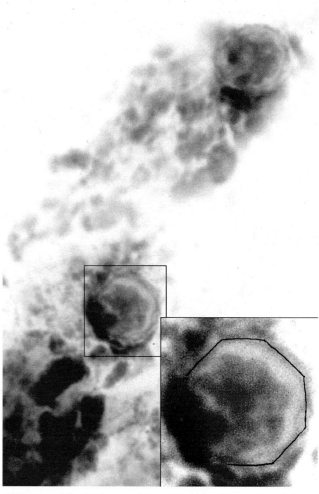

FIGURE 10-75 *Polygonal Acanthamoeba cysts with large nuclei and dark nucleoli.* The cysts have a hexagonal shape *(inset).* When the *Acanthamoeba* infection is in the epithelium (see Figures 10-66 and 10-74), a superficial scraping of the involved areas often yields cysts easily visible with hematoxylin and eosin or Gram stain. Once the organism is in the corneal stroma, it can be difficult to recover without a corneal biopsy. Culture on a nonnutrient agar plate overlaid with *Escherichia coli* bacteria can definitively establish the diagnosis.

CHAPTER 11

Interstitial Keratitis

Interstitial keratitis is a nonnecrotizing inflammation of the corneal stroma often associated with vascularization. There may be stromal infiltrates or stromal edema. Historically, the most common etiology for interstitial keratitis was syphilis; however, with improved prenatal screening, this cause of interstitial keratitis has become exceedingly rare.

Syphilitic Interstitial Keratitis

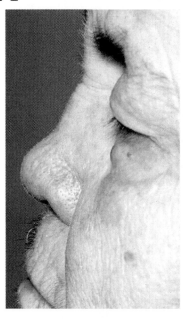

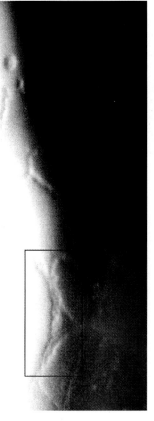

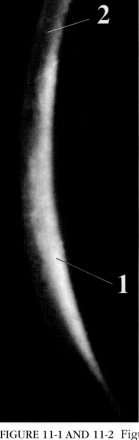

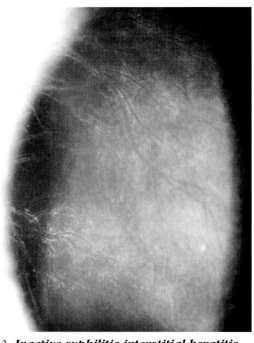

FIGURE 11-3 *Inactive syphilitic interstitial keratitis with ghost vessels and diffuse corneal scarring.* Some of the vessels actually transmit a very small column of blood.

FIGURE 11-5 Inactive syphilitic interstitial keratitis with nets of Descemet's proliferation.

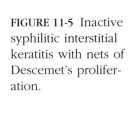

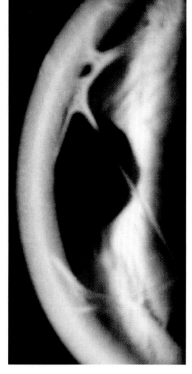

FIGURE 11-1 AND 11-2 Figure 11-1 *(above left)* shows congenital syphilitic facies, with prominence of the maxillary bone and saddle nose deformity. Figure 11-2 *(above)* is an example of inactive interstitial keratitis. Posterior stromal scarring *(1)* and ghost vessels *(2)* are seen.

FIGURE 11-4 Inactive syphilitic interstitial keratitis with proliferation of Descemet's membrane *(box).*

Nonsyphilitic Interstitial Keratitis

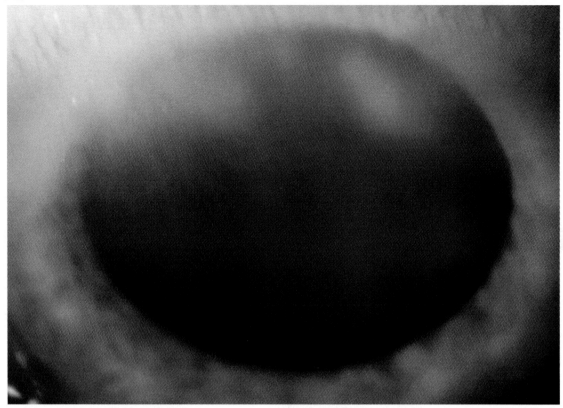

FIGURE 11-6 ***Cogan's syndrome.*** This consists of interstitial keratitis, vertigo, and hearing loss. The interstitial keratitis usually begins in the peripheral cornea with round, white stromal opacities. It is important to recognize this diagnosis because early treatment with systemic corticosteroids may prevent permanent hearing loss. Approximately 25% of patients with Cogan's syndrome have evidence of polyarteritis nodosa.

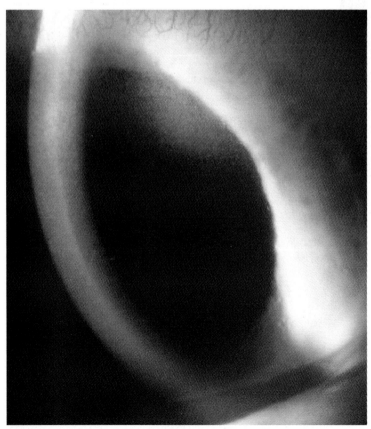

FIGURE 11-7 A slit beam view of peripheral infiltrates in Cogan's syndrome.

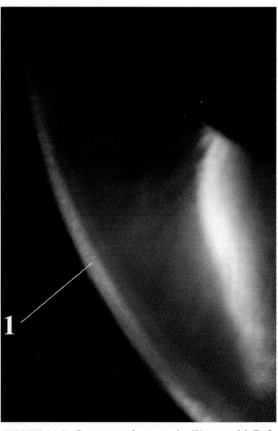

FIGURE 11-8 ***Same patient as in Figure 11-7, 2 months later.*** New inflammation is seen inferiorly (1).

CHAPTER 12

Noninfectious Keratopathy

This chapter discusses noninfectious causes of corneal pathology. Most of these disorders relate to problems with the corneal surface. Some, such as neurotrophic keratopathy, exposure keratopathy, and radiation keratopathy, require aggressive treatment or progressive corneal ulceration may ensue.

Recurrent Erosion Syndrome

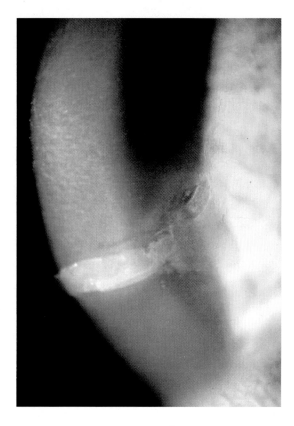

FIGURE 12-1 *Recurrent erosion syndrome.* This is characterized by the sudden onset of ocular pain that often awakens the patient from sleep, but the symptoms can occur at any time. It is associated with a history of prior trauma in the involved eye and may also be accompanied by corneal dystrophies, the two most common being epithelial basement membrane dystrophy and lattice corneal dystrophy. The pathogenesis of traumatic recurrent erosion relates to thickened basement membrane with poor hemidesmosomal attachment to the anterior corneal stroma. In the acute stages the epithelium may be irregular and loose (as seen here) or absent.

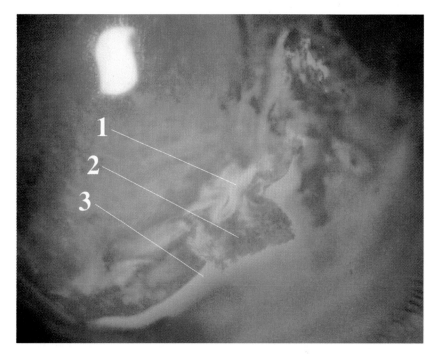

FIGURE 12-2 *Posttraumatic recurrent erosion in same patient as in Figure 12-1.* Areas of epithelial loss (positive staining) *(1)*, lack of fluorescein over elevated epithelium (negative staining) *(2)*, and pooling of fluorescein *(3)* are seen.

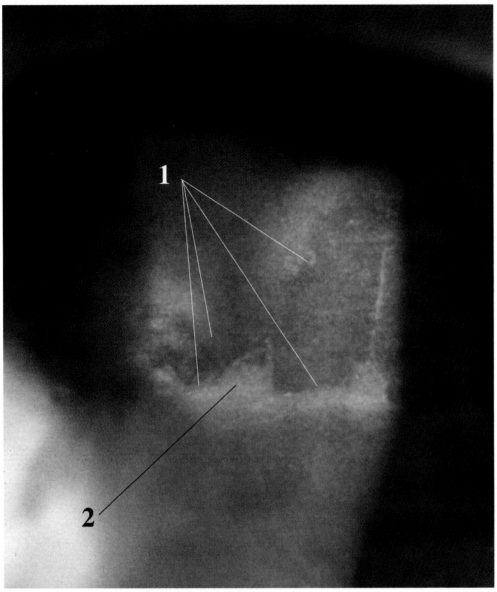

FIGURE 12-3 *Posttraumatic recurrent erosion.* Surrounding the edges of the erosion (1) is a white infiltrate (2). These infiltrates are usually sterile but occasionally may be associated with infections.

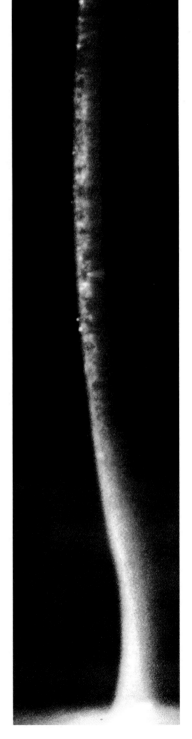

FIGURE 12-4 *Posttraumatic recurrent erosion.* This thin slit beam view demonstrates anterior stromal haze, which is often associated with chronic recurrent erosions.

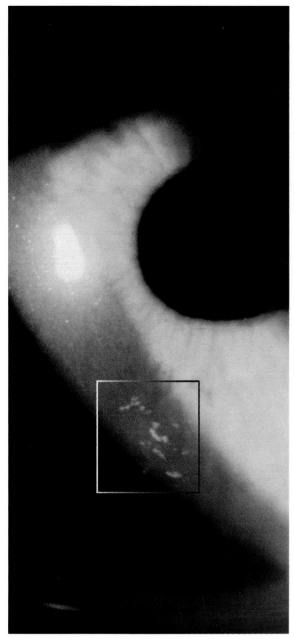

FIGURE 12-5 Direct view of posttraumatic recurrent erosion with intraepithelial debris *(box)*.

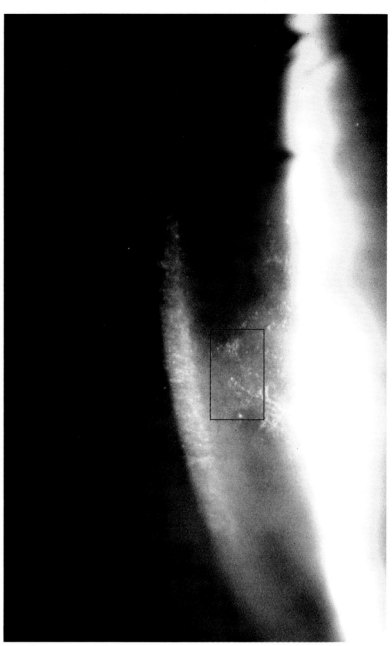

FIGURE 12-6 Indirect view of posttraumatic recurrent erosion with intraepithelial debris *(box)*.

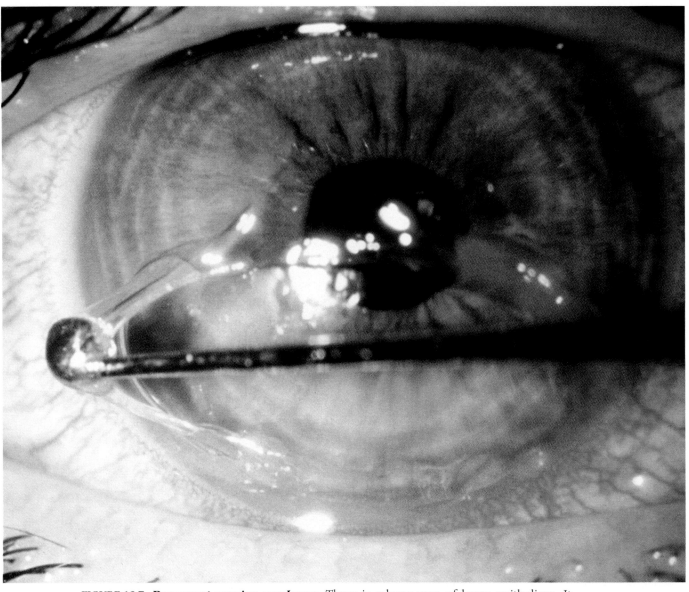

FIGURE 12-7 **Recurrent erosion syndrome.** There is a large area of loose epithelium. It extends well beyond the region of the acute erosion and can sometimes be delineated with a moist cotton swab.

Filamentary Keratitis

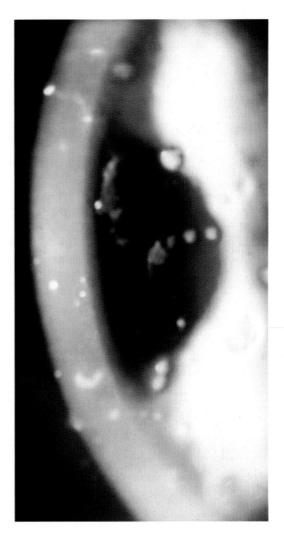

FIGURE 12-8 *Filamentary keratitis.* Filaments are accumulations of mucus attached to loose epithelium. As opposed to free mucus in the tear film, filaments cause a foreign body sensation, remain adherent to the cornea with each blink, and cause a small epithelial defect when removed. Filaments are associated with various conditions, including patching of the eyelids (as seen here), ptosis, dry eye, recurrent erosion, fifth nerve paresis, seventh nerve paresis, chronic bullous keratopathy, superior limbic keratoconjunctivitis, herpes simplex keratitis, and toxicity from topical medications. Administration of 10% acetylcysteine (Mucomyst) dissolves the mucus and can be effective in the treatment of chronic filamentary keratitis.

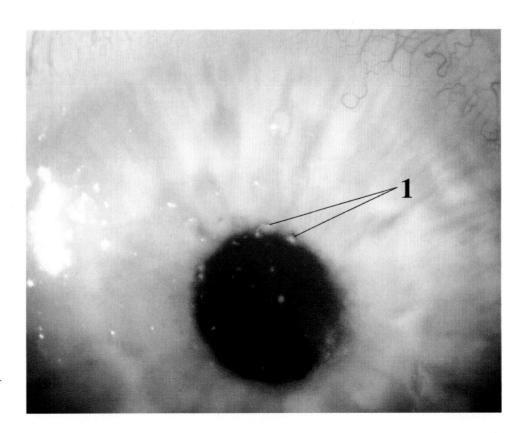

FIGURE 12-9 *Filamentary keratitis.* This patient had a third nerve palsy and resultant ptosis. There are small (micro) filaments *(1)* on the cornea.

Thygeson's Superficial Punctate Keratitis

Thygeson's superficial punctate keratitis is a chronic, usually bilateral disorder characterized by focal epithelial lesions without stromal involvement. It can affect all ages but is more common in children and young adults. Patients complain mainly of foreign body sensation and photophobia. The conjunctiva is uninflammed.

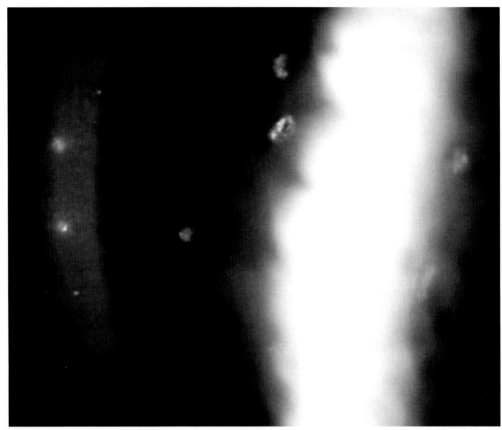

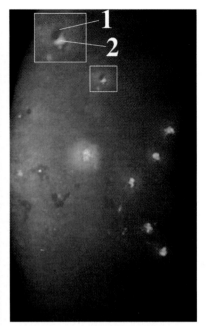

FIGURE 12-10 Direct and indirect view of Thygeson's superficial punctate keratitis.

FIGURE 12-11 *Fluorescein staining of Thygeson's superficial punctate keratitis.* Dark areas where fluorescein rolls off elevated edges of lesions (negative staining) *(1)* and elevated white pearls evident with central fluorescein staining (positive staining) *(2)* are shown.

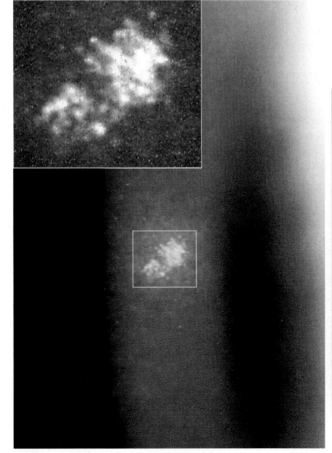

FIGURE 12-12 Early Thygeson's superficial punctate keratitis with elevated pearls *(inset).*

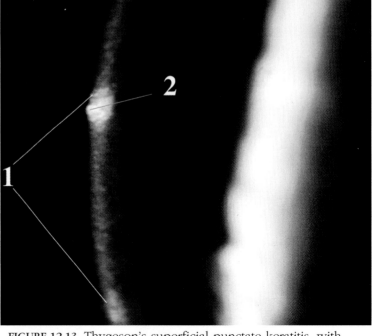

FIGURE 12-13 Thygeson's superficial punctate keratitis, with subepithelial *(1)* and elevated pearly *(2)* components.

Neurotrophic Keratopathy

FIGURE 12-14 *Neurotrophic keratopathy.* This is the right eye of a patient with Prader-Willi syndrome and congenital insensitivity to pain. He developed a neurotrophic corneal ulcer in the eye at age 2 years. There is an inferior paracentral epithelial defect.

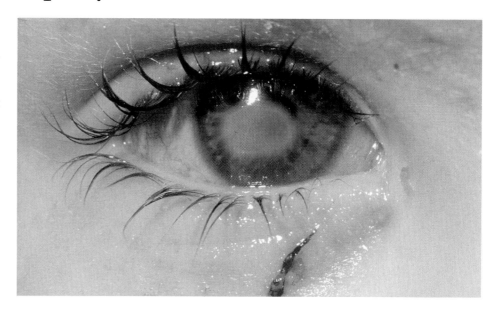

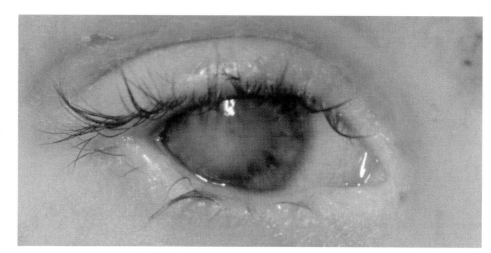

FIGURE 12-15 *Same patient as in Figure 12-14, with a corneal scar.* The epithelium has healed after treatment with a tarsorrhaphy, punctal occlusion, and aggressive lubrication.

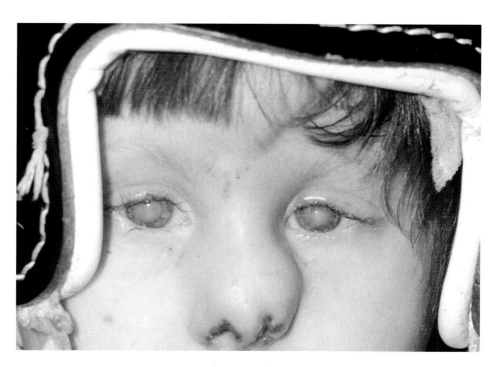

FIGURE 12-16 *Same patient as in Figures 12-14 and 12-15.* There are bilateral corneal scars. The nose deformity is from repetitive trauma. The protective helmet is to prevent skull fractures.

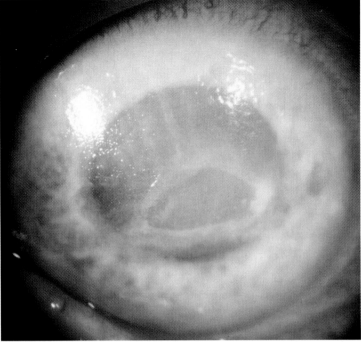

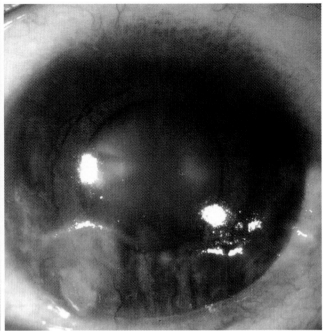

FIGURE 12-17 *Neurotrophic ulcer after surgical intervention for trigeminal neuralgia.* Characteristically, the ulcer is in the inferior paracentral cornea and has thick, rolled epithelial edges. Tarsorrhaphy is often needed to prevent further ulceration and perforation.

FIGURE 12-18 *Neurotrophic keratopathy.* This patient had a chronic inferior keratitis and corneal thinning. There was absent sensation in the ipsilateral distribution of cranial nerve five, divisions one through three. Neuroimaging disclosed an acoustic neuroma.

Dellen

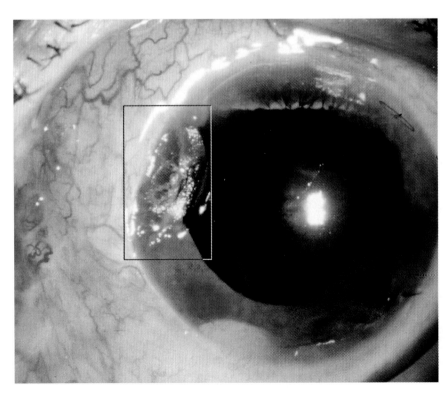

FIGURE 12-19 *Dellen.* These are localized areas of corneal thinning with intact epithelium and lack of corneal infiltration. They occur next to areas of elevated tissue and are caused by localized drying of the cornea. The dellen in the box was caused by an elevation of the conjunctiva after scleral buckle surgery. The lesion resolved when the conjunctival swelling abated.

Neurogenic Keratopathy

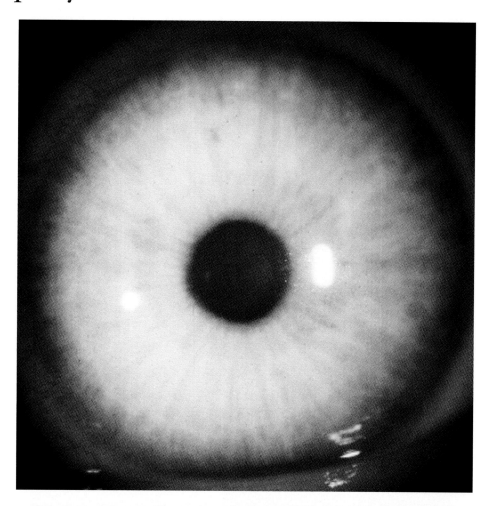

FIGURE 12-20 **Neurogenic keratopathy.** This 34-year-old man noticed decreased vision in his right eye when he went hunting during the winter. This is the appearance of the cornea at room temperature.

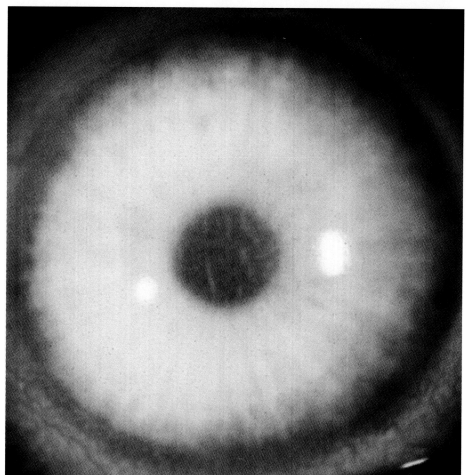

FIGURE 12-21 **Same patient as in Figure 12-20.** After exposure to a cold environment (a meat freezer), there was diffuse stromal edema with Descemet's folds, as seen here. The etiology was related to trigeminal nerve dysfunction caused by a meningioma.

Exposure Keratopathy

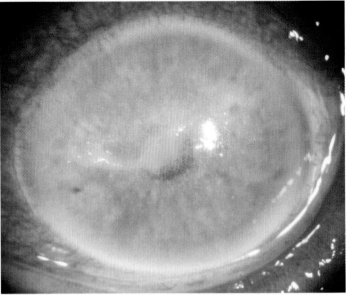

FIGURE 12-22 *Chronic corneal exposure from thyroid eye disease.* Exophthalmos and lid retraction contributed to this complication.

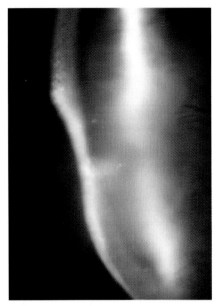

FIGURE 12-23 *Chronic progressive external ophthalmoplegia.* This patient developed exposure keratopathy, thinning, and scarring. Predisposing factors included overcorrection after ptosis surgery and lack of a Bell's phenomena with eyelid closure.

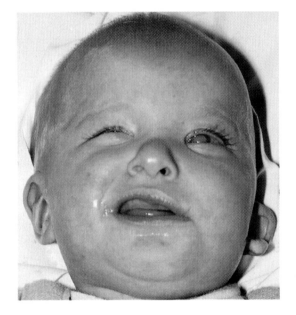

FIGURE 12-24 Exposure corneal ulcer in an infant from a left seventh nerve paralysis.

Radiation Keratopathy

FIGURE 12-25 *Radiation keratopathy after radiation treatment for a malignant fibrous histiocytoma of the orbit.* The cornea is scarred and vascularized. There is mucus in the tear film from an associated dry eye. The patient also had radiation retinopathy.

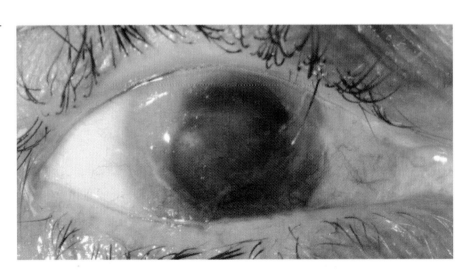

Toxicity

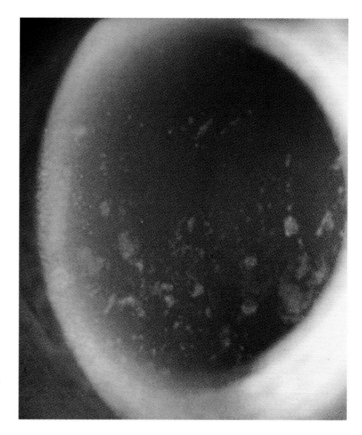

FIGURE 12-26 ***Toxic reaction.*** It is common to see a diffuse irregular epitheliopathy after topical anesthetic instillation. The surface is most affected in the interpalpebral region.

Factitious Disease

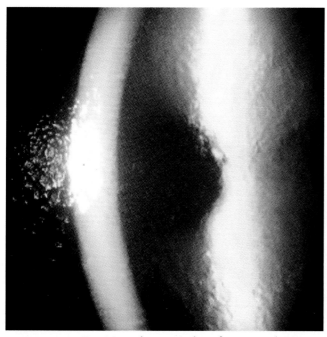

FIGURE 12-27 Factitious keratopathy after topical anesthetic abuse.

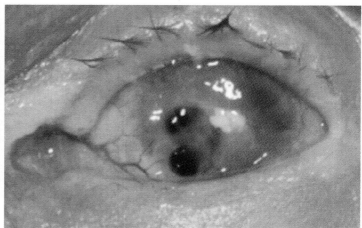

FIGURE 12-28 ***Factitious disease.*** A retired physician admitted to using topical lidocaine in his left eye. The corneal stroma is necrotic, and there are two areas of perforation with protruding uvea.

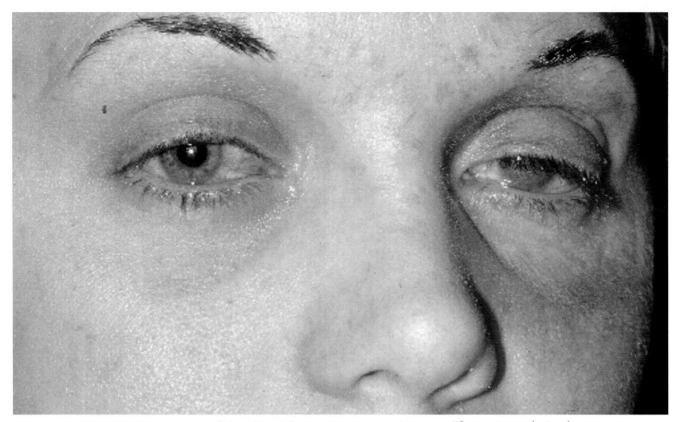

FIGURE 12-29 *Scarring of the skin, lids, conjunctiva, and cornea.* The patient admitted under hypnosis that she was putting caustic chemicals in her eyes.

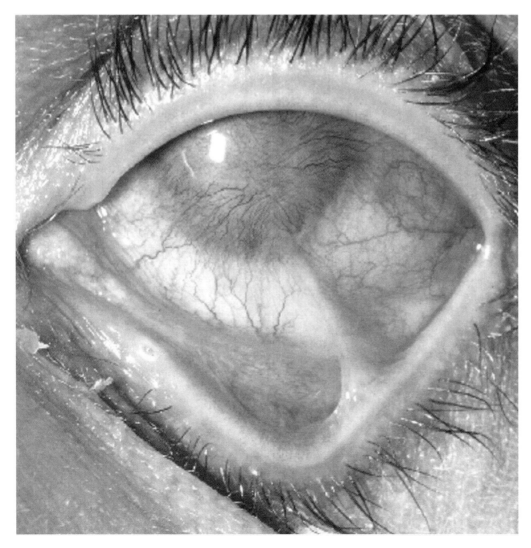

FIGURE 12-30 *Same patient as in Figure 12-29.* There is extensive conjunctival and corneal scarring.

Immunologic Disorders Of The Cornea

Some immunologic disorders are unique to the cornea, but many are associated with systemic diseases. The abundance of collagen and blood vessels in the sclera and corneal limbus predispose the sclera and cornea to manifestations of collagen vascular diseases. Some of these disorders, such as rheumatoid arthritis, affect the cornea after long-standing systemic disease, whereas others, such as Wegener's granulomatosis and polyarteritis nodosa, may have their initial manifestations in the sclera and cornea.

Rheumatoid Arthritis

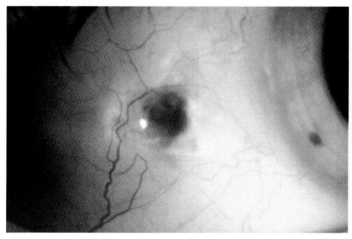

FIGURE 13-1 *Scleromalacia perforans.* This is a slow thinning of the sclera unassociated with pain or episodes of acute inflammation. This patient with rheumatoid arthritis was noted to have an early area of scleromalacia perforans. The sclera is excavated in this region, and the underlying uvea is well seen.

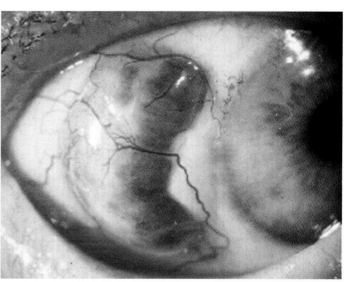

FIGURE 13-2 *Advanced scleromalacia perforans in rheumatoid arthritis.* The sclera is diffusely thin, and uveal tissue protrudes as a staphyloma. Minor trauma can be associated with ocular perforation.

FIGURE 13-3 *Necrotizing scleritis in rheumatoid arthritis.* In contrast to scleromalacia perforans, these lesions are painful and are associated with acute inflammation. Systemic immunosuppression is usually required to treat these patients.

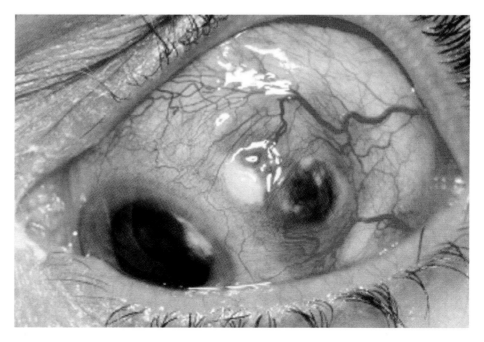

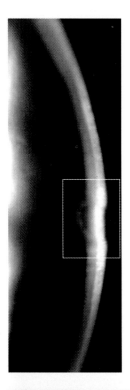

FIGURE 13-4 **Central corneal ulceration in rheumatoid arthritis.** These central ulcers *(box)* tend to occur in extremely dry eyes and can progress very rapidly to perforation without significant pain.

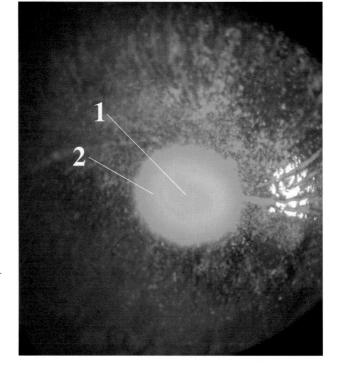

FIGURE 13-5 **Same patient as in Figure 13-4.** An area of true fluorescein staining devoid of all epithelium *(1),* and an area of unhealthy epithelium, which soaks up fluorescein and stains less intensely *(2),* are shown.

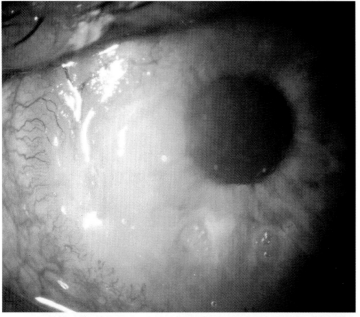

FIGURE 13-6 **Peripheral ulceration in rheumatoid arthritis.** In contrast to the central ulcer just seen, peripheral ulcers in rheumatoid arthritis usually occur at the edge of peripheral corneal vascularization. These eyes tend to be less dry than those with central ulceration, and there is usually an associated scleritis with some degree of pain.

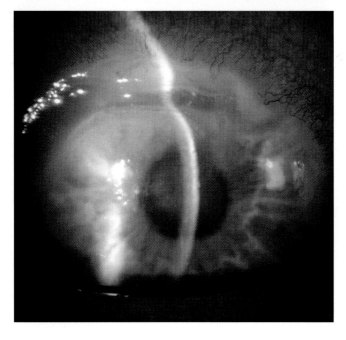

FIGURE 13-7 **Peripheral corneal ulcer in rheumatoid arthritis.** The cornea is thinned superiorly at the edge of a region of corneal vascularization. These ulcers may progress to perforation and often require some form of systemic immunosuppression for treatment.

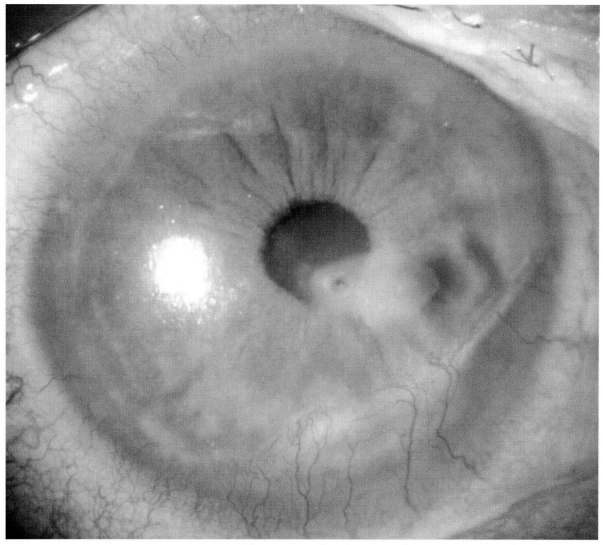

FIGURE 13-8 ***Rheumatoid arthritis.*** There is peripheral scarring from previous peripheral ulcerations. In addition, there is a central ulceration with perforation.

FIGURE 13-9 ***Same patient as in Figure 13-8.*** The area of perforation is Seidel positive.

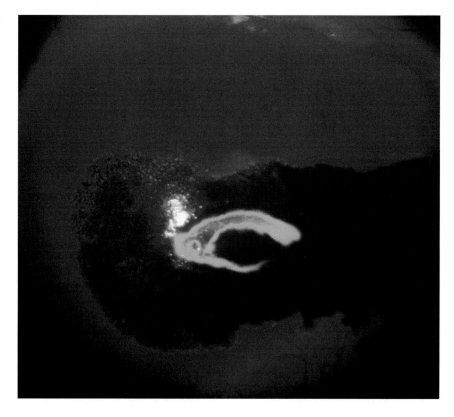

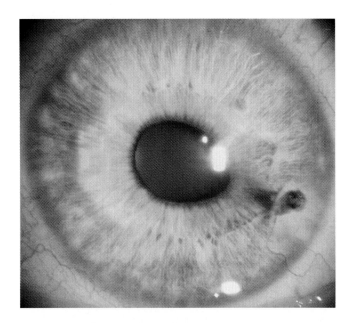

FIGURE 13-10 **Rheumatoid arthritis.** This patient had an old peripheral perforation that plugged with iris tissue. The epithelium healed over the iris and a corneal scar formed.

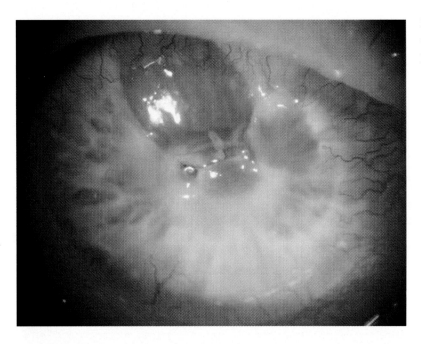

FIGURE 13-11 **Rheumatoid arthritis.** There is extensive melting of the central cornea with perforation.

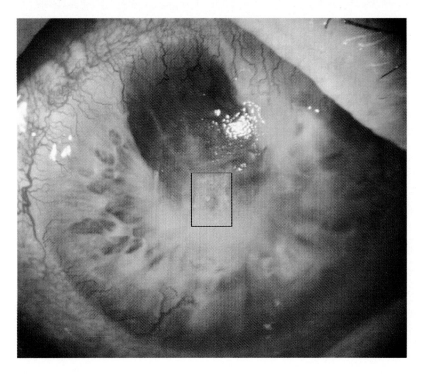

FIGURE 13-12 **Same patient as in Figure 13-11, with tissue adhesive closing the perforation site.** Eventually epithelium and vascular tissue will grow beneath the glue *(box)* to heal the area of perforation, and the glue will become dislodged.

Nonrheumatoid Collagen Vascular Disease

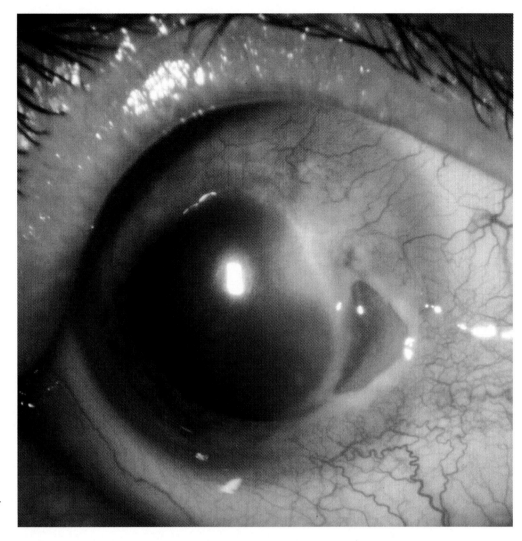

FIGURE 13-13 **Polyarteritis nodosa.** This systemic vasculitis affects small and medium-sized arteries. Anterior segment manifestations include episcleritis, diffuse scleritis, necrotizing scleritis, and peripheral necrotizing keratitis (as seen here). Ocular findings may be the initial manifestation of this disease.

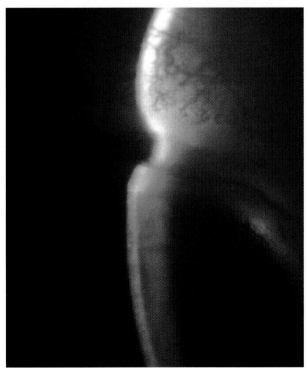

FIGURE 13-14 **Systemic lupus erythematosis.** Marginal corneal ulcer in a patient with systemic lupus erythematosus.

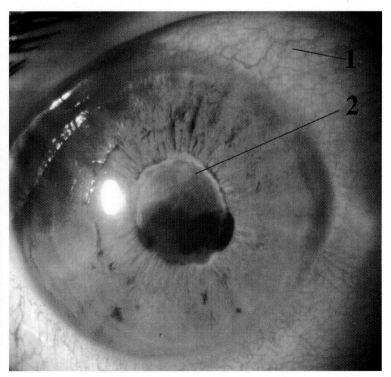

FIGURE 13-15 **Systemic lupus erythematosus.** This patient has scleritis (1) and an associated uveitis with a fibrinous pupillary membrane (2).

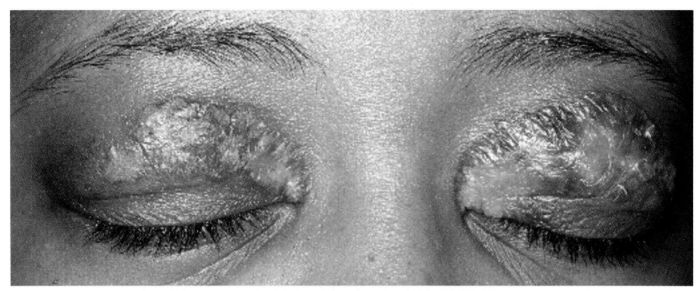

FIGURE 13-16 ***Discoid lupus erythematosus.*** Eyelid involvement may be the initial manifestation. The lesions are characteristically erythematous, raised plaques with superficial scaling. A small percentage of patients with discoid lupus may progress to systemic lupus, and 20% of patients with systemic lupus may have the skin lesions of discoid lupus.

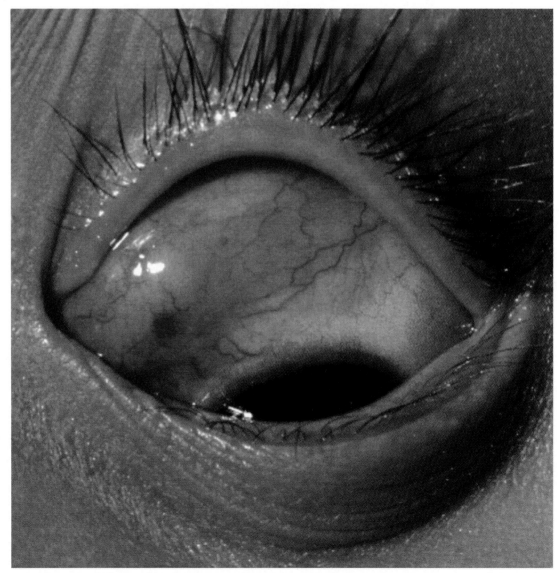

FIGURE 13-17 ***Wegener's granulomatosis.*** This necrotizing granulomatous reaction frequently involves the upper and lower respiratory tracts and the kidneys. The initial sign in this patient with Wegener's granulomatosis was a conjunctival mass.

FIGURE 13-18 *Necrotizing scleritis in Wegener's granulomatosis.* There is central absence of scleral tissue, and the uvea is easily visualized. Surrounding this central area is a ring of avascular, necrotic sclera. The conjunctival epithelium over this area is absent.

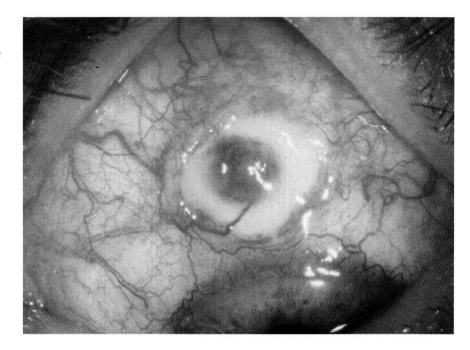

FIGURE 13-19 Same patient as in Figure 13-18, 2 months after treatment with systemic cyclophosphamide.

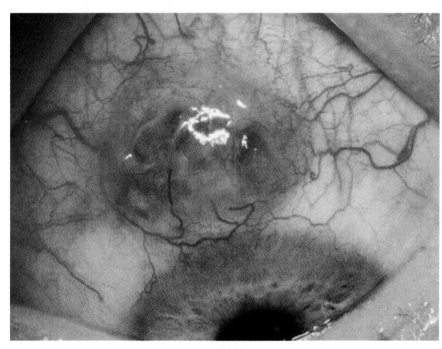

FIGURE 13-20 *Same patient as in Figures 13-18 and 13-19, 4 months after treatment with systemic cyclophosphamide.* The conjunctival epithelium is healed, and the sclera is well vascularized and scarred.

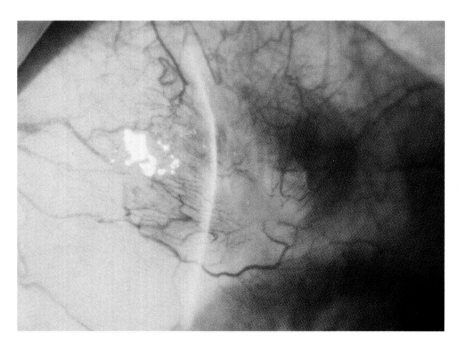

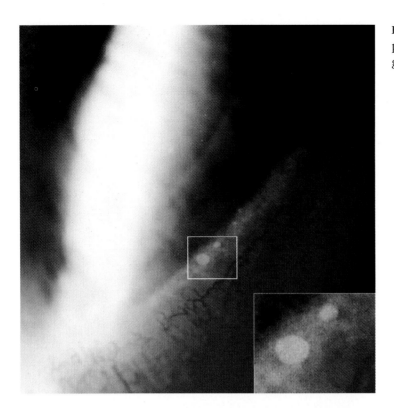

FIGURE 13-21 *Wegener's granulomatosis.* Early peripheral corneal infiltration *(inset)* in Wegener's granulomatosis.

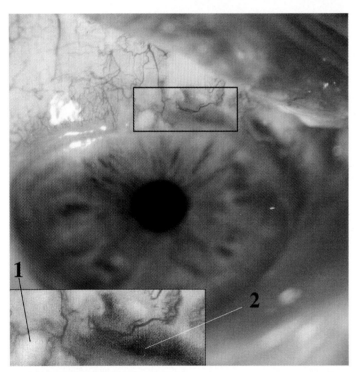

FIGURE 13-22 *Wegener's granulomatosis with a limbal ulcer (inset).* There is an area of active infiltration *(1)*; the cornea is thinned in this region *(2).*

1

2

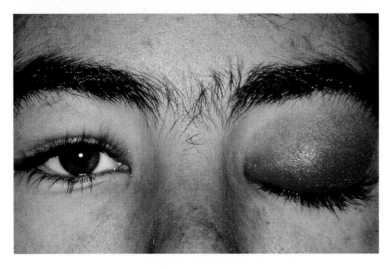

FIGURE 13-23 *Dermatomyositis.* This is an inflammatory disease of skeletal muscles associated with cutaneous lesions. A butterfly rash and violaceous discoloration may occur on the upper eyelids (heliotrope rash).

Staphylococcal Disease

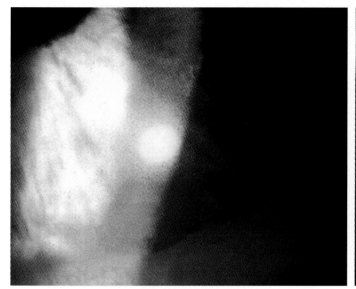

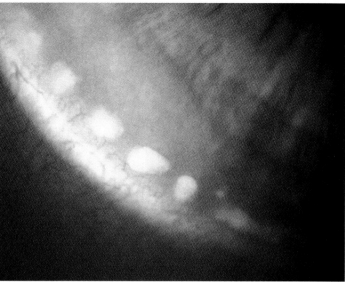

FIGURE 13-24 *Staphylococcal marginal infiltrate.* These infiltrates are hypersensitivity reactions to staphylococcal antigen. Characteristically, there is a clear area between the infiltrate and limbus. Patients often present with ocular pain and redness. These lesions respond well to topical corticosteroids.

FIGURE 13-25 Multiple staphylococcal marginal infiltrates near the limbus.

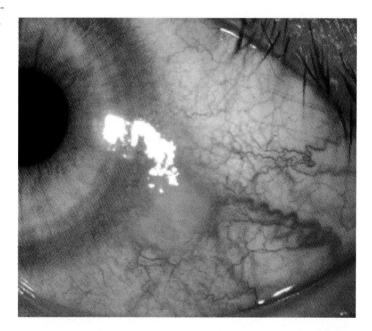

FIGURE 13-26 *Conjunctival phlyctenule.* A phlyctenule is a type-IV hypersensitivity reaction usually associated with a response to staphylococcal antigen; however, it can occur in the presence of tuberculosis. The word *phlycten* means "blister." These lesions start as an elevation of the conjunctiva, progressively become ulcerated, and eventually form a localized scar over a 2-week interval. Mild ocular discomfort can occur, and the symptoms are relieved by topical corticosteroids.

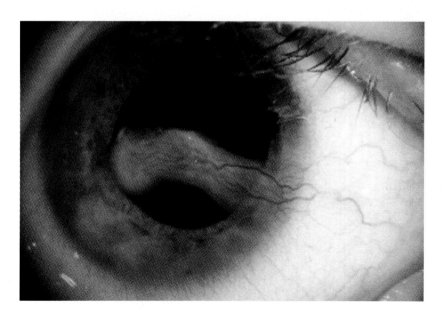

FIGURE 13-27 *Corneal phlyctenule.* These lesions can "march" across the cornea with progressive vascularization and scarring.

Mooren's Ulcer

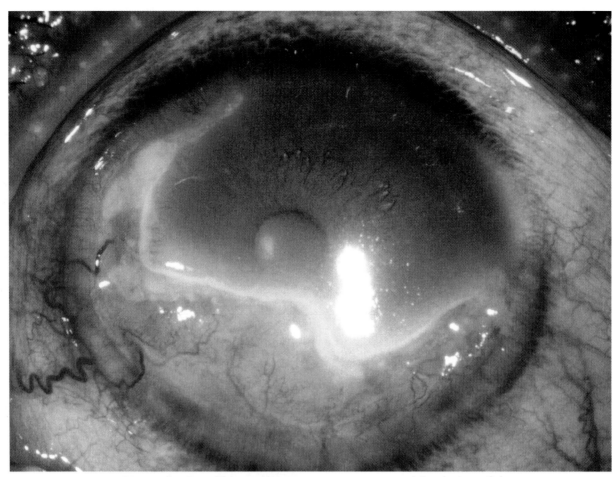

FIGURE 13-28 *Mooren's ulcer.* This condition presents as a necrotizing lesion of the cornea. It is a diagnosis of exclusion, since many other conditions can present somewhat similarly. It is characterized by corneal thinning and ulceration extending inward from the limbus centrally. The epithelium is absent in areas of active ulceration; however, there may be a vascularized pannus leading up to areas of active ulceration. Typically, there is an abrupt transition between involved and uninvolved cornea with an overhanging edge. The disease can sometimes be characterized by extreme pain.

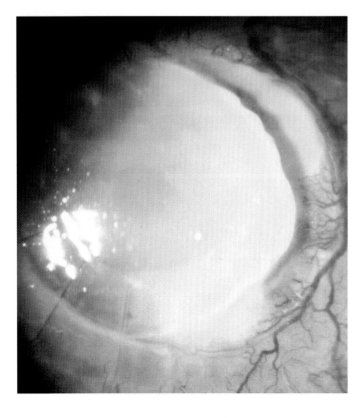

FIGURE 13-29 *Mooren's ulcer.* A penetrating keratoplasty was performed. There was recurrence of Mooren's ulcer in the cornea, with the characteristic overhanging edge between areas of involved and uninvolved cornea.

CHAPTER 14

Corneal Trauma

Because the cornea is the most powerful refractive element of the eye and one of the most sensitive tissues of the body, even minor injury can produce significant visual and symptomatic problems. Prompt diagnosis and appropriate treatment are essential.

Foreign Body, Mechanical, Thermal, and Radiation Trauma

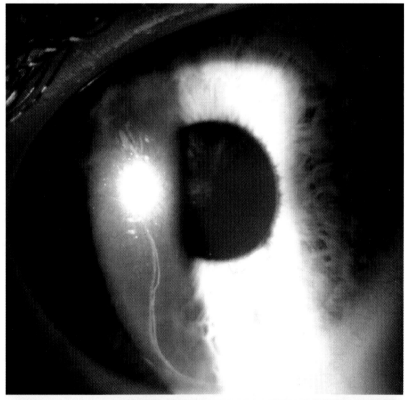

FIGURE 14-1 *Corneal abrasions.* These are common after minor trauma. Here a fingernail injury caused a vertically oriented abrasion.

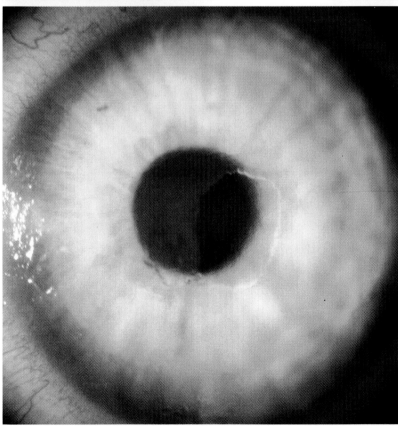

FIGURE 14-2 *Corneal abrasion after a chemical (detergent) injury.* Chemical injuries usually affect the interpalpebral region, since this area is the first to come in contact with the chemical. These defects usually heal rapidly with pressure patching and antibiotic ointments. If a secondary infection is suspected, treatment with frequent topical antibiotics rather than pressure patching should be initiated.

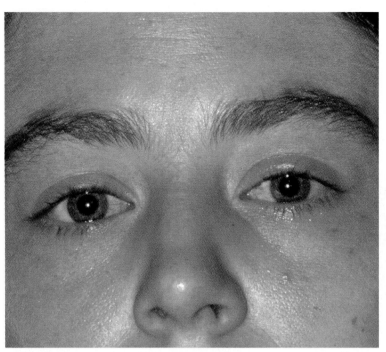

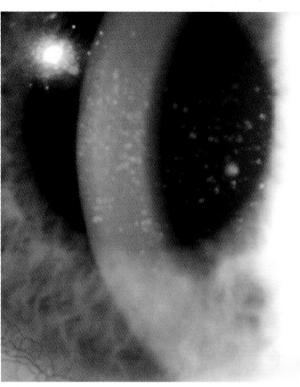

FIGURE 14-3 *Dermatitis and keratoconjunctivitis from ultraviolet sterilizing operating room equipment.* The reaction of the skin is similar to that seen after excessive exposure to sunlight (sunburn).

FIGURE 14-4 *Same patient as in Figure 14-3.* There is a diffuse punctate keratopathy caused by excessive exposure to ultraviolet light. The keratitis begins several hours after exposure and is extremely painful.

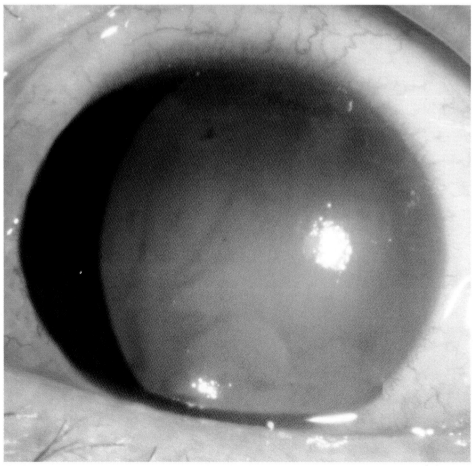

FIGURE 14-5 *Blunt trauma to the eye from an elastic cord.* There was a 360° iridodialysis, and the iris fell en bloc into the vitreous cavity. The lens was dislocated temporally and posteriorly.

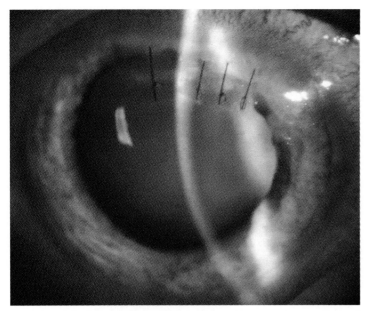

FIGURE 14-6 *Corneal laceration.* It has been re-approximated with 10-0 nylon sutures.

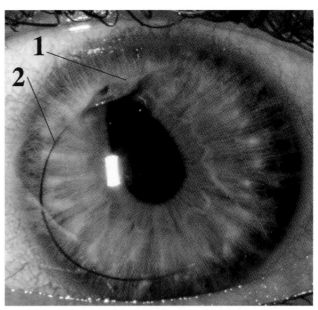

FIGURE 14-7 Acute corneal laceration with prolapsed iris and resultant peaked pupil *(1).* An eyelash has entered into the anterior chamber *(2).*

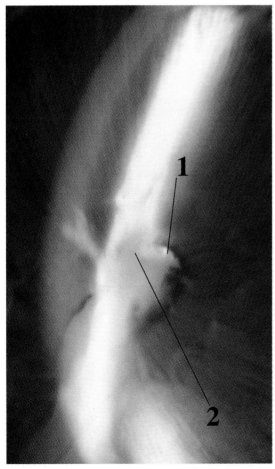

FIGURE 14-8 *Penetrating corneal trauma.* A central white cataract *(1)* is shown. Lens material and iris adhere to the posterior cornea *(2).*

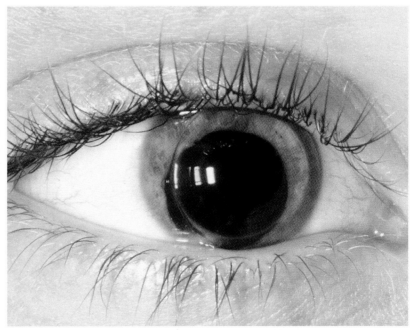

FIGURE 14-9 *Same patient as in Figure 14-8.* The postoperative appearance after corneal transplant, lensectomy, and vitrectomy is evident. The patient is wearing an aphakic contact lens.

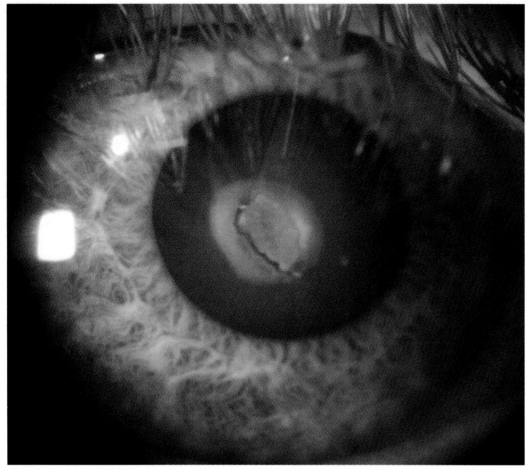

FIGURE 14-10 Necrotic corneal perforating wound from a stick injury in a 5-year-old boy.

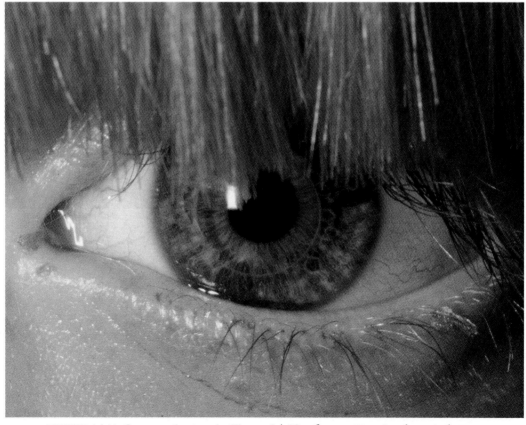

FIGURE 14-11 Same patient as in Figure 14-10, after penetrating keratoplasty.

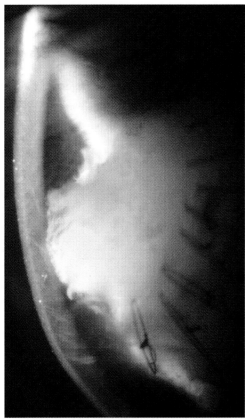

FIGURE 14-12 *Traumatic cataract and corneal laceration.* The lens material is against the corneal endothelium and was removed with a second operation.

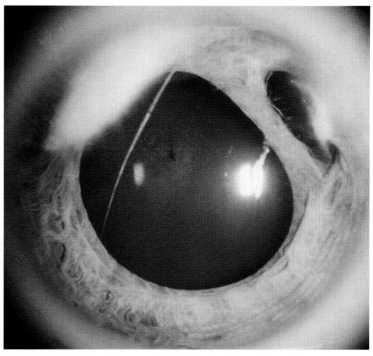

FIGURE 14-13 *Previous corneal laceration.* A scar is seen superiorly. There is a lash in the anterior chamber.

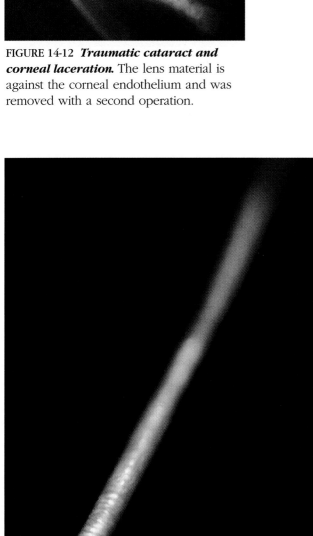

FIGURE 14-14 Same patient as in Figure 14-13, showing intraocular cilia wrapped in Descemet's proliferation.

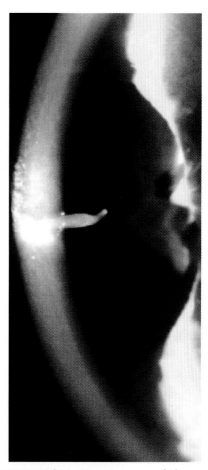

FIGURE 14-15 *Appearance of the cornea 12 years after a penetrating dart injury.* There is a wick of Descemet's proliferation extending from the posterior cornea. A localized traumatic cataract with posterior synechiae is present.

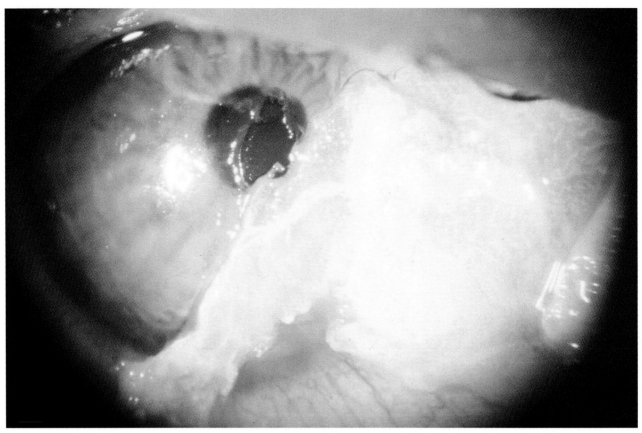

FIGURE 14-16 *Epoxy glue injury to the cornea.* Fortunately, the glue is usually stuck only to the epithelium and does not cause severe scarring.

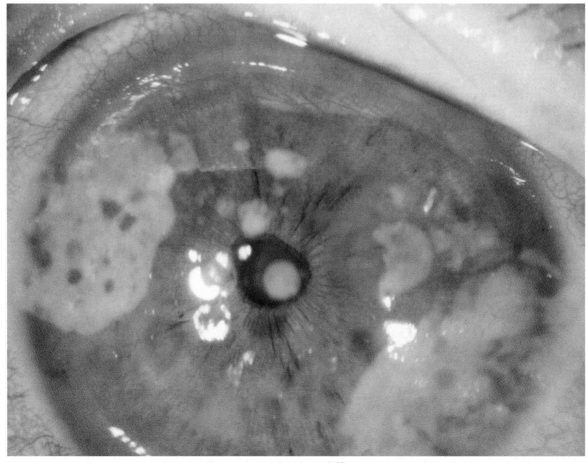

FIGURE 14-17 *Epoxy glue on the cornea.* This is a different patient than that seen in Figure 14-16.

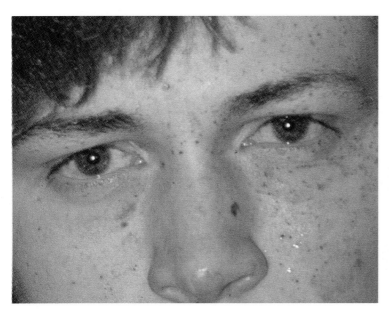

FIGURE 14-18 *Multiple skin and corneal foreign bodies after a blast injury.* The superficial foreign bodies should be carefully removed; deep foreign bodies may need to be left behind.

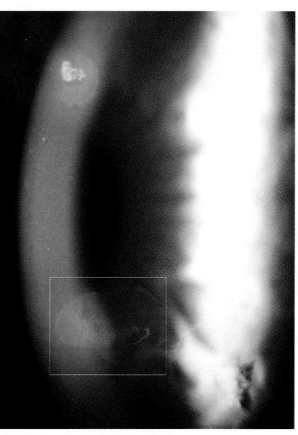

FIGURE 14-19 *Same patient as in Figure 14-18.* An anterior corneal foreign body has been removed. There is a traumatic endothelial ring *(right side of box).* The ring is formed from a concussive effect of the foreign body and is composed of swollen endothelial cells and deposits of fibrin and leukocytes on the endothelium. The ring resolved several days after the injury.

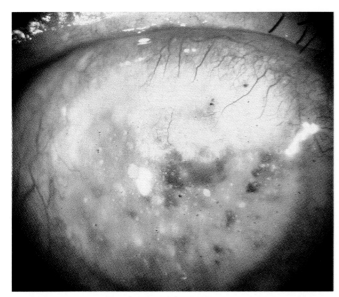

FIGURE 14-20 *Multiple foreign bodies in the cornea and conjunctiva after an old blast injury.* The cornea has diffuse scarring and vascularization.

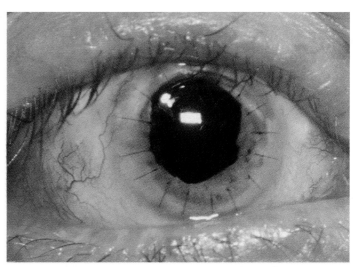

FIGURE 14-21 Same patient as in Figure 14-20, after penetrating keratoplasty.

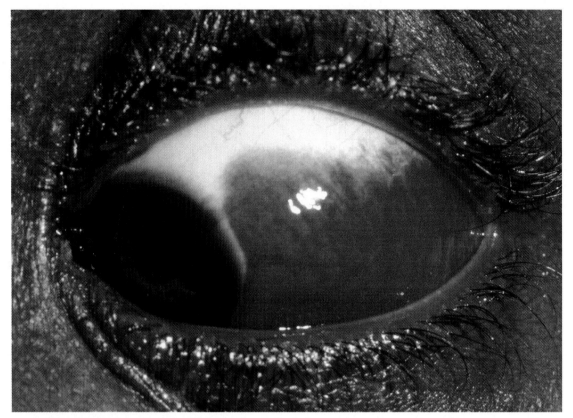

FIGURE 14-22 *Subconjunctival hemorrhage.* Such hemorrhages can occur after trauma, with Valsalva maneuvers or coughing, or from a broken blood vessel caused by hypertension. Rarely, systemic hematologic disorders can be manifested by subconjunctival hemorrhages. Most commonly, they are spontaneous, with no identifiable cause.

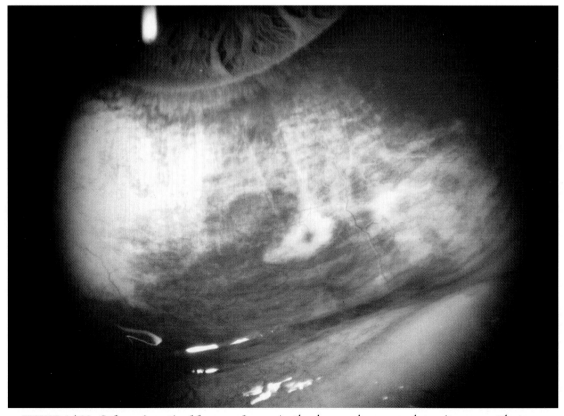

FIGURE 14-23 *Subconjunctival hemorrhage.* As the hemorrhage resolves, it may settle to the most dependent area of the eye and assume a yellow color as the blood is broken down and absorbed.

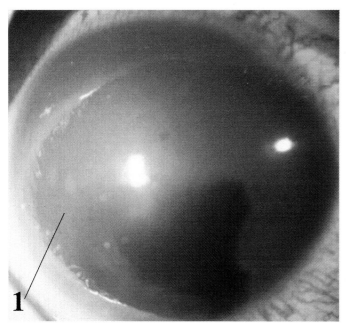

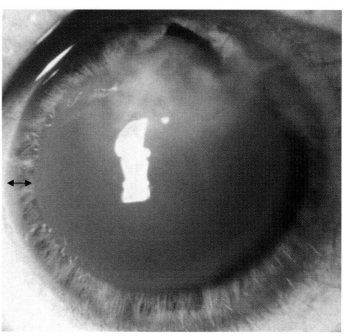

FIGURE 14-24 **Early blood staining in the cornea caused by a traumatic hyphema.** This appears as a deep brown discoloration of the posterior cornea *(1)*. Corneal blood staining is an indication for surgical removal of the hyphema.

FIGURE 14-25 **Late corneal blood staining.** With time the blood in the cornea becomes yellow. The blood clears over several years, beginning at the limbus and progressing centrally.

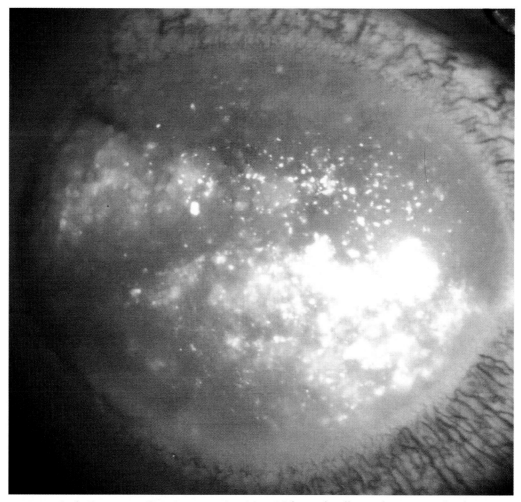

FIGURE 14-26 **Long-standing intraocular blood.** The red cell membranes are broken down into cholesterol. Multiple refractile crystals of cholesterol can form within the eye (cholesterolosis bulbi).

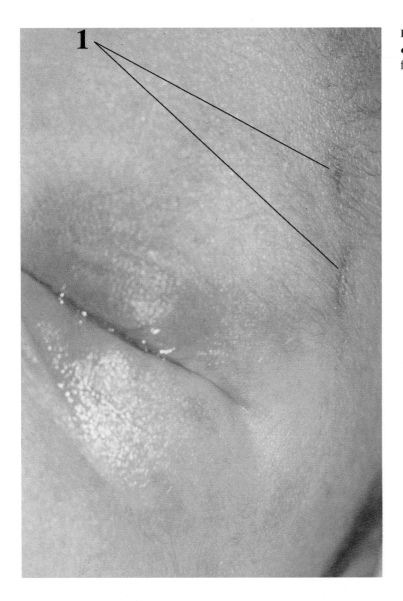

FIGURE 14-27 *Forceps injury in a 1-day-old infant.* There are skin lesions from the forceps *(1)*.

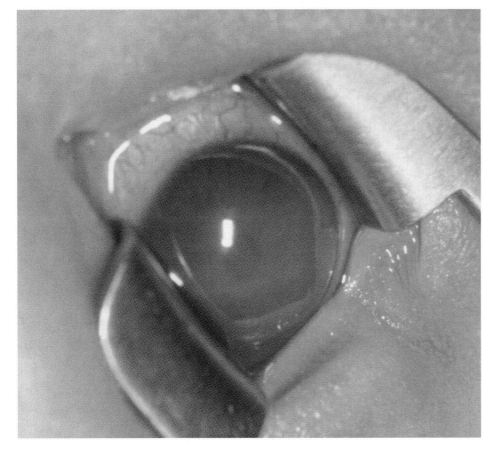

FIGURE 14-28 *Same patient as in Figure 14-27.* There is acute corneal edema from the forceps injury.

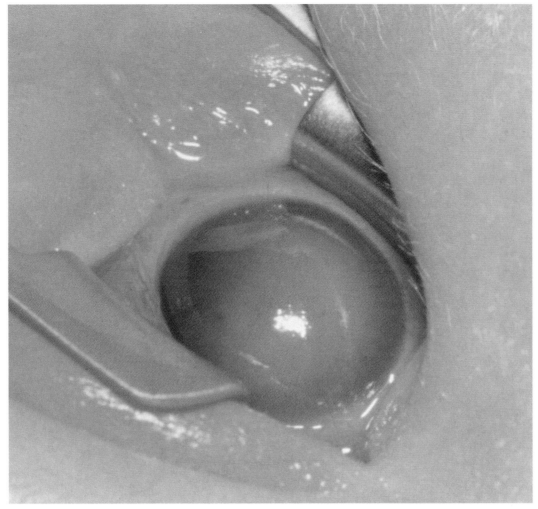

FIGURE 14-29 *A second case of forceps injury in a 1-day-old infant.* Again, there is acute corneal edema.

FIGURE 14-30 *Same patient as in Figure 14-29, at age 3 months.* The central cornea has cleared, and there are vertically oriented breaks in Descemet's membrane *(1)*.

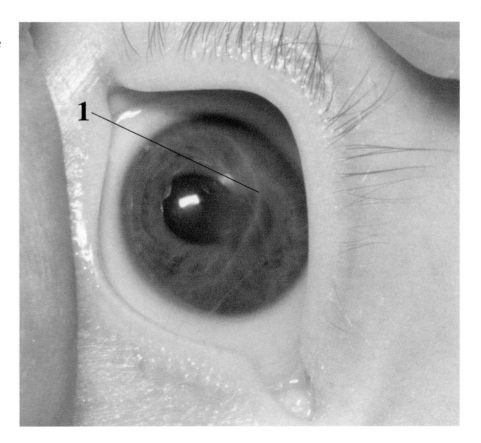

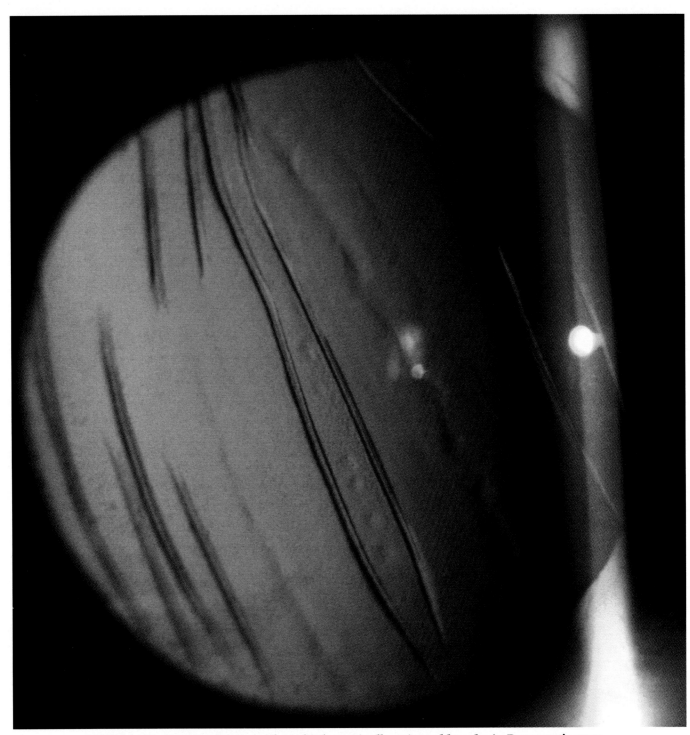

FIGURE 14-31 *Forceps injury with multiple vertically oriented breaks in Descemet's membrane.* The breaks have a railroad track appearance on retro-illumination. Endothelial cells migrate into the area of injury.

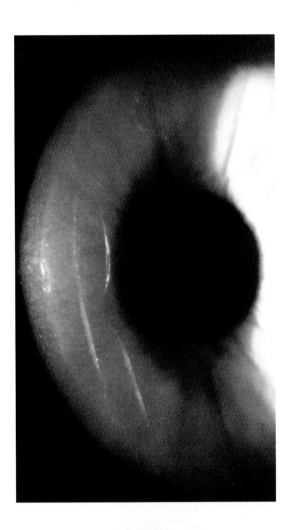

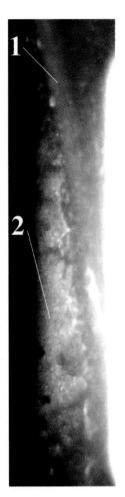

FIGURE 14-32 Direct beam view of forceps injury with breaks in Descemet's membrane.

FIGURE 14-33 *Specular photomicrograph of the same patient as in Figure 14-32.* There is a rolled-up edge of Descemet's membrane *(1).* Endothelial cells are enlarged *(2)* and have migrated from the adjacent tissue into the area of injury.

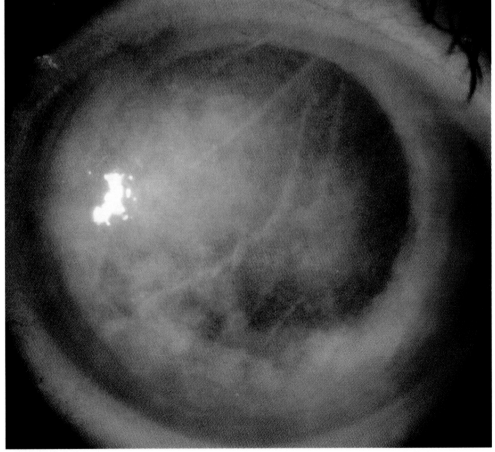

FIGURE 14-34 *Delayed-onset corneal edema after a forceps injury.* This 57-year-old man developed new-onset corneal decompensation and required penetrating keratoplasty. The breaks in Descemet's membrane can be visualized through the corneal edema.

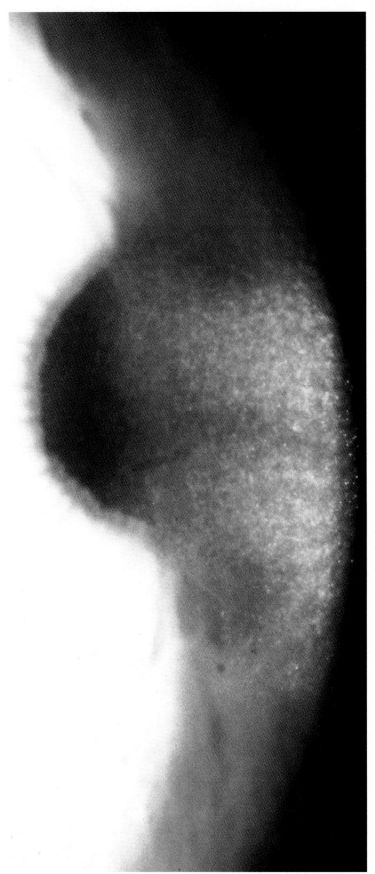

FIGURE 14-35 *A 27-year-old man was struck by lightning.* He developed a broad area of corneal scarring from the injury.

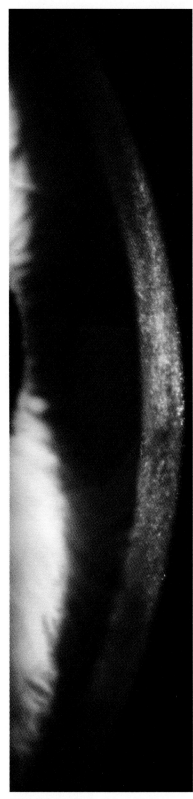

FIGURE 14-36 *A thin slit beam view of the same patient as in Figure 14-35.* There is scarring in all layers of the stroma. Cataracts may also develop after a lightning injury, sometimes many years after the acute event.

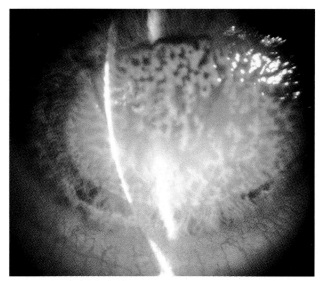

FIGURE 14-37 *Thermal injury.* In this case the injury to the corneal epithelium was caused by a curling iron.

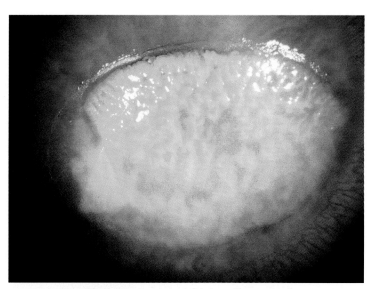

FIGURE 14-38 Fluorescein stain of injured area in the same patient as in Figure 14-37.

FIGURE 14-39 Necrotic inferior corneal ulcer from a thermal injury with hot metal.

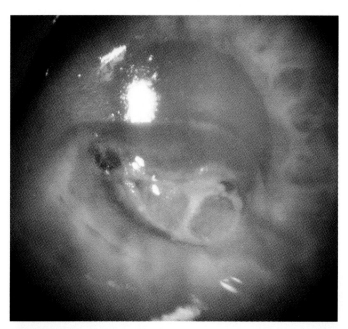

FIGURE 14-40 *Thermal injury.* Argon laser photocoagulation can injure the cornea. In this case, there are extensive corneal scars *(1)* and calcific degeneration *(2).*

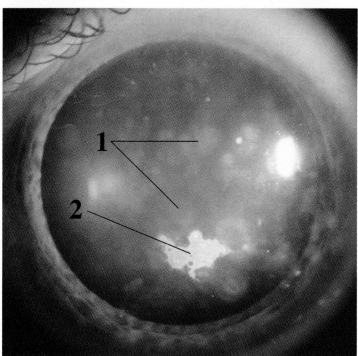

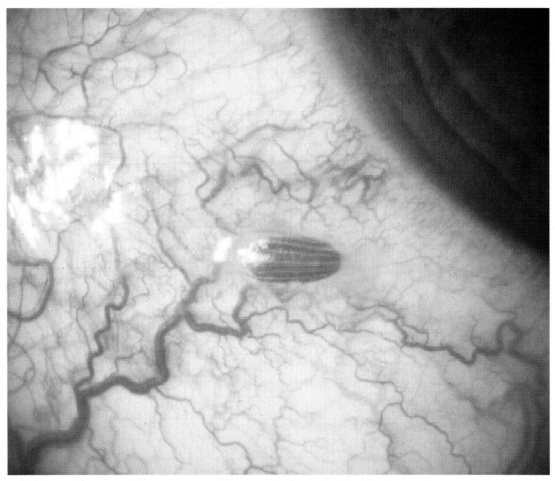

FIGURE 14-41 A corn husk foreign body embedded in the conjunctiva.

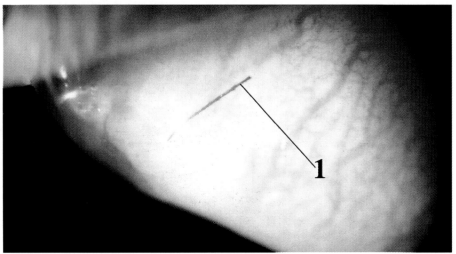

FIGURE 14-42 A grasshopper leg *(1)* embedded in the conjunctiva.

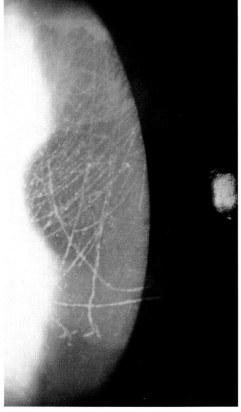

FIGURE 14-43 *Same patient as in Figure 14-42.* There are multiple vertical epithelial abrasions (from blinking) from the grasshopper leg embedded in the superior tarsal conjunctiva. This pattern of corneal abrasion should always prompt the examiner to evert the lids and look carefully for a foreign body.

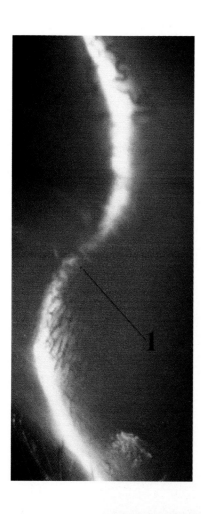

FIGURE 14-44 A small metallic foreign body *(1)* embedded in the lower palpebral conjunctiva.

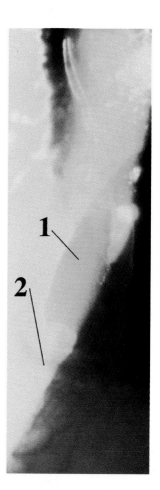

FIGURE 14-45 **_Same patient as in Figure 14-44._** There was an unhealed corneal abrasion *(1)* present for 3 days. The conjunctival foreign body was not noted on the initial examination. The limbus *(2)* is identified for orientation.

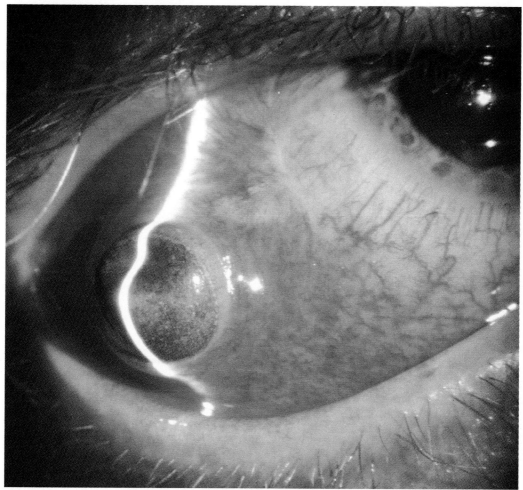

FIGURE 14-46 This patient shot an empty shotgun shell casing with a bullet. The casing exploded, and the primer cap embedded in his conjunctiva. There was no deep penetrating injury to the globe.

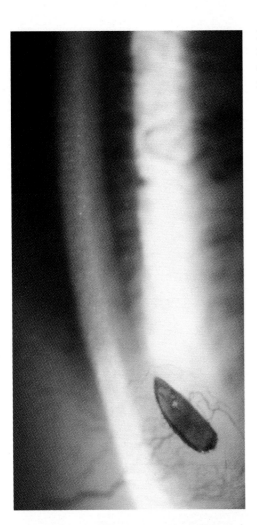

FIGURE 14-47 *A corn husk foreign body embedded in the cornea.* There is no sign of infection in this case, but patients should always be observed carefully for the development of fungal keratitis after injury with vegetable matter.

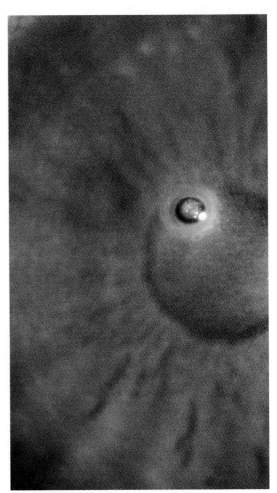

FIGURE 14-48 *An iron foreign body in the cornea with an early rust ring.* The foreign body and rust ring can be gently removed with a hypodermic needle or small forceps. Care should be taken not to penetrate deep into the stroma because this may cause unnecessary scarring. This was particularly true here, since the foreign body is near the visual axis.

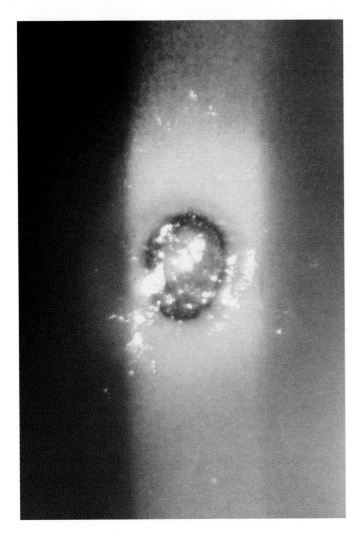

FIGURE 14-49 *A rust ring with surrounding infiltrate several days after the iron foreign body had been removed.* There was a toxic inflammatory response to the rust ring that resolved when the ring was removed. Patients with foreign bodies may develop infectious keratitis and should be treated with antibiotics until the epithelial defect and inflammation have resolved.

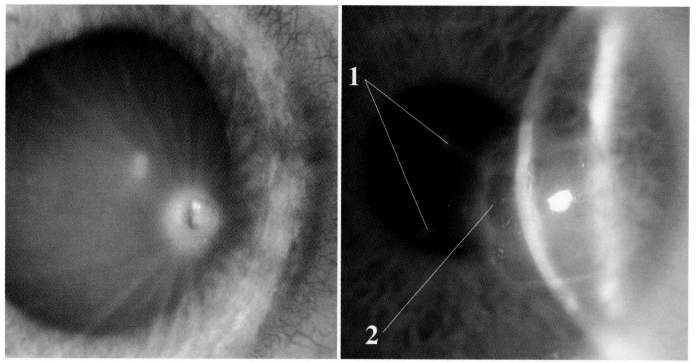

FIGURE 14-50 *A deep iron corneal foreign body that was not initially removed.* Necrosis of the surrounding tissue resulted in a perforation. There are corneal striae surrounding the foreign body, suggesting low pressure because of leaking aqueous.

FIGURE 14-51 *Same patient as in Figure 14-50 after a freehand lamellar keratoplasty.* The scar is in the visual axis *(1)*, and the edge of the graft encroaches on the visual axis *(2)*.

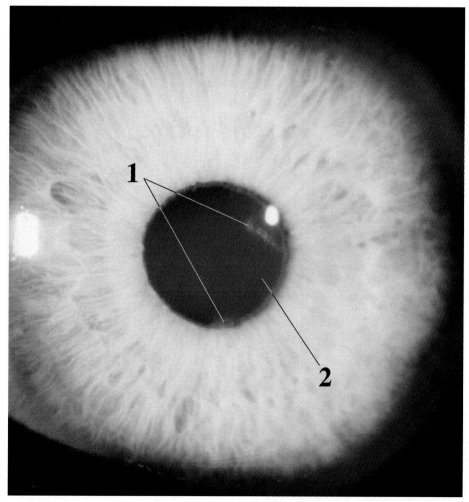

FIGURE 14-52 *Same patient as in Figures 14-50 and 14-51, 2 years later.* Visual acuity is 20/20. There is some scarring in the visual axis *(1)*; however, most of the visual axis remains clear *(2)*.

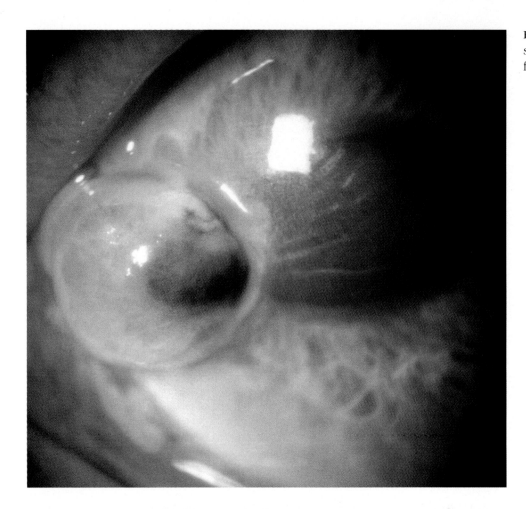

FIGURE 14-53 A perforated staphyloma from an old corneal foreign body.

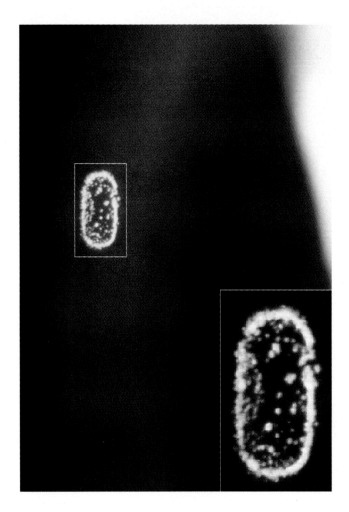

FIGURE 14-54 *Coat's white ring.* This is composed of iron and probably develops when a rust ring from an iron foreign body is not entirely removed. It is located in the superficial cornea. Inside the ring are small white opacities *(inset).*

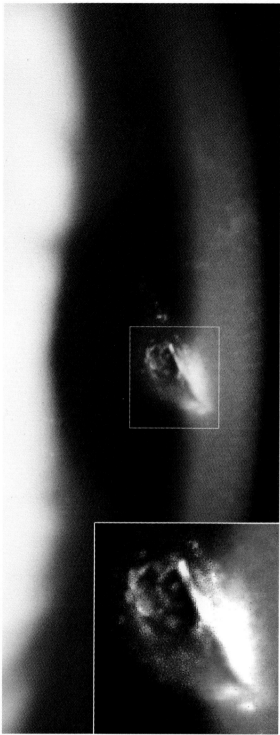

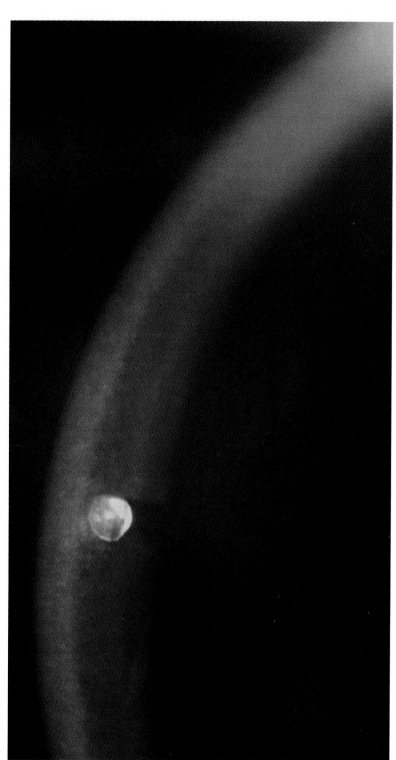

FIGURE 14-55 *An old glass foreign body in the corneal stroma with an associated scar (inset).* Glass is inert, and deep glass foreign bodies can be left in the stroma if their removal is difficult and could potentially cause more corneal damage.

FIGURE 14-56 *An old corneal foreign body from an explosion injury.* Similar to the glass foreign body seen in Figure 14-55, aggressive attempts at removal are not necessary.

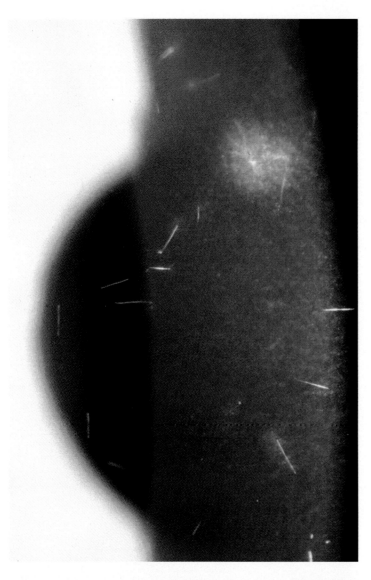

FIGURE 14-57 *Tarantula hairs in the cornea.* A 22-year-old man rubbed his left eye after playing with his pet tarantula. He immediately experienced redness, burning, and a foreign body sensation. Slit lamp examination showed multiple tarantula hairs in the corneal stroma. Some of the anterior tarantula hairs had associated subepithelial infiltrates. (One of these is seen superiorly.)

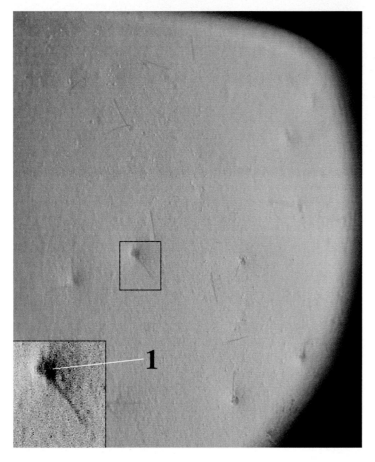

FIGURE 14-58 *Same patient as in Figure 14-57.* The red reflex view highlights the tarantula hairs. An individual hair *(1)* is seen in the inset. These hairs have many barbs (similar to fish hooks) and can penetrate deep into the corneal stroma and anterior chamber. There is one reported case of tarantula hairs penetrating through the sclera and causing a peripheral choroiditis. The hairs cannot be removed, and treatment is symptomatic with topical corticosteroids.

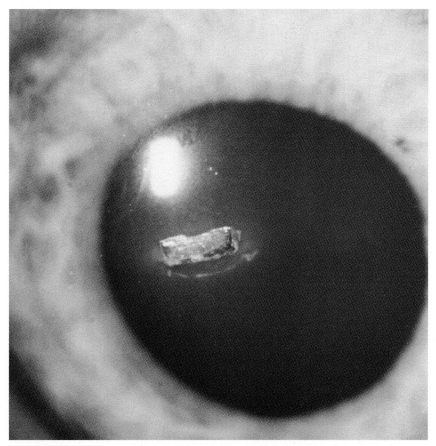

FIGURE 14-59 *Vegetable foreign matter in the corneal stroma.* The depth of penetration cannot be appreciated in this view.

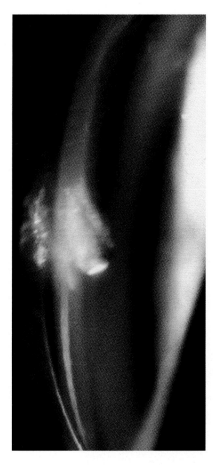

FIGURE 14-60 *Same patient as in Figure 14-59.* Gonioscopy shows that the foreign body penetrates the cornea and is surrounded by an inflammatory reaction.

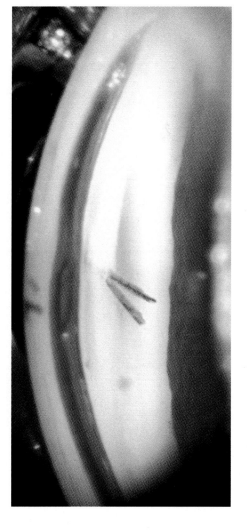

FIGURE 14-61 *Vegetable foreign matter in the cornal stroma.* Penetrating injury from vegetable foreign matter is seen by gonioscopy in another patient.

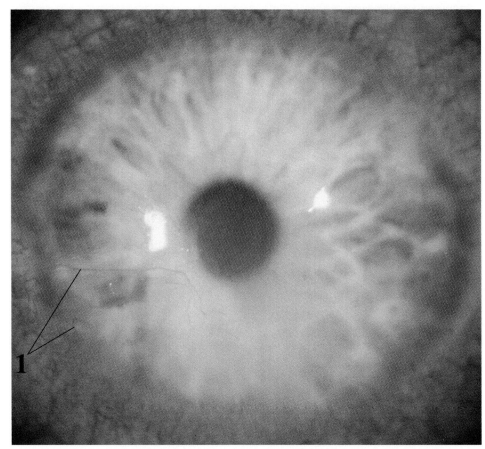

FIGURE 14-62 *Intraocular glass foreign body.* Corneal edema may develop from a retained intraocular foreign body. Here there was an intraocular glass foreign body in the angle that could only be appreciated by gonioscopy. There is vascularization *(1)* from chronic corneal edema. Unexplained inferior corneal edema should raise suspicion about a foreign body in the inferior anterior chamber angle.

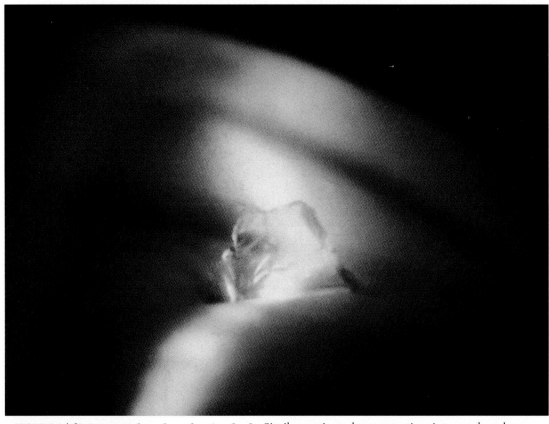

FIGURE 14-63 *Intraocular glass foreign body.* Similar patient demonstrating intraocular glass as seen by gonioscopy.

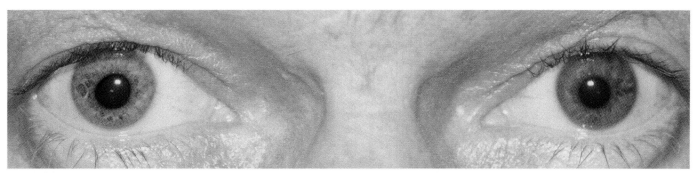

FIGURE 14-64 *Intraocular iron foreign body.* An intraocular iron foreign body in the left eye caused heterochromia in this patient.

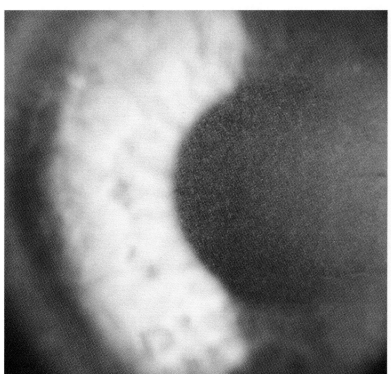

FIGURE 14-65 *Same patient as in Figure 14-64.* There are brown deposits in the deep corneal stroma from the iron foreign body.

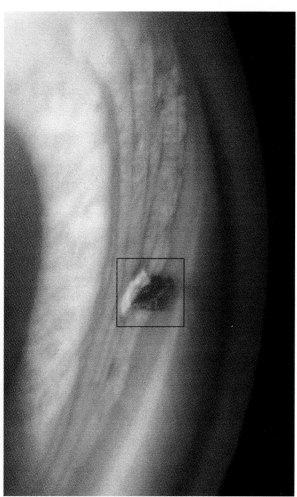

FIGURE 14-66 *Same patient as in Figures 14-64 and 14-65.* The iron foreign body *(box)* was in the angle and could only be appreciated by gonioscopy.

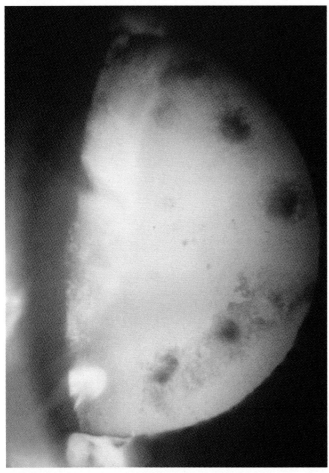

FIGURE 14-67 *Intraocular iron foreign body.* Brown deposits are seen in the lens, and there is a mature cataract.

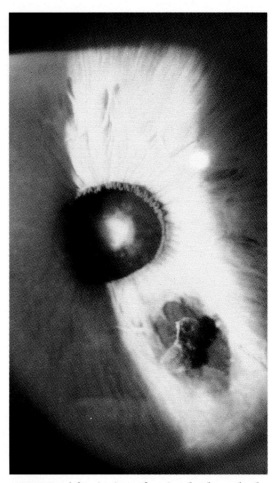

FIGURE 14-68 *An iron foreign body embedded in the iris.* A small central cataract is present.

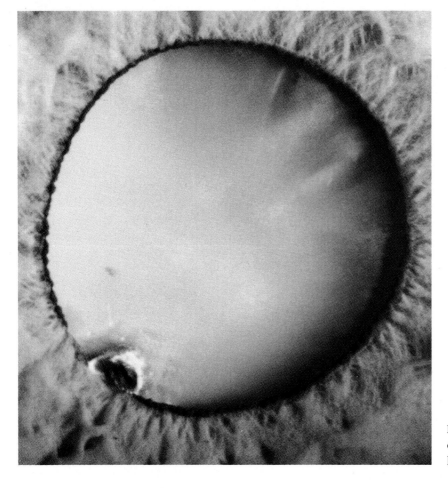

FIGURE 14-69 A traumatic cataract that developed from an iron foreign body that had penetrated the anterior lens capsule.

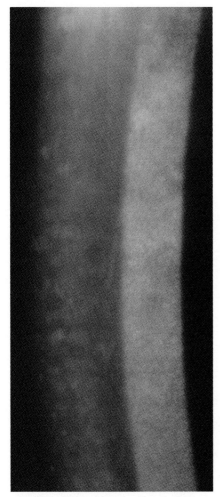

FIGURE 14-70 *Intraocular copper foreign body (chalcosis).* This resulted in a green-yellow discoloration in Descemet's membrane.

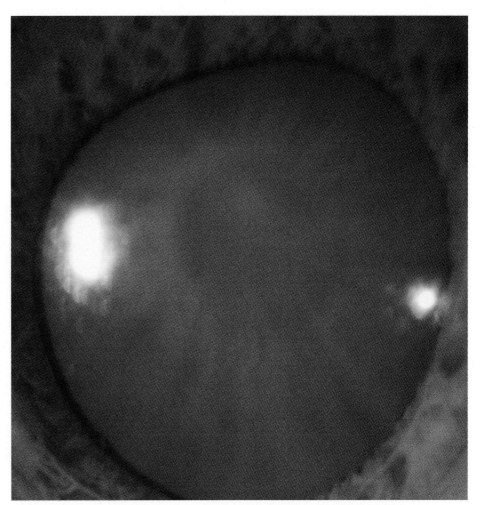

FIGURE 14-71 *An intraocular copper foreign body causing a sunflower cataract.* Foreign bodies that cause chalcosis are usually composed of less than 85% copper. Pure copper causes a suppurative endophthalmitis.

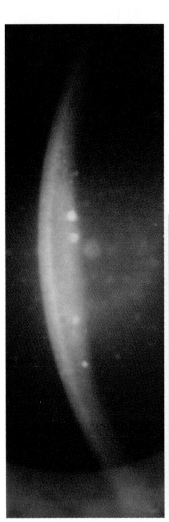

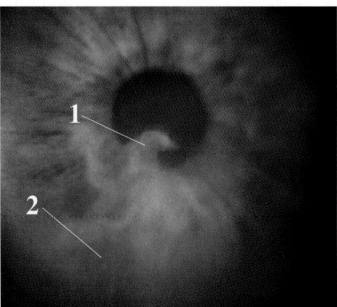

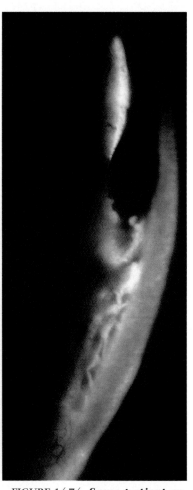

FIGURE 14-72 *Herpetic keratitis.* This 9-year-old girl gave a history of an insect bite on her right eyelid several days before developing disciform keratitis. She had several recurrences that were successfully treated with topical corticosteroids and topical antivirals for a presumed herpetic etiology. Occasionally, patients with herpetic keratitis relate their injury to an episode of trauma.

FIGURE 14-73 *Iridoschisis.* This patient had typical iris changes *(1)* and inferior corneal edema *(2).* The iris was chronically rubbing on the corneal endothelium.

FIGURE 14-74 *Same patient as in Figure 14-73.* A thin slit beam view shows corneal edema and iridocorneal touch.

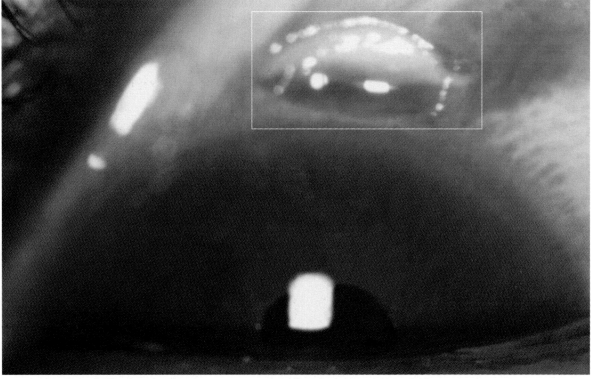

FIGURE 14-75 *Limbal perforation after blunt trauma.* The sclera is thin at the limbus *(box)* and under the rectus muscle insertions, and scleral ruptures occur more commonly in these areas.

Surgical Trauma

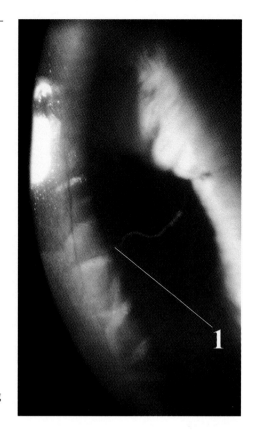

FIGURE 14-76 Corneal edema secondary to chronic trauma from a lint foreign body (introduced during cataract surgery) rubbing on the endothelium *(1)*.

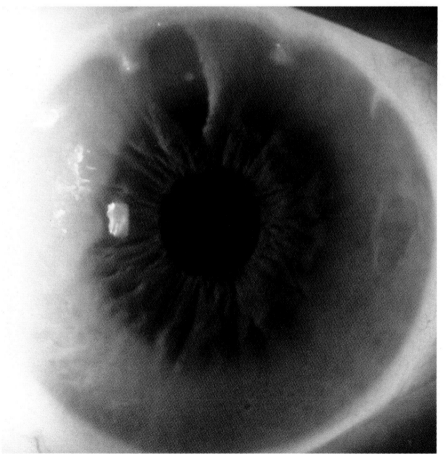

FIGURE 14-77 ***Brown-McLean syndrome.*** This is characterized by peripheral corneal edema with a relatively clear cornea centrally. The syndrome is seen primarily in aphakic eyes. Many of these eyes have floppy irides, and it is postulated that the mechanical irritation from the iris damages the peripheral endothelium. Peripheral corneal edema is not as extensive in the area overlying a peripheral iridectomy (as seen here).

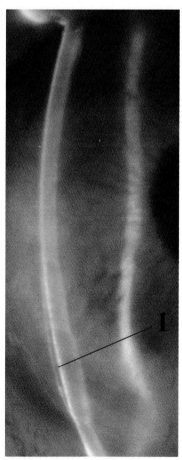

FIGURE 14-78 A thin slit beam view of the Brown-McLean syndrome showing peripheral corneal edema and a large bullae *(1)*.

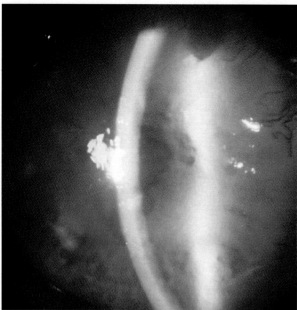

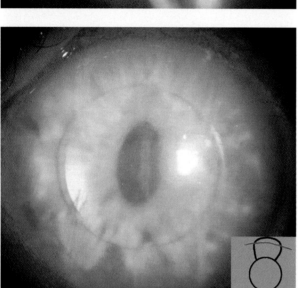

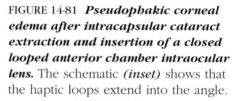

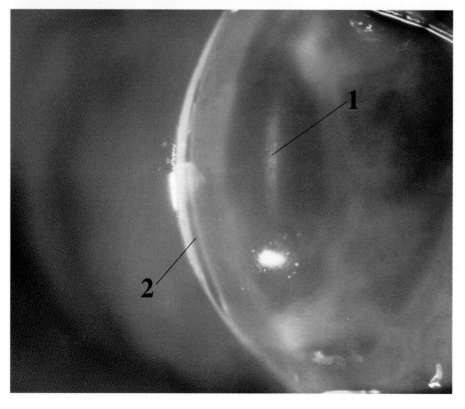

FIGURE 14-79 Aphakic bullous keratopathy many years after intracapsular cataract extraction.

FIGURE 14-80 Pseudophakic corneal edema after intracapsular cataract extraction and insertion of a four-loop iris-fixated intraocular lens.

FIGURE 14-81 *Pseudophakic corneal edema after intracapsular cataract extraction and insertion of a closed looped anterior chamber intraocular lens.* The schematic *(inset)* shows that the haptic loops extend into the angle.

FIGURE 14-82 *Pseudophakic corneal edema after extracapsular cataract extraction and insertion of a posterior chamber intraocular lens.* The posterior chamber intraocular lens *(1)* is seen behind the iris. There is a large edema cleft within the epithelium *(2)*.

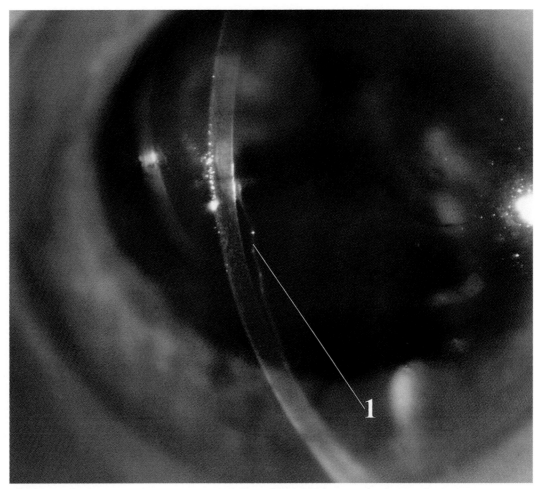

FIGURE 14-83 Mild corneal edema after cataract extraction from a detached Descemet's membrane *(1)*.

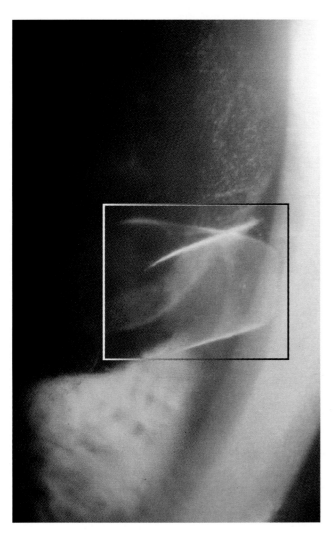

FIGURE 14-84 Scrolled Descemet's membrane *(box)* associated with trauma from cataract surgery.

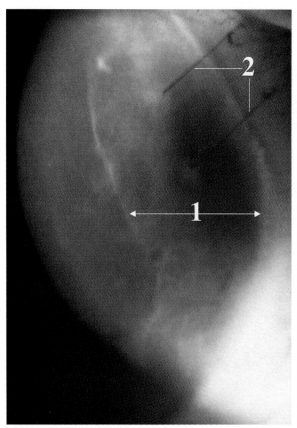

FIGURE 14-85 *Epithelial ingrowth after cataract surgery.* An epithelial membrane can be seen beginning at the limbus and growing on the back of the cornea *(1).* Cataract wound sutures *(2)* are also shown.

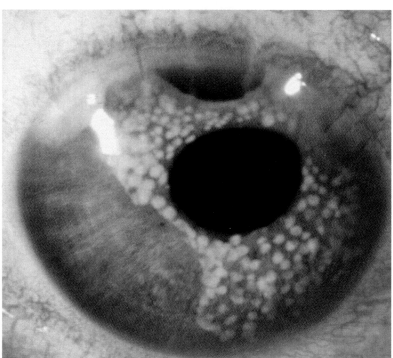

FIGURE 14-86 *Same patient as in Figure 14-85.* Argon laser photocoagulation has been applied to the surface of the iris to delineate the extent of epithelial growth. Epithelium will turn white when treated with the argon laser. The prognosis with extensive epithelial downgrowth is usually poor.

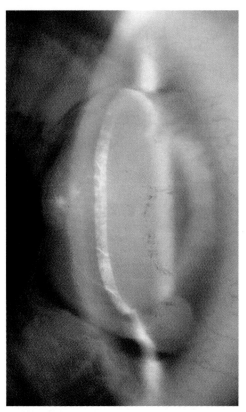

FIGURE 14-87 *Anterior chamber epithelial inclusion cyst.* This was noted several months after penetrating trauma.

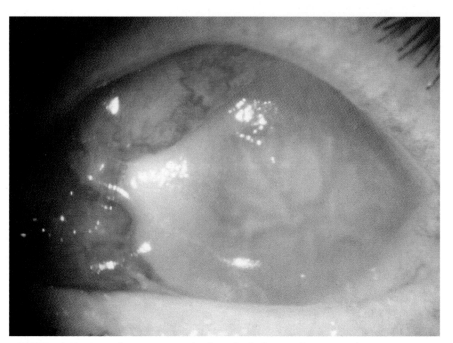

FIGURE 14-88 *Anterior segment ischemia 3 days after muscle surgery on three rectus muscles.* The early signs of anterior segment ischemia include corneal edema and anterior uveitis.

Acid Burns

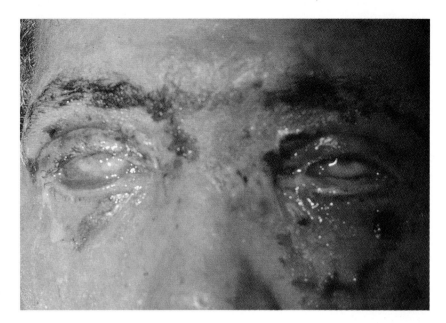

FIGURE 14-89 **_Severe acid burn to the face and eyes._** The scarring in the skin has caused a cicatricial ectropion. There is ischemic ulceration of the cornea and sclera in both eyes.

Alkali Burns

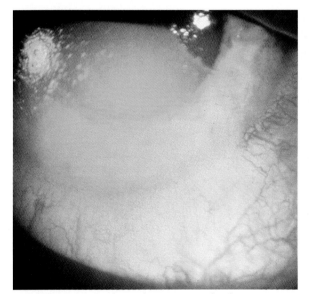

FIGURE 14-90 Moderately severe anhydrous ammonia burn to the conjunctiva and cornea.

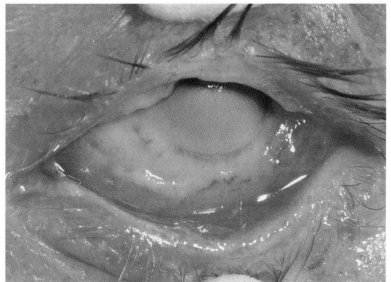

FIGURE 14-91 Severe alkali burn with conjunctival and scleral ischemia and marked corneal edema.

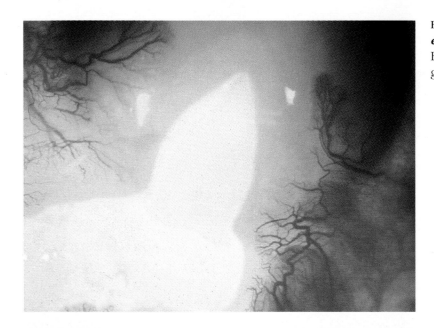

FIGURE 14-92 ***Alkali burn with nonhealing epithelial defect resulting from ischemia.*** Eyes with severe alkali burns often develop glaucoma and cataracts.

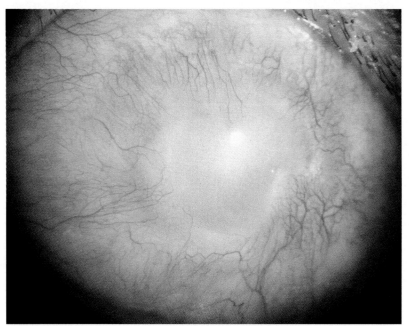

FIGURE 14-93 ***Severe alkali burn after 1 year.*** The cornea is scarred, and there is extensive vascularization. The prognosis for keratoplasty in these patients is poor because of the high risk of rejection from increased stromal vascularization and poor ability to maintain a normal epithelial surface because of damaged conjunctival and corneal stem cells.

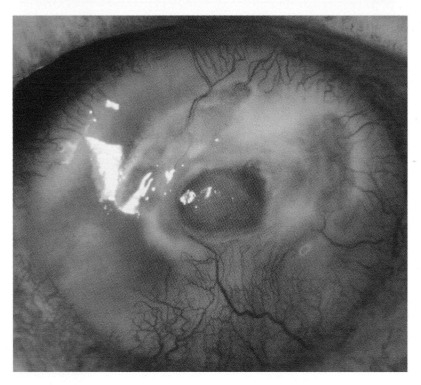

FIGURE 14-94 ***Alkali burn with stromal necrosis and perforation.*** Alkaline compounds are lipophilic and penetrate deep into the corneal stroma. They cause saponification of fatty acids in cell membranes, which leads to rapid cell death.

CHAPTER 15

Contact Lens Complications

Contact lens complications are related to three basic mechanisms: (1) mechanical trauma to the conjunctiva and cornea, (2) chronic and acute hypoxia from decreased transmissibility of oxygen in the presence of a contact lens, and (3) allergic reactions from protein deposits in the contact lenses. Many contact lens patients have dry eyes and/or blepharitis, which further compromises the conjunctival and corneal surface, increasing the chances of complications.

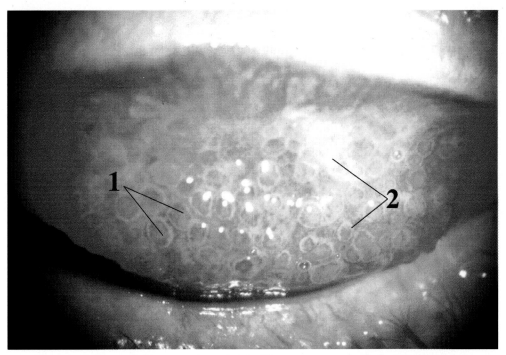

FIGURE 15-1 *Giant papillary conjunctivitis.* The symptoms include itching and mucous discharge. Giant papillae *(1)* are present on the upper tarsal conjunctiva. Mucus *(2)* may surround the papillae as seen below or may be floating freely as seen above. The pathophysiology of this disorder is multifactorial and probably relates to chronic trauma from the contact lens and an allergic reaction to proteins that accumulate in the contact lens.

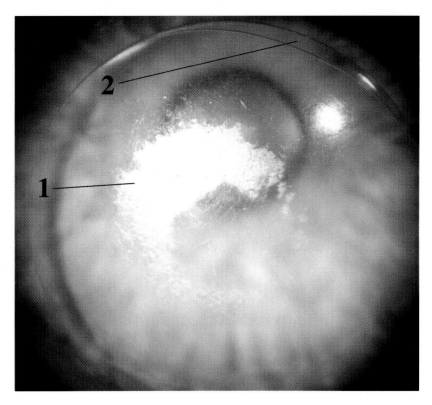

FIGURE 15-2 Debris *(1)* may accumulate on the surface of the contact lens or between the contact lens and the epithelium. If it is on the back of the lens, the debris can rub on the epithelium and increase the risk of infectious keratitis. The superior portion of the lens is lifted away from the cornea, causing a space filled by air *(2)*.

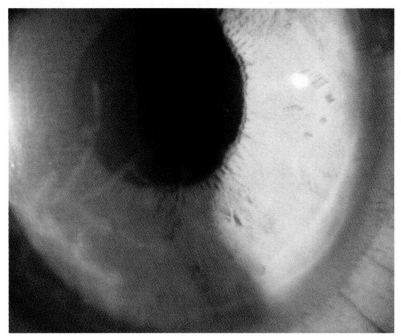

FIGURE 15-3 Mechanical irritation from soft contact lenses may produce dendritic epithelial patterns in the corneal epithelium. These patterns should be distinguished from herpes simplex dendrites (see Figure 10-13) and dendritic forms from Acanthamoeba keratitis (see Figure 10-66).

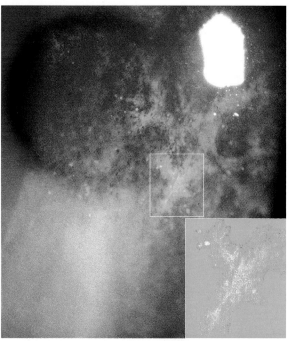

FIGURE 15-4 *Fluorescein staining of dendritic epithelial patterns in a soft contact lens wearer.* In contrast, herpes simplex epithelial keratitis produces an actual ulceration into the superficial cornea.

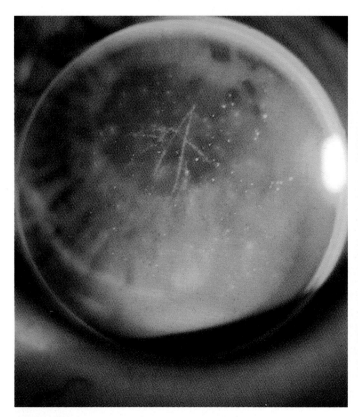

FIGURE 15-5 *Dust trail linear abrasions from a rigid contact lens.* These occur when a foreign body lodges between the contact lens and the patient's cornea.

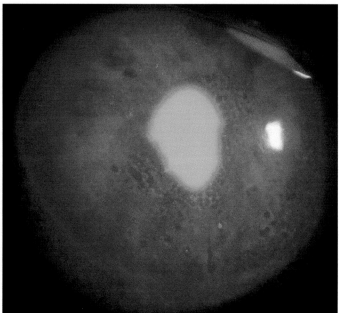

FIGURE 15-6 *Corneal erosions from a soft contact lens.* These should be treated with topical antibiotics rather than pressure patching because the risk of developing infectious keratitis is high.

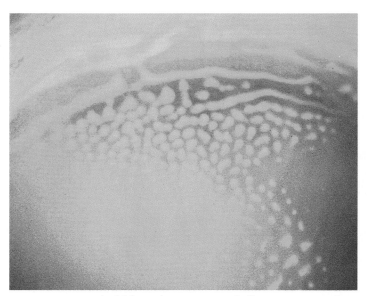

FIGURE 15-7 Air bubble indentations with fluorescein pooling in a contact lens wearer.

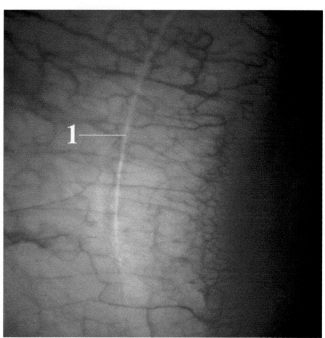

FIGURE 15-8 *A tight-fitting soft contact lens producing a groove in the conjunctiva (1).* Tight lenses decrease the oxygen diffusion to the cornea and can be associated with vascularization, edema, and infiltrates.

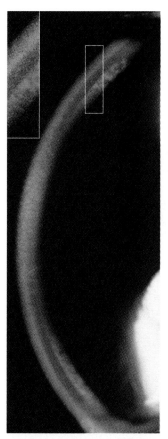

FIGURE 15-9 *Cyan mottling of the posterior cornea in a soft contact lens wearer.* The etiology of this lesion *(inset)* is unknown.

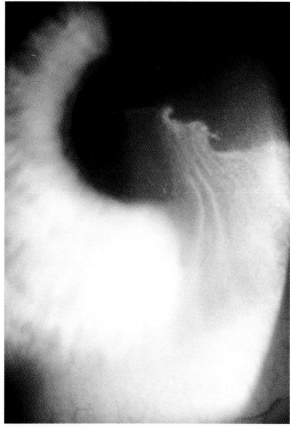

FIGURE 15-10 *Epithelial dysplasia.* Chronic mechanical irritation from a contact lens can induce epithelial dysplasia, as seen here. This is a benign condition, although treatment is very difficult and may require surgery such as a conjunctival transplant or keratoepithelialplasty.

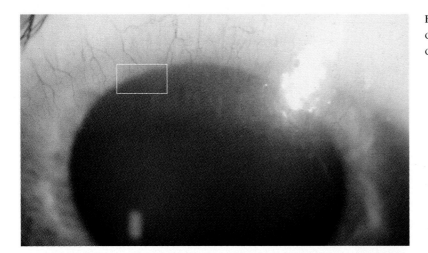

FIGURE 15-11 Superficial pannus in a soft contact lens wearer resulting from chronic hypoxia.

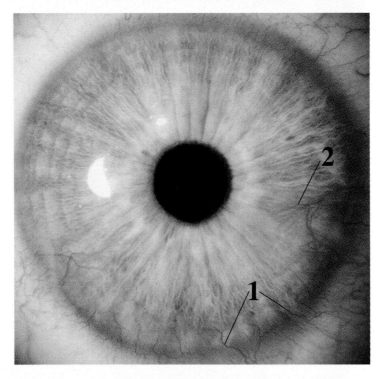

FIGURE 15-12 Superficial *(1)* and stromal *(2)* vascularization from a low-riding, rigid contact lens.

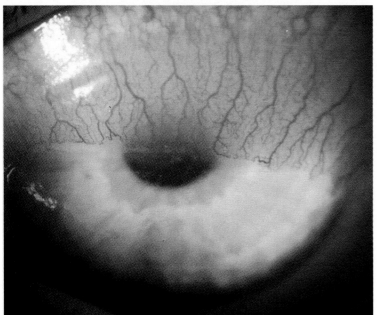

FIGURE 15-13 Severe corneal vascularization from a poorly fit, soft contact lens.

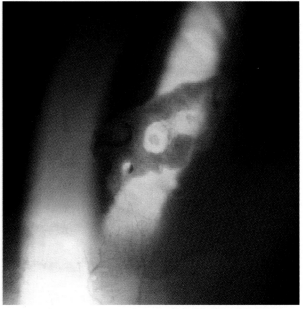

FIGURE 15-14 Occasionally a blood vessel in the cornea breaks from contact lens–related trauma. This is an example of a subepithelial hemorrhage in a soft contact lens wearer. Intrastromal hemorrhages can also occur.

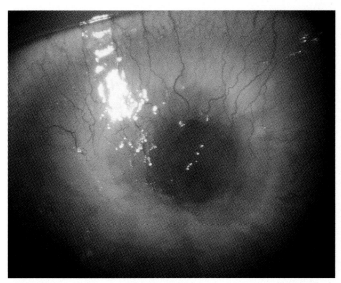

FIGURE 15-15 **_Corneal vascularization and epithelial dysplasia in a soft contact lens wearer._** Chronic contact lens wear has altered the epithelium.

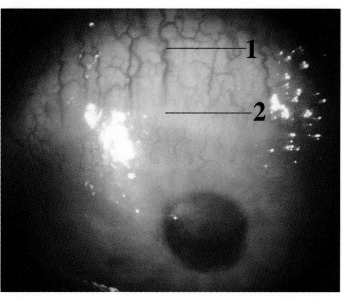

FIGURE 15-16 **_Superior limbic keratoconjunctivitis syndrome in a soft contact lens wearer._** There is superficial conjunctival vascularization *(1)* and limbal thickening *(2)*. Thimerosal preservatives in contact lens solutions can produce a similar clinical picture.

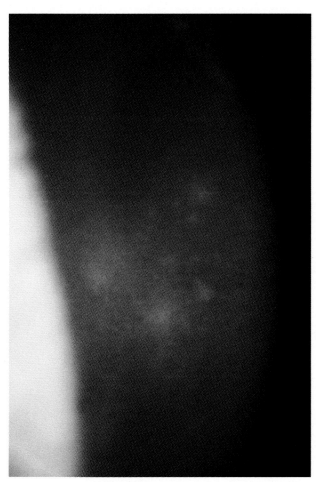

FIGURE 15-17 **_Mild diffuse anterior stromal infiltrate in a soft contact lens wearer._** This infiltrate is sterile and caused by corneal hypoxia.

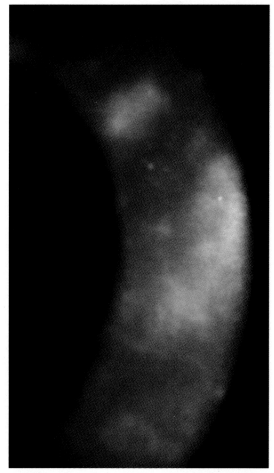

FIGURE 15-18 Severe diffuse anterior stromal infiltrates in a soft contact lens wearer.

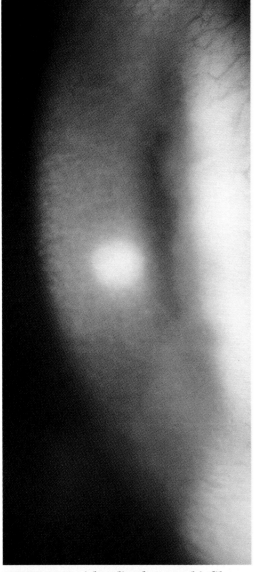

FIGURE 15-19 *A localized stromal infil-trate in a soft contact lens wearer.* There is no epithelial defect, and this infiltrate was a sterile reaction. Frequent antibiotic instillation without a laboratory work-up and follow-up examination the next day are indicated.

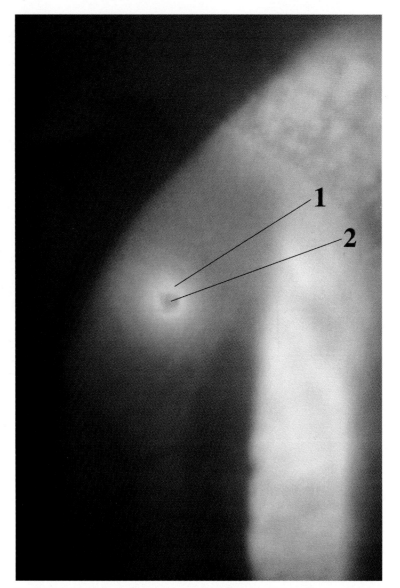

FIGURE 15-20 *A localized stromal infiltrate (1) with an overly-ing epithelial defect (2) in a soft contact lens wearer.* When an epithelial defect is present, there should be a high index of suspicion for infectious keratitis, and a laboratory work-up is indicated.

FIGURE 15-21 *Extensive pseudomonas bacterial corneal ulcer associated with soft contact lens use.* A laboratory work-up is performed. Frequent fortified antibiotics are indicated.

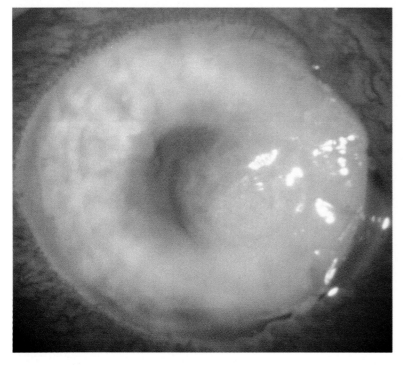

CHAPTER 16

Disorders Of The Sclera

Collagen vascular diseases associated with scleritis and keratitis are discussed in Chapter 13. The purpose of this chapter is to demonstrate the clinical features of the different forms of episcleritis and scleritis.

Episcleritis

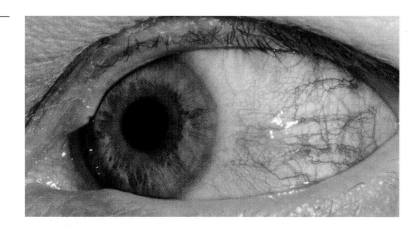

FIGURE 16-1 *Nodular episcleritis in a patient with gout.* The symptoms of episcleritis include redness and mild ocular irritation. There is some blanching of the vessels after the instillation of topical phenylephrine. In many cases, there is no known systemic association.

Scleritis

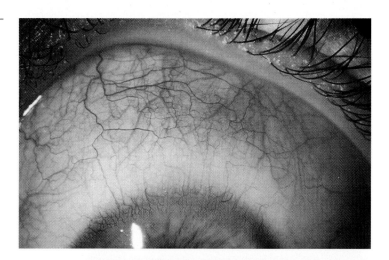

FIGURE 16-2 *Diffuse scleritis.* The hallmark of scleritis is severe ocular and orbital pain. Often there is an associated iritis. There is injection of the conjunctiva and deep episcleral vessels; the inflammation extends into the sclera. Scleritis is often associated with systemic conditions, and systemic treatment is usually required to control the pain and inflammation.

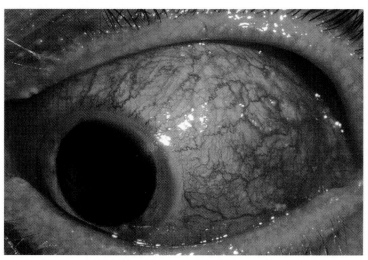

FIGURE 16-3 *A second more severe case of diffuse scleritis.* Dilation of the deep episcleral vessels gives the lesion a bluish-red discoloration.

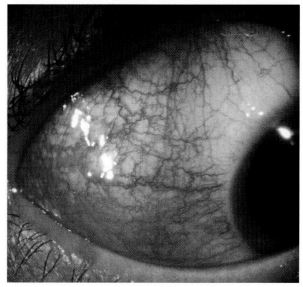

FIGURE 16-4 *Nodular scleritis.* In this variety of scleritis, there is an elevated inflamed mass within the area of inflammation.

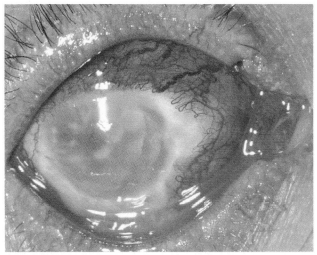

FIGURE 16-5 *Necrotizing scleritis.* There are avascular areas with tissue loss adjacent to areas of active inflammation. This is the most severe form of scleritis and requires aggressive treatment. In this patient the underlying diagnosis was rheumatoid arthritis.

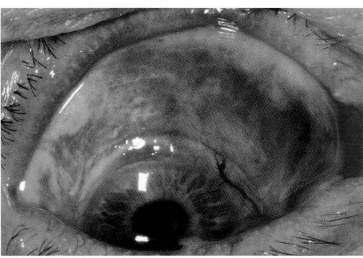

FIGURE 16-6 *Scleromalacia perforans.* This usually occurs in the setting of long-standing rheumatoid arthritis. It is a painless, progressive thinning of the sclera not associated with episodes of acute inflammation. Minor trauma may result in scleral perforation.

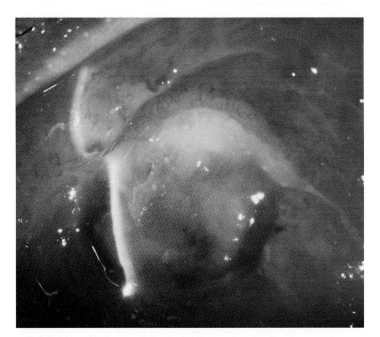

FIGURE 16-7 *Pseudomonas scleritis that began as a localized keratitis.* In all cases of scleritis, it is important to exclude infectious etiologies. *Pseudomonas* scleritis is extremely difficult to treat, and the prognosis is poor.

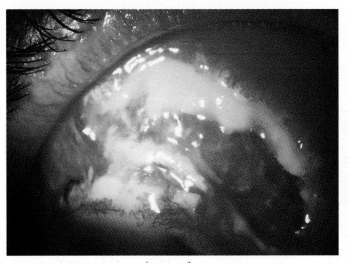

FIGURE 16-8 *Nocardia* scleritis after cataract surgery.

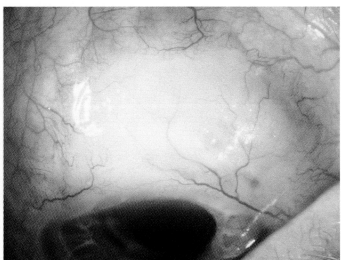

FIGURE 16-9 *Same patient as in Figure 16-8, after intensive treatment with topical trimethoprim-sulfamethoxazole.* The sclera has thinned, and the patient developed marked against-the-rule astigmatism.

CHAPTER 17

Anterior Uveitis

Anterior uveitis can occur alone or combined with a keratitis or scleritis. This chapter focuses on primary causes of anterior uveitis related to specific etiologies. However, many cases of anterior uveitis are idiopathic and cannot be attributed to any systemic or local disease process.

Sarcoidosis

Sarcoidosis is a systemic inflammatory condition that affects multiple organ systems, including the eyes, skin, central nervous system, and pulmonary system. Sarcoid granulomas can occur in the conjunctiva (see Figures 5-28 and 5-29).

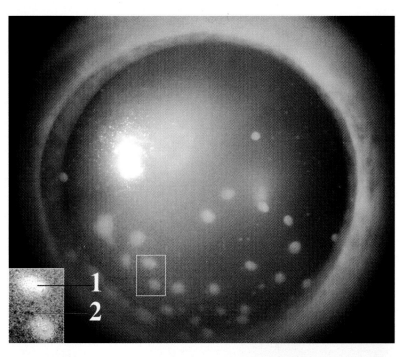

FIGURE 17-1 *Acute uveitis from sarcoidosis.* There are multiple "mutton-fat" keratic precipitates *(1)*, as well as microcystic corneal edema *(2)* caused by a rapid increase in intraocular pressure to 50 mm Hg. A chronic granulomatous iridocyclitis is the most common ocular finding in sarcoidosis, although occasionally a nongranulomatous uveitis may occur.

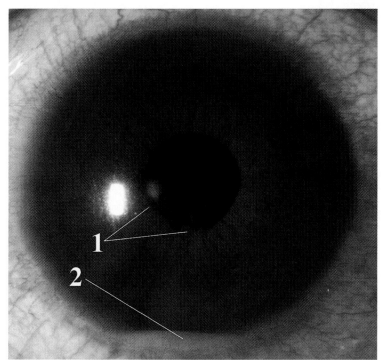

FIGURE 17-2 Posterior synechiae *(1)* and a hemorrhagic hypopyon *(2)* from an episode of acute sarcoid iridocyclitis.

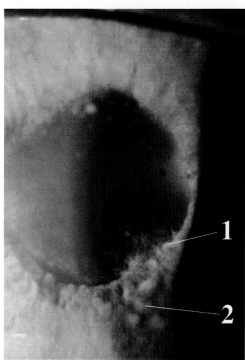

FIGURE 17-3 *Iridocyclitis secondary to sarcoidosis.* Koeppe nodules *(1)* occur at the pupillary margin, and Busacca nodules *(2)* occur on the iris surface.

Fuchs' Heterochromic Iridocyclitis

Fuchs' heterochromic iridocyclitis is a unilateral chronic iridocyclitis that causes heterochromia as a result of iris stromal thinning and iris pigment epithelial loss.

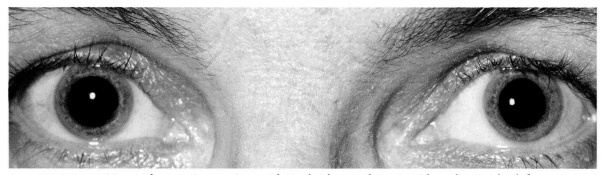

FIGURE 17-4 Heterochromia in a patient with Fuchs' heterochromic iridocyclitis in the left eye.

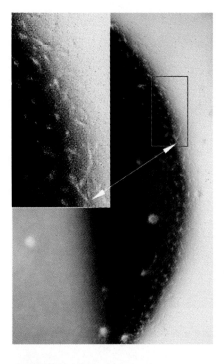

FIGURE 17-5 **Fuchs' heterochromic iridocyclitis.** There are small, white, stellate keratic precipitates on the back of the cornea *(inset)*.

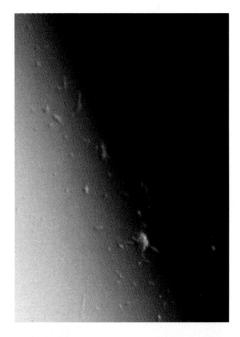

FIGURE 17-6 **Fuchs' heterochromic iridocyclitis.** Stellate precipitates are seen under high magnification. These precipitates are most likely composed of inflammatory cells and fibrin. Usually minimal aqueous cell and almost no flare are associated with these precipitates. Anterior chamber cells do not decrease with corticosteroids.

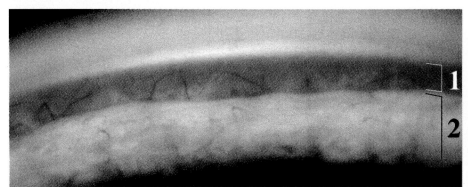

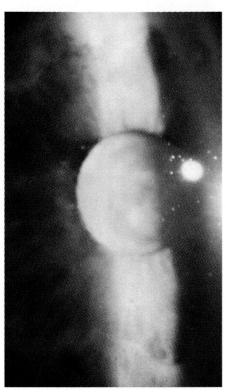

FIGURE 17-7 **Gonioscopy in Fuchs' heterochromic iridocyclitis.** Fine blood vessels course over the trabecular meshwork *(1)* and iris *(2)*. A paracentesis characteristically produces bleeding from these vessels.

FIGURE 17-8 **Fuchs' heterochromic iridocyclitis.** A posterior subcapsular cataract may be present, which can progress to a mature white cataract (as seen here). Peripheral anterior synechiae and posterior synechiae do not usually develop in this disorder. Cataract surgery is very successful in this condition.

Behçet's Disease

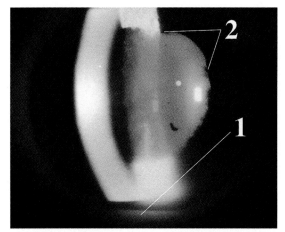

FIGURE 17-9 Uveitis with hypopyon *(1)*, characteristic of Behçet's disease. Posterior synechiae *(2)* are present.

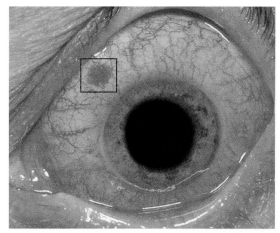

FIGURE 17-10 Scleritis in Behçet's disease with a localized erythematous nodule *(box)*.

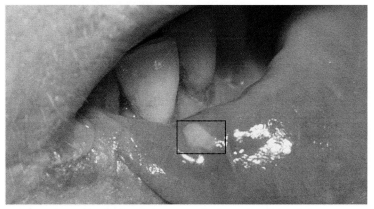

FIGURE 17-11 Typical aphthous oral ulcer *(box)* in Behçet's disease.

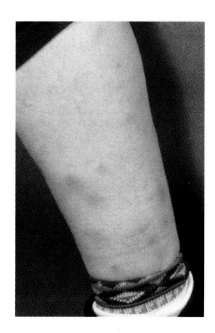

FIGURE 17-12 Subcutaneous erythematous nodules in Behçet's disease.

Vogt-Koyanagi-Harada Syndrome

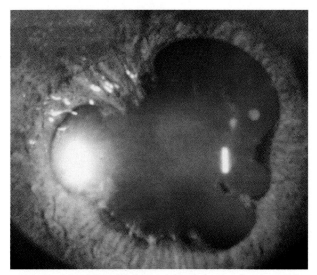

FIGURE 17-13 Vogt-Koyanagi-Harada syndrome with posterior synechiae from an anterior uveitis.

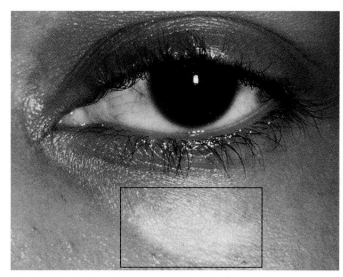

FIGURE 17-14 Vogt-Koyanagi-Harada syndrome with vitiligo *(box)*.

Juvenile Rheumatoid Arthritis

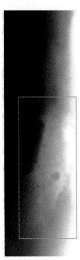

FIGURE 17-15 **Band keratopathy.** This finding may occur in the presence or absence of active inflammation in juvenile rheumatoid arthritis.

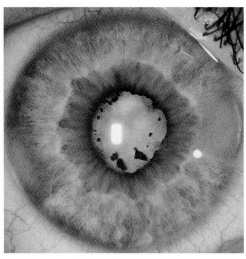

FIGURE 17-16 **Mature white cataracts and extensive posterior synechiae.** These findings may occur in juvenile rheumatoid arthritis.

Syphilitic Uveitis

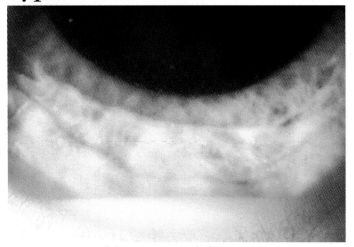

FIGURE 17-17 Syphilitic uveitis with hypopyon in a patient with AIDS.

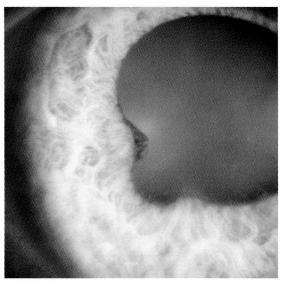

FIGURE 17-18 Fellow eye of same patient as in Figure 17-17, with posterior synechiae.

HLA-B27–Related Uveitis

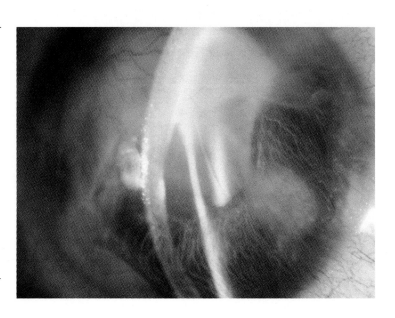

FIGURE 17-19 HLA-B27–associated disorders include Reiter's syndrome, ankylosing spondylitis, inflammatory bowel disease, and psoriatic arthritis. This patient with uveitis and ankylosing spondylitis developed a severe inflammatory response after cataract surgery. There is corneal edema associated with a retrocorneal membrane superiorly. The posterior chamber intraocular lens is encased in fibrin.

CHAPTER 18

Penetrating Keratoplasty

In 1906, Edward Zirm reported the first successful penetrating keratoplasty. Since that time, advances in surgical techniques have greatly improved the prognosis of corneal transplantation. The clinician must recognize the spectrum of postoperative complications that can occur after penetrating keratoplasty.

Preoperative and Postoperative Appearance

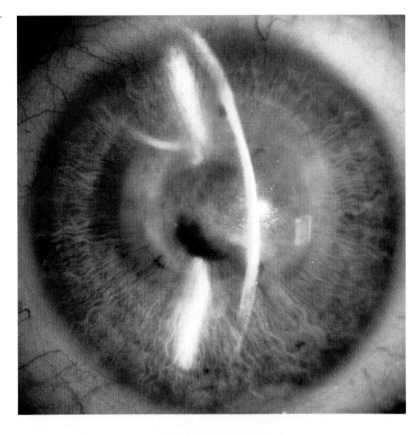

FIGURE 18-1 Preoperative view of central corneal scar from a varicella infection.

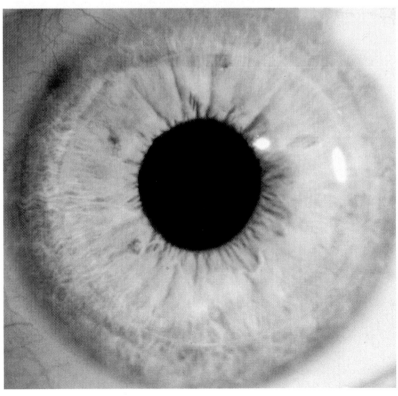

FIGURE 18-2 *Postoperative appearance of same patient as in Figure 18-1, 17 months after a penetrating keratoplasty.* The graft is clear.

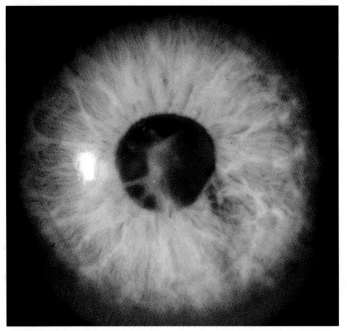

FIGURE 18-3 Preoperative appearance of central corneal scar secondary to trauma.

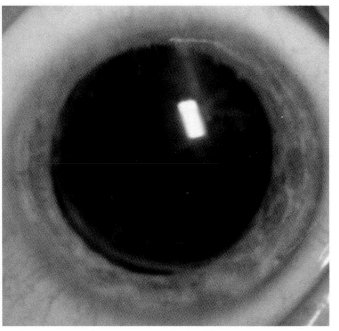

FIGURE 18-4 Postoperative appearance 16 months after a rotating penetrating keratoplasty was performed, rotating the scar superiorly.

Intraoperative and Early Postoperative Complications

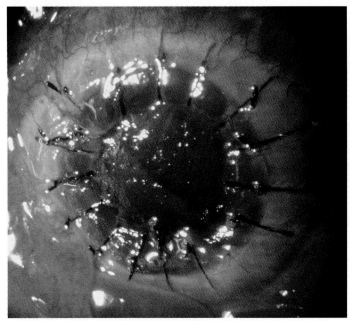

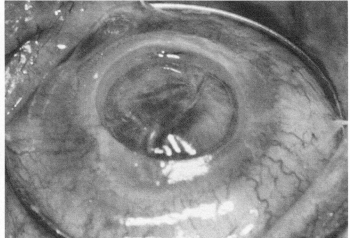

FIGURE 18-6 *Intraoperative complication.* This patient with syphilitic interstitial keratitis underwent penetrating keratoplasty. A retained Descemet's membrane was noted. This membrane must be removed before suturing the donor cornea.

FIGURE 18-5 *A suprachoroidal hemorrhage that developed intraoperatively.* The graft was sutured into place with 8-0 black silk suture becauses this suture is larger and more visible and therefore easier to work with in an emergency situation.

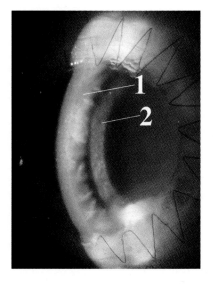

FIGURE 18-7 *Intraoperative complication.* A penetrating keratoplasty was performed for Fuchs' dystrophy. The donor cornea is seen *(1)* as well as Descemet's membrane from the host cornea *(2),* which was inadvertently left behind.

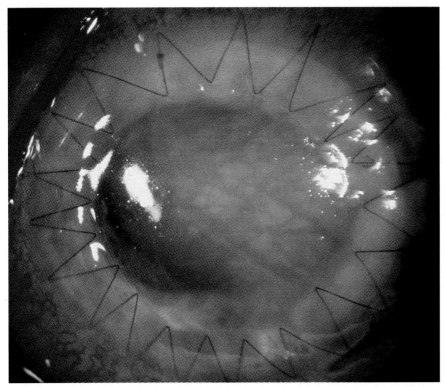

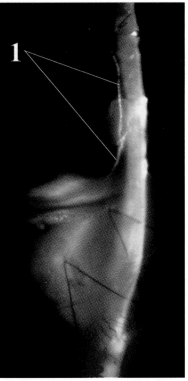

FIGURE 18-8 *Postoperative complication.* A large detachment of Descemet's membrane developed after penetrating keratoplasty. There is diffuse stromal edema.

FIGURE 18-9 A thin slit beam view of the same patient as in Figure 18-8 showing detached Descemet's membrane *(1).*

FIGURE 18-10 *Same patient as in Figures 18-8 and 18-9.* Air was injected into the anterior chamber to repair the detached Descemet's membrane. The graft is clear 2 weeks after the air injection.

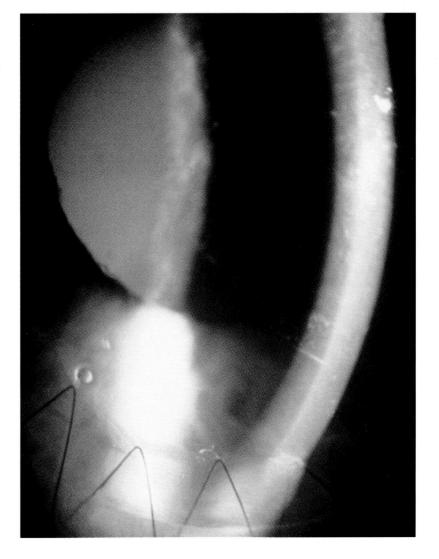

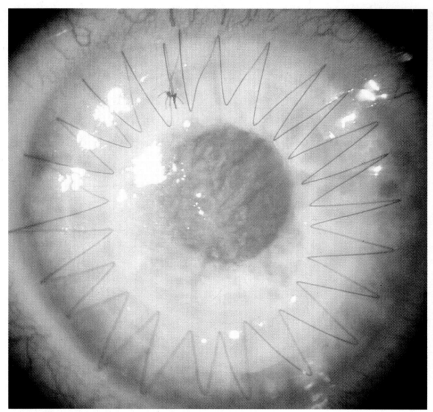

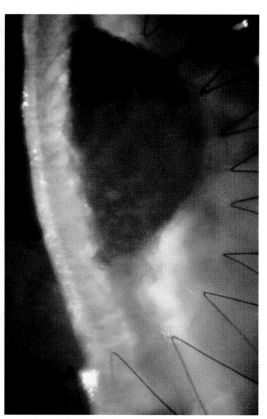

FIGURE 18-11 ***Postoperative complication.*** Primary donor failure occurs when a graft remains edematous over the entire postoperative period. It is believed to be secondary to endothelial cell dysfunction or surgical trauma. Pathologic examination usually shows the endothelium to be nearly or completely absent.

FIGURE 18-12 ***A thin slit beam view of the same patient as in Figure 18-11.*** There is diffuse stromal edema and folds in Descemet's membrane.

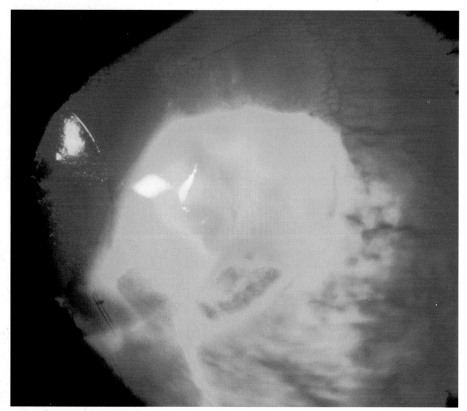

FIGURE 18-13 ***Postoperative complication.*** A wound leak developed in an area of poor tissue apposition after penetrating keratoplasty. Wound leaks may also occur along suture tracks.

FIGURE 18-14 ***Postoperative complication.*** A severe fibrin response in the anterior chamber developed in a patient with a history of Mooren's ulcer who underwent a penetrating keratoplasty.

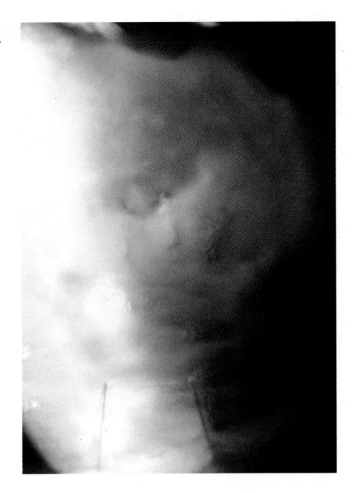

FIGURE 18-15 ***Same patient as in Figure 18-14.*** Several hours after the injection of 6 micrograms of tissue plasminogen activator into the anterior chamber, the eye showed marked resolution of the anterior chamber fibrin and the intraocular lens can now be visualized.

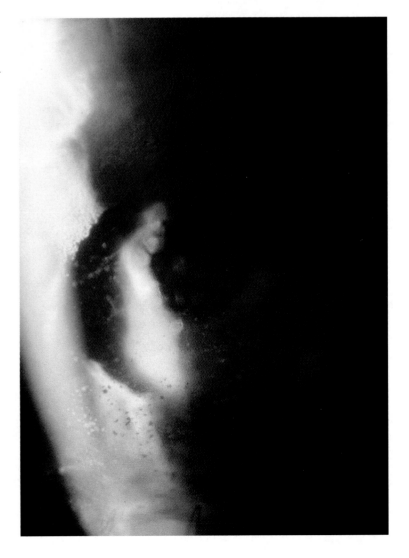

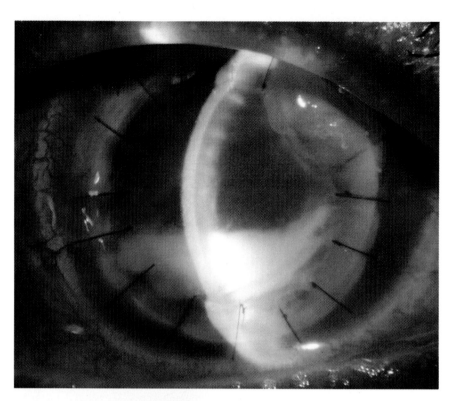

FIGURE 18-16 **Postoperative complication.** Endophthalmitis is a rare but serious complication after penetrating kerato-plasty. The causative agent was *Streptococcus pneumoniae.*

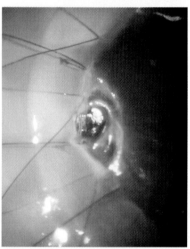

FIGURE 18-17 **Postoperative complication.** A delle has developed on the host tissue secondary to an edematous elevated wound margin.

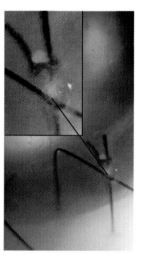

FIGURE 18-18 **Filaments.** These are commonly found attached to sutures *(inset).* They should be removed with forceps because they can induce a foreign body sensation and may predispose to infection.

FIGURE 18-19 Multiple sterile abscesses surrounding corneal sutures *(2).* A high magnification view is seen *(inset) (1).* These infiltrates are often composed of eosinophils and are more common in young patients with marked peripheral inflammation.

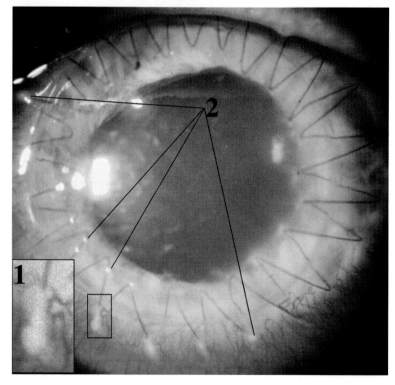

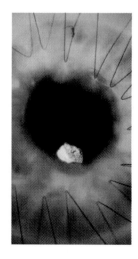

FIGURE 18-20 **Postoperative complication.** A metallic foreign body was found in this graft during a routine examination. The patient did not feel it because of decreased sensation in the graft. Corneal sensation in grafts returns slowly over the course of 2 years but typically does not reach normal levels.

Late Complications

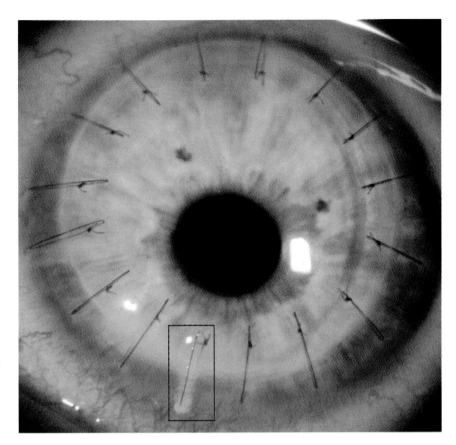

FIGURE 18-21 ***Suture erosion, a common late complication of penetrating keratoplasty.*** In this case an inferior suture has become loose and is covered with mucus *(box)*.

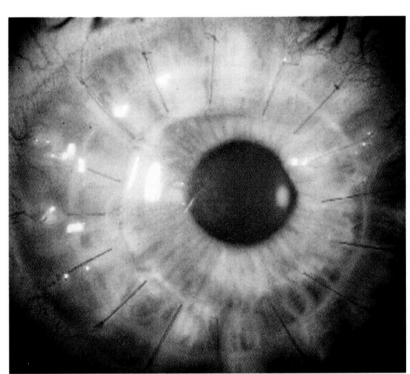

FIGURE 18-22 ***Eroded sutures.*** These can induce localized inflammation and vascularization. This graft is clear; however, it is not unusual for patients to have multiple eroded sutures, corneal vascularization, and acute allograft rejection.

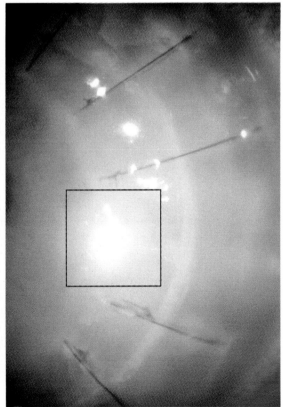

FIGURE 18-23 Suture abscess caused by ***Staphylococcus aureus*** infection *(box)*. Sutures can provide an entry tract for microorganisms into the stroma.

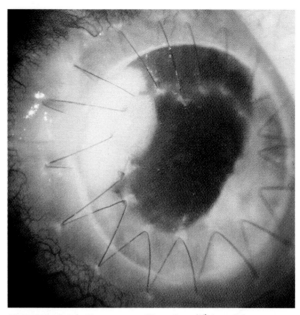

FIGURE 18-24 *Late complication.* This patient developed a *Streptococcus pneumoniae* infection several years after penetrating keratoplasty.

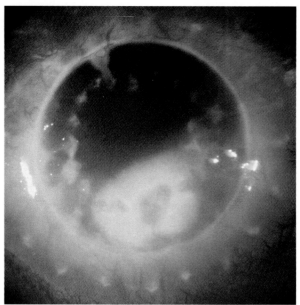

FIGURE 18-25 *The fellow eye of the same patient as in Figure 18-25.* There is an infiltrate resulting from *Proteus* species in the inferior graft. This infection occurred several months after the infection shown in Figure 18-24.

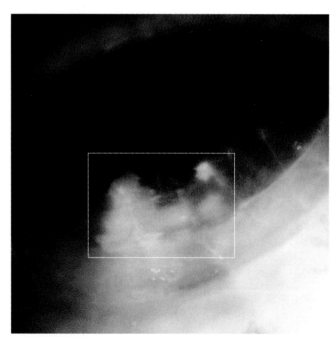

FIGURE 18-26 *Infectious crystalline keratopathy.* This most commonly results from an infection with *Streptococcus viridans* group (specifically nutritionally variant streptococci). The organism forms a crystalline pattern in the corneal stroma *(box)*, and the overlying epithelium is often intact. There is minimal host response to the infection, and for this reason, the stroma surrounding the infiltrate is relatively clear. The infection is typically located at the wound site. This condition is associated with chronic immunosuppression with topical corticosteroids.

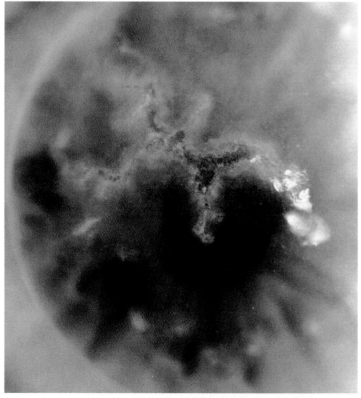

FIGURE 18-27 *Recurrence of active herpes simplex infection in a graft performed for scarring secondary to herpes simplex keratitis.* Antiviral agents should be used along with topical corticosteroids after penetrating keratoplasty to lessen the risk of recurrent herpes simplex infection. Systemic acyclovir may decrease the chance of this occurrence.

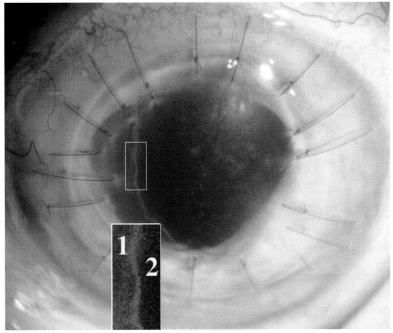

FIGURE 18-28 *Epithelial ingrowth.* This is a rare but devastating complication of penetrating keratoplasty. The inset demonstrates an area of epithelium on the posterior cornea *(1)* next to an area of normal endothelium *(2)*.

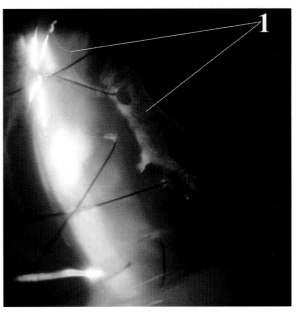

FIGURE 18-29 *Calcium deposits found near sutures after penetrating keratoplasty.* In some cases, phosphate rather than acetate corticosteroids may be responsible.

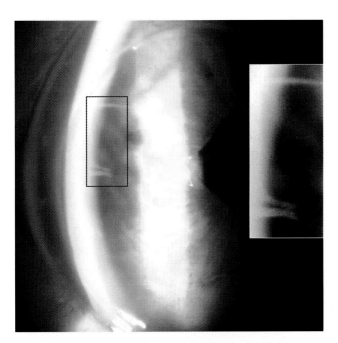

FIGURE 18-30 *Late complication.* This patient with cystoid macular edema had strands of vitreous extending to the keratoplasty wound *(inset)*. The pupil is peaked toward the wound.

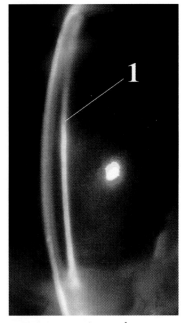

FIGURE 18-31 Avascular retrocorneal membrane *(1)*.

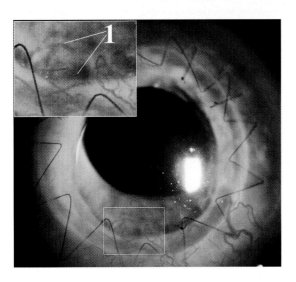

FIGURE 18-32 *Late complication.* A dense, circumscribed, white retrocorneal membrane is present for 360° inside the keratoplasty wound. Fine vessels *(1)* extend into the membrane. Poor wound apposition may predispose to this complication. The membrane grows slower than epithelial ingrowth, and the prognosis is better.

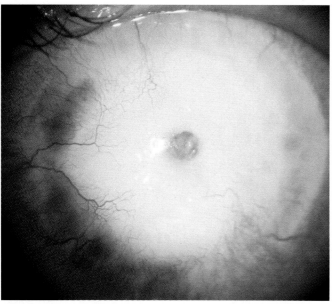

FIGURE 18-33 *Failed graft with a central filtering cica-trix.* This complication can develop when a scarred graft slowly thins over time.

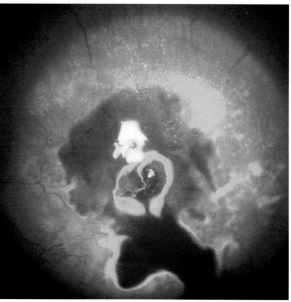

FIGURE 18-34 *Same patient as in Figure 18-33.* When fluorescein dye is applied, the central area is Seidel positive.

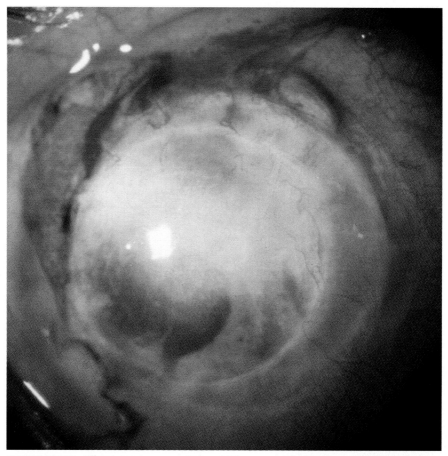

FIGURE 18-35 *Blunt trauma sustained 22 years after a penetrating keratoplasty.* Uveal tissue is protruding from the outer keratoplasty wound. The inner wound is intact. (This patient had two penetrating keratoplasties.)

Rejection Reactions

Allograft rejection occurs in up to a third of eyes undergoing corneal transplantation. Most commonly it occurs in the first 6 months after transplantation, but it can occur any time in the life of the graft. Corneal vascularization dramatically increases the risk of rejection. Fortunately, most rejection reactions can be reversed with local and systemic corticosteroids. Rejection must be recognized early, and patients should seek immediate attention if they experience one of the three danger signals—decreased vision (the most common and frequently recognized signal), redness, or discomfort.

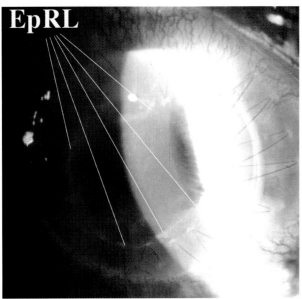

FIGURE 18-36 *Epithelial rejection.* An epithelial rejection line (EpRL) occurs as the recipient epithelium replaces the donor epithelium. In this case an EpRL was seen 3 weeks postoperatively.

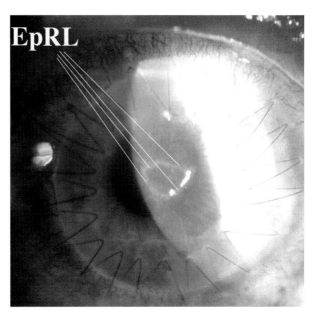

FIGURE 18-37 *Same patient as in Figure 18-36, 4 days later.* The EpRL is smaller.

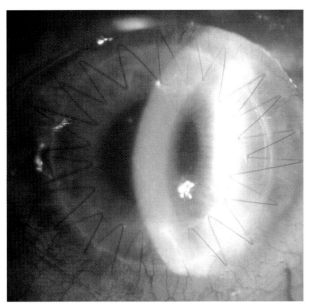

FIGURE 18-38 *Same patient as in Figures 18-36 and 18-37, 11 days later.* The epithelial rejection has cleared. Host epithelium covers the graft.

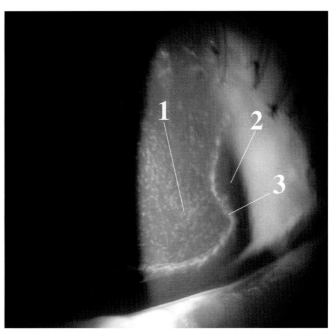

FIGURE 18-39 *EpRL.* Donor epithelium *(1)*, host epithelium *(2)*, EpRL composed of inflammatory cells and donor epithelium *(3)* are shown.

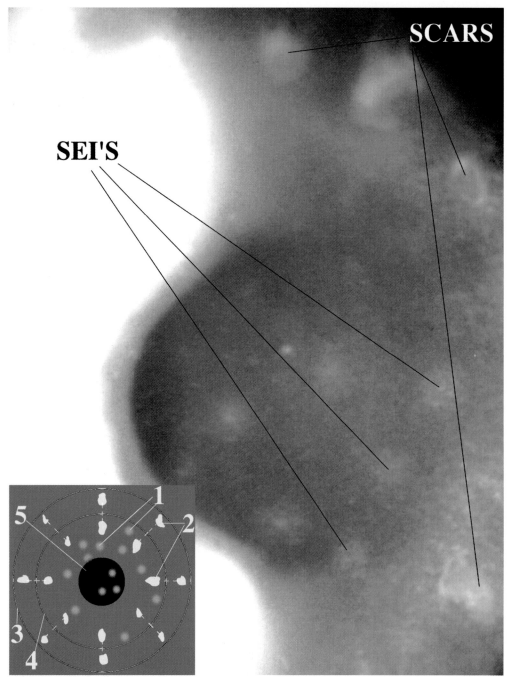

SCARS

SEI'S

FIGURE 18-40 *Subepithelial infiltrates (SEIs).* These can occur as an isolated form of graft rejection or accompany other forms. They resemble the SEIs seen after adenoviral infection. As an isolated finding, they represent a mild form of graft rejection and usually clear with moderate doses of topical corticosteroids. The schematic demonstrates the location of several findings: SEIs *(1)*, suture tract scars *(2)*, limbus *(3)*, penetrating keratoplasty wound *(4)*, and pupil *(5)*.

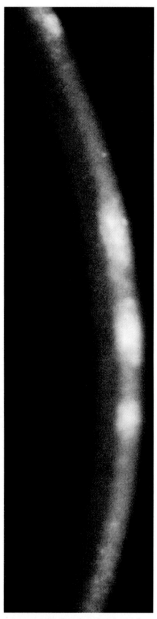

FIGURE 18-41 A thin slit beam view showing SEIs in the anterior stroma.

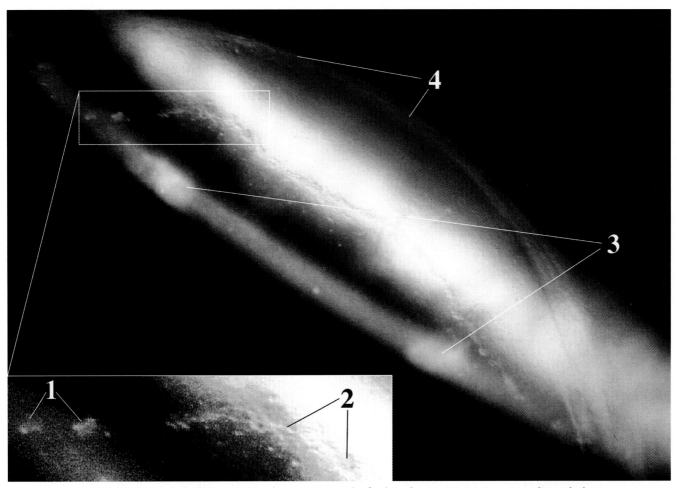

FIGURE 18-42 Endothelial rejection line composed of white keratic precipitates in direct light *(1)*. The endothelial rejection line is translucent in indirect light *(2)*. Suture tract scars *(3)* and penetrating keratoplasty wound *(4)* are also seen.

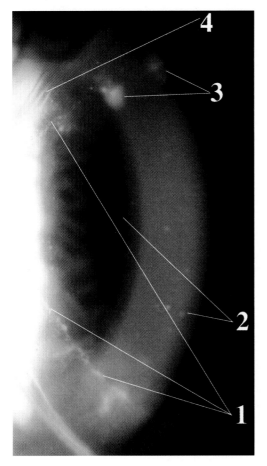

FIGURE 18-43 Endothelial rejection line *(1)*, keratic precipitates *(2)*, suture tract scars *(3)*, and penetrating keratoplasty wound *(4)* are shown.

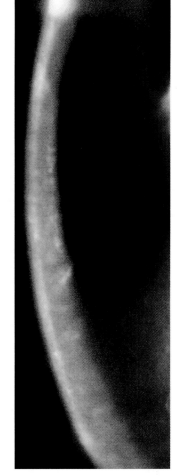

FIGURE 18-44 ***Endothelial rejection line.*** As the endothelial rejection line progresses across the endothelium, corneal edema develops. Here the rejection line began inferiorly and has extended near the central cornea. Stromal edema is seen inferiorly, which corresponds to the path of the rejection line.

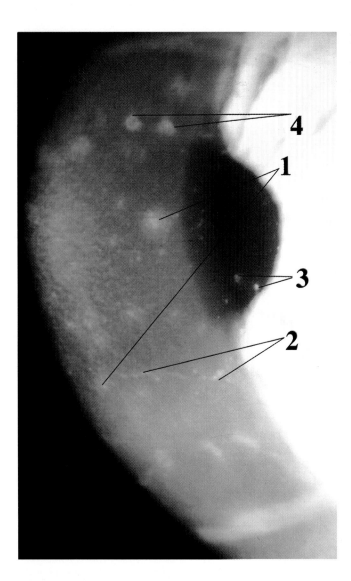

FIGURE 18-45 SEIs *(1)*, endothelial rejection line *(2)*, keratic precipitates *(3)*, and corneal scars *(4)* are shown. This case demonstrates the simultaneous occurrence of two forms of rejection—endothelial and SEIs.

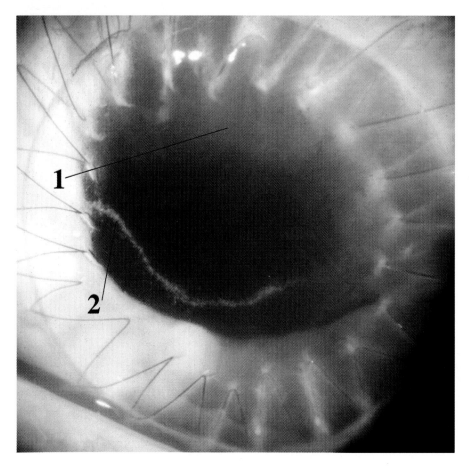

FIGURE 18-46 *Stromal rejection (1).* This appears as a diffuse stromal haze or infiltrate usually associated with stromal vascularization. If the rejection occurs without endothelial involvement, as in this case, the corneal thickness remains relatively normal. An epithelial rejection line *(2)* is present.

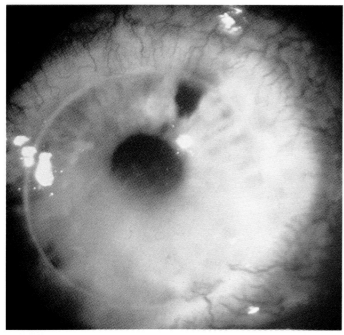

FIGURE 18-47 Diffuse endothelial rejection with corneal edema.

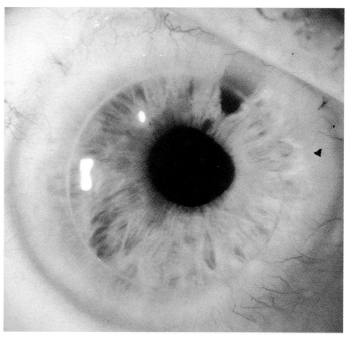

FIGURE 18-48 *Same patient as in Figure 18-47 after intensive treatment with topical and systemic corticosteroids.* The rejection has resolved, and the graft is clear.

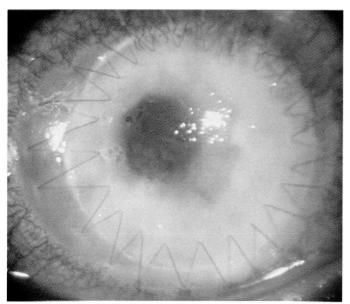

FIGURE 18-49 Severe endothelial rejection with stromal and epithelial edema.

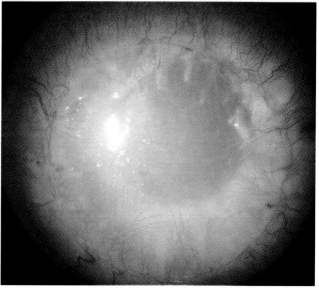

FIGURE 18-50 *Graft failure because of rejection.* There is marked stromal vascularization.

High Astigmatism

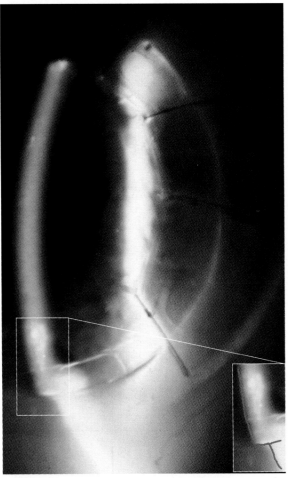

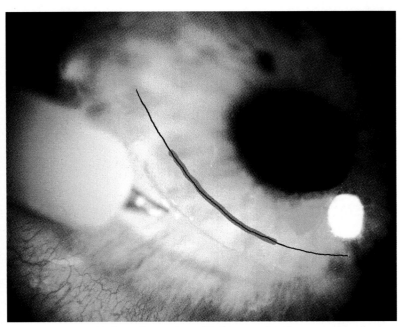

FIGURE 18-52 *High astigmatism (6 diopters) after penetrating keratoplasty.* A relaxing incision was performed within the wound. The relaxing incision is performed in the meridian of greatest corneal curvature. The area of the incision is represented by a gray band, and the wound is represented by a black line above and to the right of the actual incision and wound.

FIGURE 18-51 *High astigmatism.* There is severe anterior displacement of the graft inferiorly *(inset).* This leads to flattening of the graft in the meridian of the anterior wound displacement.

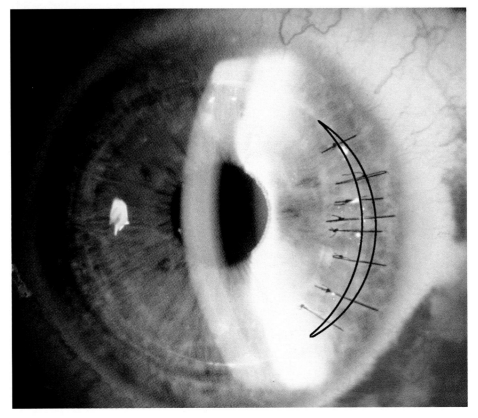

FIGURE 18-53 *Extremely high astigmatism (10 diopters) after penetrating keratoplasty.* A wedge resection was performed in this case. The area of resected tissue is outlined in black, and the sutures have re-approximated the new wound edges. The wedge resection is performed in the meridian of least corneal curvature.

CHAPTER 19

Therapeutic And Reconstructive Procedures

This chapter discusses conjunctival and corneal surgical procedures other than penetrating keratoplasty.

Conjunctival Flaps

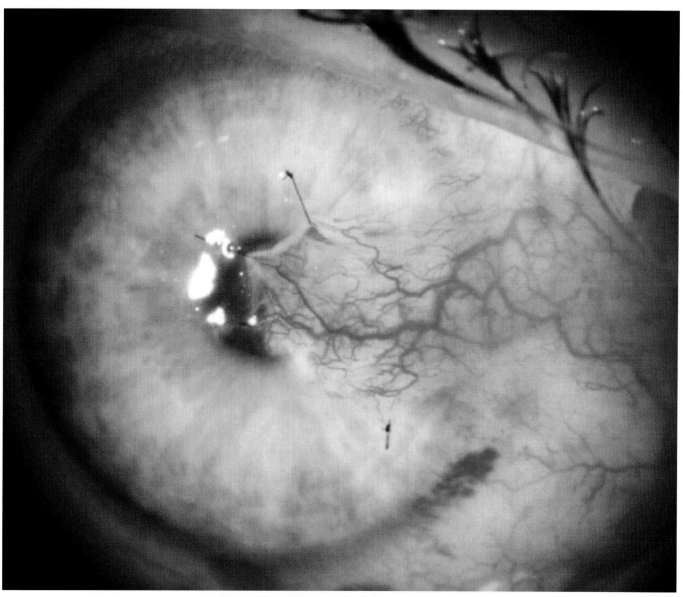

FIGURE 19-1 *Conjunctival flap.* This patient with chronic progressive external ophthalmoplegia developed an exposure ulcer near the nasal limbus. The etiology of the ulcer was related to poor lid closure from an overcorrected ptosis repair and an absent Bell's reflex. (The preoperative appearance is seen in Figure 12-23.) The area of ulceration was controlled with a small conjunctival pedicle flap, as seen here. The flap retracted slightly with time, and the visual acuity returned to the preoperative level once the sutures were removed.

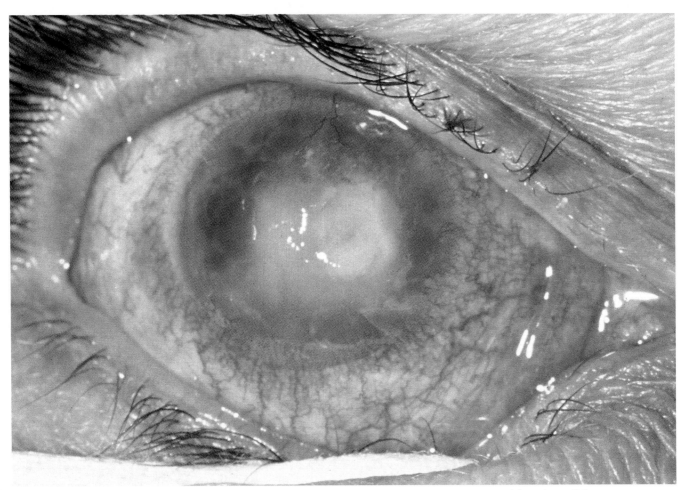

FIGURE 19-2 *Herpes simplex keratitis with a chronic neurotrophic ulcer.* The ulcer did not respond to conservative therapy. This is the appearance of the eye before a Gunderson conjunctival flap procedure.

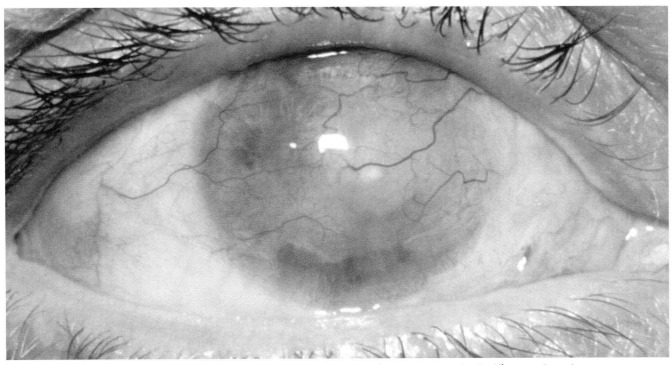

FIGURE 19-3 *Same patient as in Figure 19-2, 10 months postoperatively.* The eye is quiet, and the conjunctival flap has healed.

Surgery for Pterygia

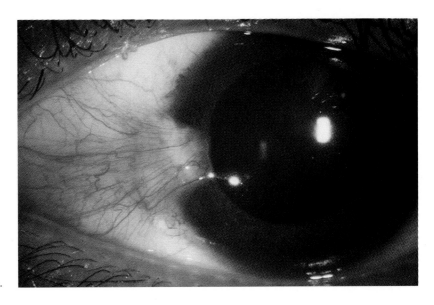

FIGURE 19-4 Pterygium before excision.

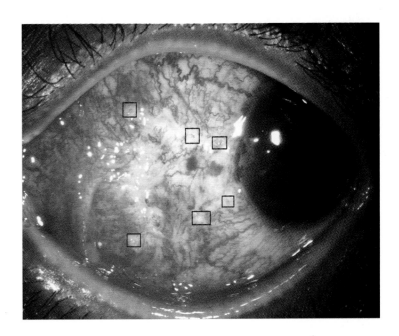

FIGURE 19-5 *Same patient as in Figure 19-4, 1 week postoperatively with conjunctival autograft.* The boxes show the position of the buried sutures.

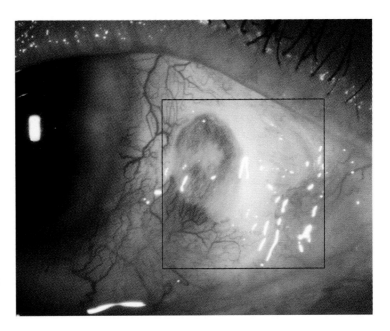

FIGURE 19-6 *Pterygium excision with mitomycin application to the scleral bed.* Approximately 1 year after the excision, there was continued scleral melting and a lack of vascularity in the necrotic scleral bed. Uveal tissue is seen at the base of the ulcer.

Keratoepithelialplasty

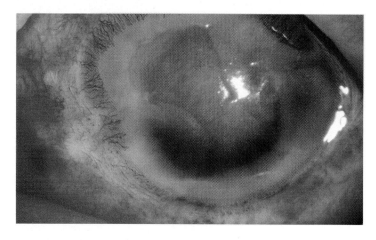

FIGURE 19-7 *Chronic nonhealing corneal ulcer after an alkali burn.* Preoperative appearance of the eye before a keratoepithelialplasty.

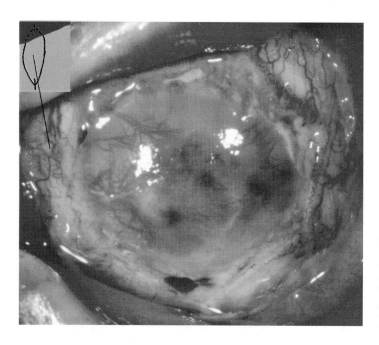

FIGURE 19-8 *Same patient as in Figure 19-7.* Early postoperative appearance shows six donor corneal lenticules sutured near the limbus. (The superior lenticule is under the lid.) The lenticules are cut from the donor cornea near the limbus. The inset diagrams the lenticule and shows the location of the two sutures.

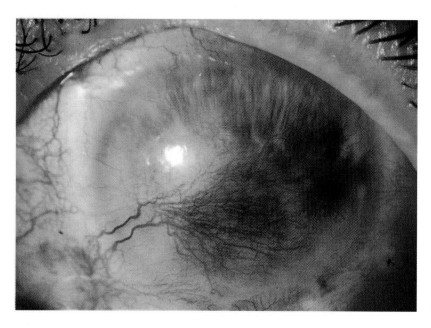

FIGURE 19-9 *Same patient as in Figures 19-7 and 19-8, 6 months postoperatively.* The epithelial surface is vascularized and scarred, and there is no active ulceration.

Surgery for Recurrent Erosions

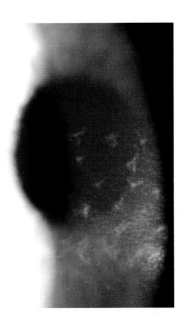

FIGURE 19-10 ***Recurrent erosion syndrome.*** There is defective adhesion of the epithelium and basement membrane complex to the underlying corneal stroma. (See Figures 12-1 through 12-7 for clinical description.) With anterior stromal puncture, a hypodermic needle is passed through the epithelium into the anterior stroma to create a focal area of scarring. Multiple punctures are performed, and the scars formed serve to "spot weld" the epithelium to the underlying stroma.

Lamellar Keratoplasty

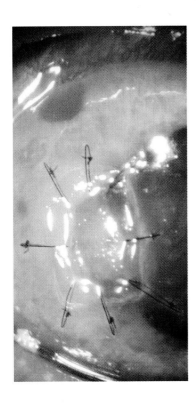

FIGURE 19-11 A rectangular lamellar graft for a peripheral perforation in a patient with rheumatoid arthritis.

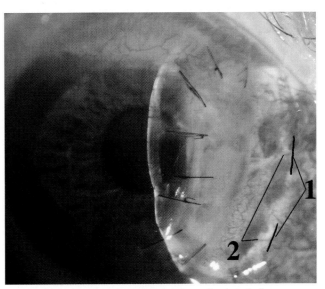

FIGURE 19-12 A crescentic lamellar graft for an impending perforation in polyarteritis nodosa (see Figure 13-13 for preoperative appearance.) The peripheral edge of the graft is identified *(1)* as well as two peripheral sutures *(2)*.

Anterior Segment Reconstruction

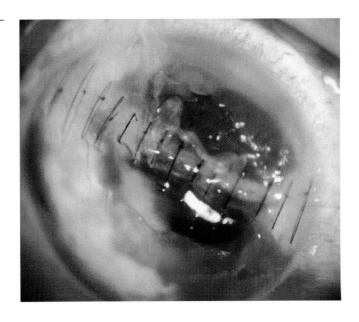

FIGURE 19-13 ***Repaired corneal laceration.*** Peripheral long powerful sutures and shorter central sutures are used to minimize the potential for central corneal flattening.

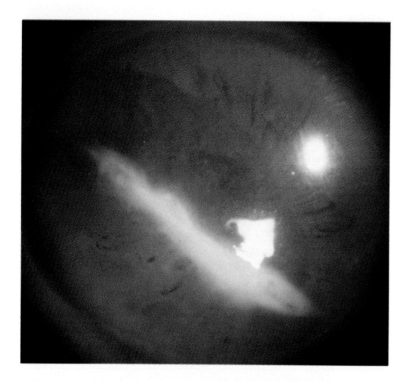

FIGURE 19-14 **Corneal laceration.** This is the appearance 20 years after a traumatic self-sealing laceration with scarring and extensive iris incorporation into the wound.

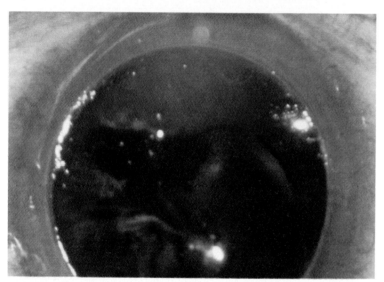

FIGURE 19-15 **Same patient as in Figure 19-14.** This photograph was taken during penetrating keratoplasty and shows extensive loss of iris tissue.

FIGURE 19-16 Same patient as in Figures 19-14 and 19-15 after penetrating keratoplasty with iris repair.

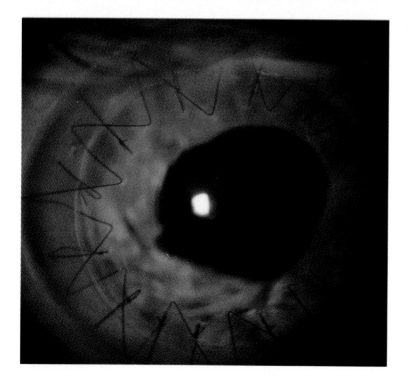

Keratoprosthesis

Prosthokeratoplasty should be considered in patients who have exhausted all other therapeutic options, including multiple attempts with penetrating kerato-plasty, or in cases where keratoplasty would certainly fail. Indications for prosthokeratoplasty include severe chemical burns, ocular cicatricial pem-phigoid, Stevens-Johnson syndrome, and recurrent graft failure. Preoperative visual function should be bare ambulatory or nonambulatory in both eyes.

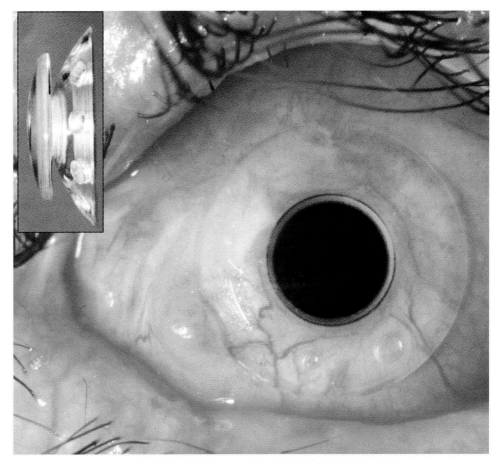

FIGURE 19-17 *Dohlman-Doane type-I intracorneal kerato-prosthesis performed 30 years after an explosion injury.* The cornea between the anterior and posterior support-ing plates of the keratoprosthe-sis is well vascularized, and there is no sign of necrosis around the optical cylinder. The visual acuity has improved to 20/20 with 20 months of follow-up. The inset shows the pros-thesis before insertion.

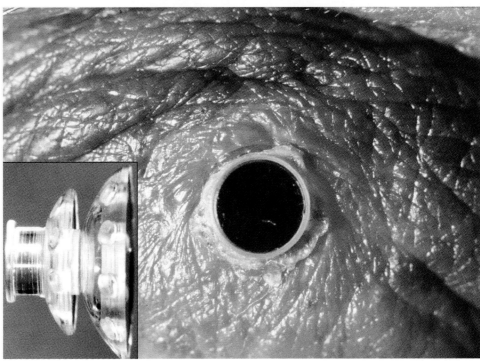

FIGURE 19-18 *Dohlman-Doane type-II keratoprosthesis per-formed for Stevens-Johnson syndrome.* The prosthesis is similar in design to the type-I prosthesis, but there is a longer optical cylinder that protrudes through the lid skin. Here, total ankyloblepharon necessitated the use of a through-the-lid design. The visual acuity has improved to 20/20 with 15 months of follow-up. The inset shows the prosthesis before insertion.

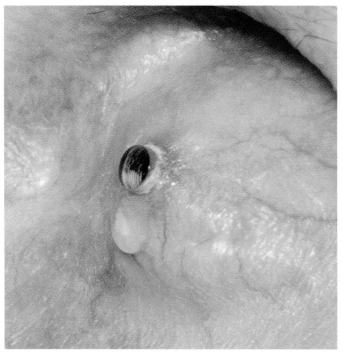

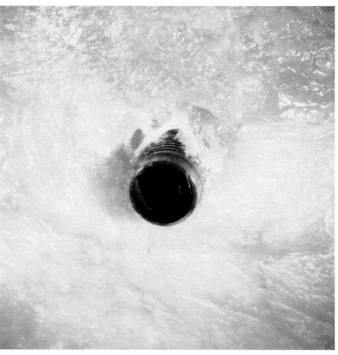

FIGURE 19-19 *A nut-and-bolt keratoprosthesis with aqueous leak around the optical cylinder.* This complication requires immediate surgical repair.

FIGURE 19-20 *A nut-and-bolt keratoprosthesis with partial unscrewing of the optical cylinder and exposed Dacron mesh superiorly.* This was successfully repaired, and the patient has maintained 20/200 vision with over 3 years of follow-up.

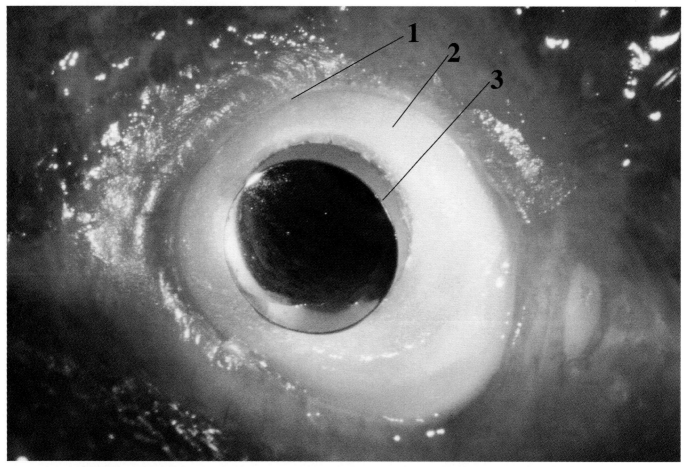

FIGURE 19-21 *Skin retraction around the optical cylinder of a nut-and-bolt keratoprosthesis.* Skin *(1)* has retracted from an underlying layer of Gortex *(2),* which was used to support the keratoprosthesis. The optical cylinder *(3)* is in relatively good position. The Gortex was removed, and the keratoprosthesis was successfully repaired. The patient has maintained 20/40 vision with over 10 years of follow-up.

CHAPTER 20

Refractive Surgery

Refractive surgery is an evolving field, and many potentially advantageous procedures are still being developed. This chapter highlights the two most common procedures performed to correct myopia: radial keratotomy and photorefractive keratectomy. These procedures may become obsolete as new and improved techniques are developed.

Incisional Refractive Surgery

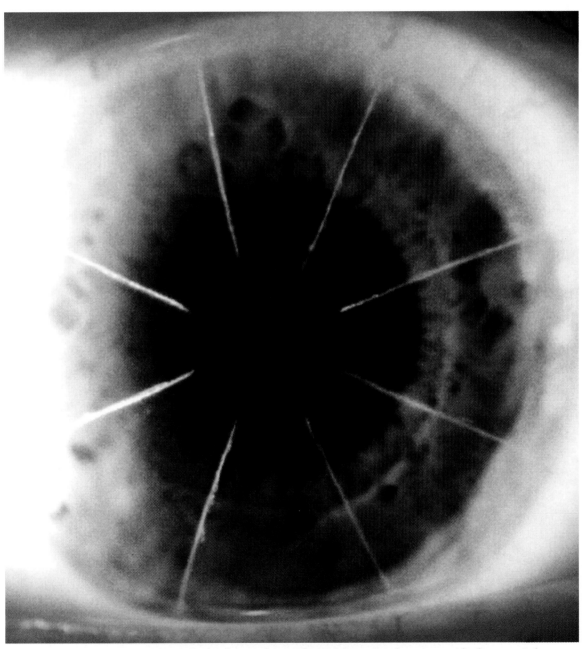

FIGURE 20-1 *Radial keratotomy.* The goal is to flatten the central cornea with deep peripheral radial incisions. The degree of flattening is related to many factors, including the number of incisions, the length of incisions, the size of the central optical zone, the depth of incisions, and wound healing. This is an excellent postoperative result following radial keratotomy. The visual acuity is 20/20 uncorrected.

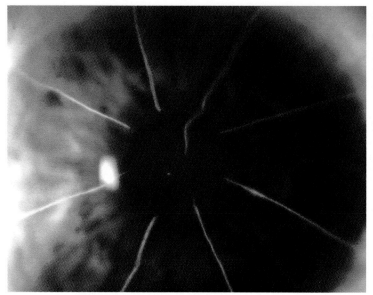

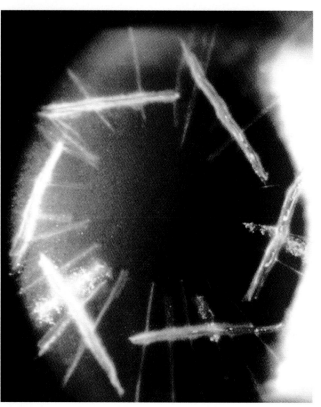

FIGURE 20-2 *Radial keratotomy.* In this eye, one of the superior radial keratotomy incisions extends into the visual axis. Newer blade designs make the chance of this complication less likely.

FIGURE 20-3 *Combined hexagonal and radial keratotomy.* Multiple crossed incisions result in irregular astigmatism with resultant poor vision.

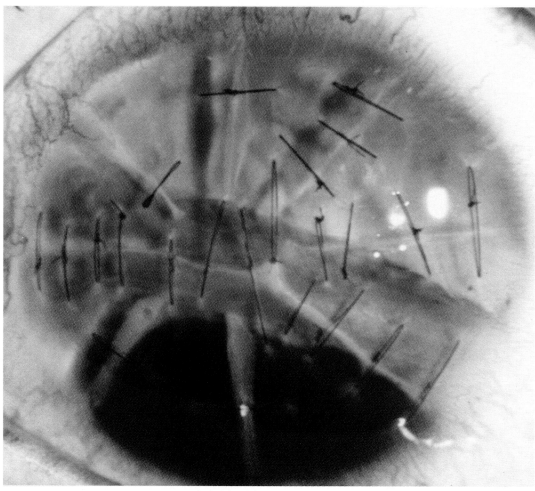

FIGURE 20-4 *Radial keratotomy.* Postoperative repair of a traumatic wound rupture follows the lines of corneal incisions and extends through the visual axis. Much of the iris was lost.

FIGURE 20-5 ***Radial keratotomy.*** This patient developed corneal scarring from herpes simplex keratitis several months after radial keratotomy. There was no prior history of herpetic infection. Stromal scarring from herpes simplex keratitis *(1)* and radial keratotomy incisions *(2)* are indicated.

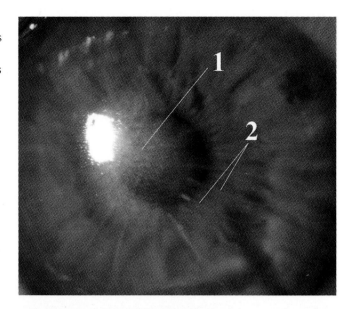

FIGURE 20-6 Radial keratotomy (2 days postoperatively) complicated by ***Streptococcus pneumoniae*** keratitis with a wound leak.

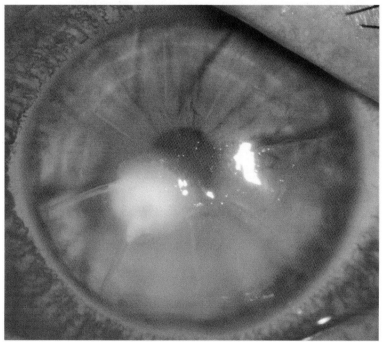

FIGURE 20-7 ***Same patient as in Figure 20-6 after penetrating keratoplasty.*** Several sutures were placed to prevent the radial keratotomy incisions from opening *(1)*.

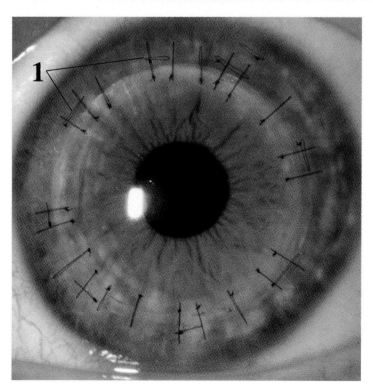

Photorefractive Surgery

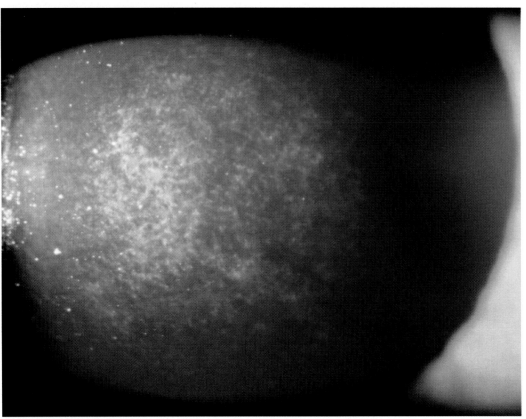

FIGURE 20-8 ***Post-excimer laser photorefractive keratectomy for myopia.*** Permanent anterior stromal scarring is demonstrated by broad oblique beam.

FIGURE 20-9 Permanent anterior stromal scarring as seen with a thin slit beam in the same case.

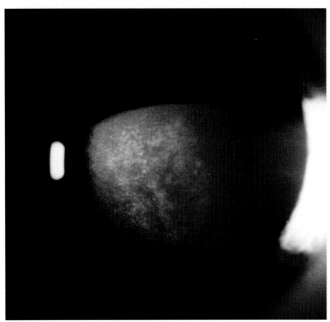

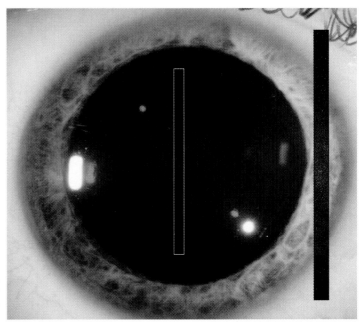

FIGURE 20-10 ***Post-excimer laser photorefractive keratectomy for myopia.*** Transient anterior stromal haze is seen only with broad oblique illumination.

FIGURE 20-11 ***Same patient as in Figure 20-10.*** The anterior stromal haze is not well visualized with diffuse light. The inset is enhanced to show that the haze is still present.

Index

EKC; *see* Epidemic keratoconjunctivitis

Embryotoxon, 83

Endocrine disorders, 106

Endophthalmitis, 54
  after penetrating keratoplasty in, 278

Endothelial dystrophy, 145, 147

Endothelial pigmentation, 176

Endothelial rejection, 287

Entropion, 3

Eosinophilic granuloma, 105

Epiblepharon, 3

Epidemic keratoconjunctivitis, 55-57

Epidermolysis bullosa, 108

Epinephrine, 113

Episcleritis, 267

Epithelial basement membrane dystrophy, 119-121

Epithelial cells in dry eyes, 30

Epithelial defect, 260, 266

Epithelial dendrites, 189

Epithelial dysplasia, 263, 265

Epithelial edema
  endothelial rejection with, 287
  Fuchs' dystrophy with, 145

Epithelial erosion, 127

Epithelial inclusion cyst, 258
  anterior chamber, 258

Epithelial ingrowth
  after cataract surgery, 258
  after penetrating keratoplasty, 281

Epithelial keratitis, 181

Epithelial lines, 169, 283, 285

Epoxy glue injury, 232

Epstein-Barr virus infection, 110

Erosions
  recurrent, 205-208
    surgery for, 293
  from soft contact lens, 262
  suture, 279

Essential iris atrophy, 160, 161

Ethylenediamine tetraacetic acid, 171

Explosion injury
  corneal foreign body from, 247
  intracorneal keratoprosthesis after, 295

Exposure keratopathy, 214

Eye, dry, 29-35

Eyelid
  anatomic abnormalities of, 1-6
    ectropion in, 1-2
    entropion in, 3
    floppy eyelid in, 6
    lagophthalmos in, 5
    trichiasis in, 4
  capillary hemangiomas of, 10
  floppy, 6
  imbrication, lower, 6
  imbrication syndrome of, 6
  inflammation of, 19-28
    allergic, 28
    bacterial infection in, 25
    blepharitis in, 19-24
    parasitic infection in, 27
    viral infection in, 26
  Kaposi's sarcoma of, 18, 45
  molluscum contagiosum lesions on, 26
  nodular malignant melanoma of, 17
  scarring of, 216
  in sebaceous cell carcinoma, 16

Eyelid—cont'd
  tumors of, 7-18
    benign, 7-13
    malignant, 14-18
  varices of, 13

F

Fabry's disease, 87-89

Facial skin herpes simplex infection, 179

Factitious conjunctivitis, 76

Factitious disease, 215-216

Familial dysautonomia, 35

Fat, prolapsed orbital, 50

Ferry line, 169

Filamentary keratitis, 209

Fish eye disease, 90

Fistula, dural-cavernous, 102-103

Flaps, conjunctival, 289-290

Fleck dystrophy, 140

Fleischer ring, 150, 152, 169

Floppy eyelid, 6

Fluorescein pooling in contact lens, 263

Fluorescein stain
  of dendritic epithelial patterns, 262
  in dry eye syndrome, 33, 34
  in herpes zoster dendrites, 189
  in punctate keratitis, 210
  in superficial punctate keratopathy, 30
  in thermal corneal injury, 241

Follicle, conjunctival, 51

Follicular conjunctivitis, 51
  toxic, 74

Forceps injury, 236-239

Foreign bodies
  conjunctival, 233
  corn husk, 242
  metallic, 243
  copper, 253
  corneal, 227-254
    abrasions in, 227
    after blast injury, 233
    copper, 253
    corn husk, 242, 244
    elastic cord in, 228
    from explosion injury, 247
    glass, 247, 250
    glue in, 232
    grasshopper leg, 242
    hair, 248
    iron, 244-245, 246, 251-252
    lacerations in, 229-231
    lint, 255
    metallic, 243, 278
    perforated staphyloma from, 246
    retained, 250
    ultraviolet light in, 228
    vegetable, 249
  of eyelid, 28

Free-band lamellar keratoplasty, 245

Fuchs' dystrophy, 145-146
  penetrating keratoplasty in, 274

Fuchs' heterochromic iridocyclitis, 270

Fungal keratitis, 195-198

Furrow degeneration, 167

Fusarium infection, 195, 196

G

Gammopathy, benign monoclonal, 105

Giant papillary conjunctivitis, 52, 68
  from contact lens, 261

Gland, Moll's, 13

Glass foreign body, 247, 250

Glass striae, 165

Glaucoma, 82

Glue injury, 232

Gold deposits, 116

Goldenbar's syndrome, 97

Gonioscopy
  in corneal injury, 249, 250, 251
  in Fuchs' heterochromic iridocyclitis, 270
  in iris-nevus syndrome, 162

Gonococcal conjunctivitis, 54
  of newborn, 62

Gout, 96

Graft
  failure of, 282, 287
  granular dystrophy in, 133
  macular dystrophy in, 136

Graft-versus-host disease, 35

Granular dystrophy, 131-133

Granuloma
  eosinophilic, 105
  pyogenic, 47

Granulomatosis, 222-224

Grasshopper leg in conjunctiva, 242

Green-yellow discoloration, 253

H

Haab's striae, 82

Hairs in cornea, 248

Hand-Schüller-Christian disease, 105

Hemangioma
  capillary, 10
  in conjunctiva, 46

Hematologic disorders, 102-105

Hemorrhage
  in soft contact lens wearer, 264
  subconjunctival, 234
  suprachoroidal, 274

Herbert's pits, 60, 61

Hereditary endothelial dystrophy, 147

Herpes blepharitis, 180

Herpes simplex, 280
  scars from, 183

Herpes simplex keratitis, 179-188
  blepharitis in, 180
  chronic, 188
  with conjunctivitis, 180
  with corneal perforation, 184
  with dendrites, 182
  disciform, 185
  epithelial, 181
  of facial skin, 179
  from insect bite, 254
  interstitial, 186
  keratouveitis in, 186, 187, 188
  of mouth, 179
  necrotizing, 187
  neurotrophic ulcer in, 184
  with peripheral inflammatory disease, 187
  scleritis in, 188
  stromal scars in, 183
  with ulcers, 182, 290

Herpes simplex scleritis, 188

Herpes simplex vesicles, 179

Herpes ulcer, 184

Herpes zoster, 191

epithelial dendrites from, 189

neurotrophic ulcer after, 193, 194

sectoral iris atrophy in, 194

Herpes zoster dendrites, 189

Herpes zoster keratitis, 189-194

Herpes zoster ophthalmicus
  corneal scarring from, 192
  with indolent corneal ulcer, 193
  with neurotrophic ulcer, 193
  subepithelial infiltrates in, 190

Herpes zoster scleritis, 194

Herpes zoster uveitis, 191

Heterochromia
  with Fuchs' heterochromic iridocyclitis, 270
  with intraocular iron foreign body, 251

Heterochromic iridocyclitis, 270

Hexagonal and radial keratotomy, 298

High astigmatism, 288

HLA-B27–related uveitis, 272

Hordeolum, 20

Horner-Trantas' dots, 66

Hudson-Stähli line, 169

Hurler's syndrome, 92

Hutchinson's sign, 189

Hydrops, 157, 158

Hyperacute conjunctivitis, 53

Hypercholesterolemia, 96

Hyperplasia of conjunctiva, 44

Hypersensitivity reaction
  of conjunctiva, 65
  of eyelids, 28

Hyphema, 235

Hypoxia, 264

I

ICE syndrome; *see* Iridocorneal endothelial syndrome

Ichthyosis, 107

IgA disease, 70

Imbrication, eyelid, 6

Immunologic disorders, 217-226
  Mooren's ulcer in, 226
  nonrheumatoid collagen vascular disease in, 221-224
  rheumatoid arthritis in, 217-220
  staphylococcal disease in, 225

Incisional refractive surgery, 297-299

Inclusion blennorrhea, 62

Inclusion conjunctivitis
  adult, 58-59
  neonatal, 62

Inclusion cyst, 258

Infection
  bacterial; *see* Bacterial infections
  chlamydial, 58-59
  corneal, 177-202; *see also* Corneal infections
  Epstein-Barr virus, 110
  eyelid, 19-28; *see also* Eyelid, inflammation of
  herpes simplex; *see* Herpes simplex
  herpes zoster; *see* Herpes zoster
  Proteus, 280
  varicella, 109, 273
  viral, 26

Infectious crystalline keratopathy, 177
  after penetrating keratoplasty, 280